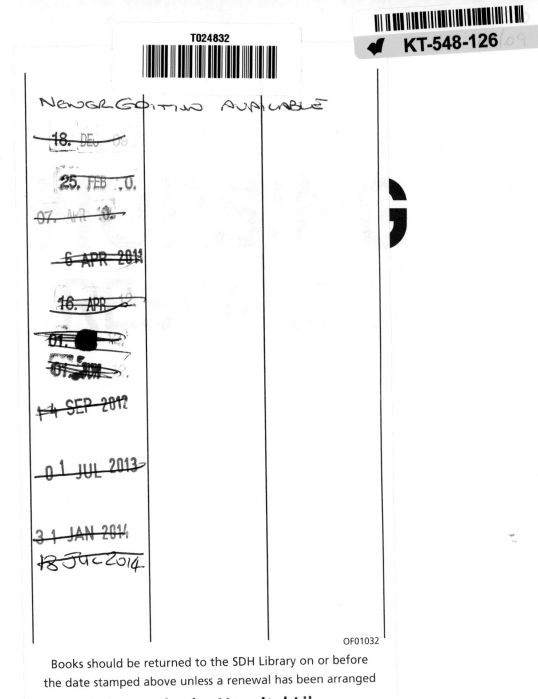

NURSING
RESEARCH

AN INTRODUCTION

PAM MOULE AND **MARGARET GOODMAN**

companion
website

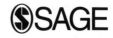

Los Angeles • London • New Delhi • Singapore • Washington DC

First published 2009

SAGE Publications Ltd
1 Oliver's Yard
55 City Road
London EC1Y 1SP

SAGE Publications Inc.
2455 Teller Road
Thousand Oaks, California 91320

SAGE Publications India Pvt Ltd
B 1/I 1 Mohan Cooperative Industrial Area
Mathura Road, Post Bag 7
New Delhi 110 044

SAGE Publications Asia-Pacific Pte Ltd
33 Pekin Street #02-01
Far East Square
Singapore 048763

Library of Congress Control Number: 2008933205

British Library Cataloguing in Publication data

A catalogue record for this book is available from
the British Library

ISBN 978-1-4129-1208-2
ISBN 978-1-4129-1209-9 (pbk)

Typeset by C&M Digitals (P) Ltd, Chennai, India
Printed and bound in Great Britain by TJ International Ltd, Padstow, Cornwall
Printed on paper from sustainable resources

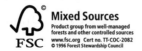

Mixed Sources
Product group from well-managed
forests and other controlled sources
www.fsc.org Cert no. TT-COC-2082
© 1996 Forest Stewardship Council
FSC

This book is dedicated to the memory of Gill Hek
who inspired many 'nurse researchers'.

CONTENTS

Contents

Contents

Contents

LIST OF FIGURES

LIST OF TABLES

LIST OF BOXES

PREFACE

Welcome to this new textbook written as a comprehensive guide to introduce student nurses and practitioners to some of the complexities of nursing research. The book leads the novice nurse researcher through the main techniques and skills required to appreciate and undertake nursing research. We have drawn on our experiences and knowledge of nursing and nursing research to develop chapters that present key theoretical information in an applied way, drawing on examples from our own research and that of others. We hope that in taking this practical and applied approach the book should help demystify research for readers and encourage appreciation and understanding of research practice and processes.

How to use this book

The book includes 25 chapters covering key aspects of nursing research that introduce the reader to issues of research design, process, dissemination and implementation. The layout is straightforward, allowing the reader to negotiate the content to meet their own learning needs. It is possible to read individual chapters without the need to constantly refer to other sections of the book, though in places we have suggested where further materials and explanations may be found.

The chapters are structured to include an introduction, learning outcomes, key terms, content with reference support, examples from practice and literature, and a summary. The key terms are explained within the comprehensive glossary provided towards the end of the text. Each chapter ends with a summary that reminds the reader of the key issues presented. Reference and further reading lists are provided and, where appropriate, websites are recommended.

Content

The initial chapters (1 and 2) discuss the position and place of research in nursing knowledge and practice development, emphasising the need for evidence-based practice. Chapter 3 introduces the research process that guides research activity and design and sets the tone for the content of the subsequent chapters. The remainder of the book is structured to follow the research process that would be undertaken by nurse researchers.

Chapters 4 and 5 cover aspects of research governance and ethics and encourage the reader to think about the processes involved in researching ethically and with potentially vulnerable populations. Ethical issues are complex and need consideration prior to developing a research design (Chapter 6). Chapters 7 to 9 give practical advice on undertaking literature searching, reviewing and developing the skills of critical appraisal. These once-coveted skills are necessary to support 'research literacy' and an ability to critically appraise and use research in practice.

Many nurses are undertaking undergraduate and postgraduate studies that require them to produce a research proposal. Others are undertaking local or funded projects as part of clinical practice or education roles. To help address these needs. Chapter 10 provides guidance and examples of how to develop a research proposal for academic study or to undertake a research project as part of current work or for a funding body. The development of a proposal is supported by understanding issues of research design, methods, data collection and sampling. These aspects of research are covered in Chapters 11 and 13 to 21. These chapters provide comprehensive information about a range of research designs, methods and data collection techniques. They explain key research terms and provide examples of use. Chapter 20 describes the use of mixed methods approaches in research that integrates both qualitative and quantitative methods in one design. Mixed methods approaches are becoming more commonplace in healthcare research as they enable the team to address different research questions within one design.

We also discuss issues of maintaining quality in the research process (Chapter 12), important for integrity, rigour and trustworthiness. This chapter discuss issues of validity and reliability, terms that can cause confusion for research consumers. Chapters 22 and 23 discuss data analysis techniques, often found difficult by many researchers. Both chapters give information on approaches to data analysis and present the processes of analysis, providing worked examples. The concluding chapters (24 and 25) address the final stages of the research process. Practical guidance regarding dissemination processes are offered in the penultimate chapter, which includes report writing, conference presentation and writing for publication. The final chapter considers how research findings might be used to support nursing practice and brings us to the conclusion of the research journey.

To further aid nurse researchers in the development of research understanding and skills we have developed an accompanying website (www.sagepub.co.uk/mouleand goodman) that provides additional materials to support learning about research. The site includes a range of materials and learning resources that can be accessed for independent study and/or used to structure formal teaching sessions. The types of resources included are: PowerPoint slides, suggested lesson plans and activities for independent learning or group use. These materials should be a useful additional resource for personal study or group facilitation.

We hope you find the book and web materials not only provide you with key knowledge and understanding of nursing research, but also stimulate you to engage with research as critical appraisers, researchers and implementers of evidence-based practice.

Pam Moule
Margaret L. Goodman

ACKNOWLEDGEMENTS

We are pleased to recognise Gill Hek's input to the conception of the book and to the fashioning of Chapters 1, 4 and 5.

We are grateful to Mollie Gilchrist (Coventry University) and Chris Wright (University of Birmingham) for contributing Chapter 22.

COMPANION WEBSITE INFORMATION

Nursing Research: An Introduction has a companion website located at (www.sagepub. co.uk/moule). The site is designed to support teachers of research methods and contains helpful information for students. The website includes teaching and learning materials linked to each of the chapters in the text. There is a suggested lesson plan, a set of associated PowerPoint slides and a suggested reading list for each of the 25 chapters.

The lesson plans suggest possible ways of structuring delivery and refer, in some cases, to papers accessible on SAGE's website (www.sagepub.co.uk) that can be used to support the session. The lesson plans suggest how the associated PowerPoint slides might be used to support delivery. The content of these slides reflects that of the associated chapter. The additional list of suggested reading materials has links to web-based journals and materials as well as to related texts.

1

RESEARCH IN NURSING

The care provided by nurses must be based on up-to-date knowledge and research that supports the delivery of the highest standards of practice possible. Nurses are developing their own professional knowledge base with strong foundations built on research. Nurses have a responsibility in some way to contribute to the development of the profession's knowledge through research.

The term 'research literate' or 'research aware' is used by many to describe the way that nurses should be in the 21st century. This means:

- having the capacity for critical thought
- possessing analytical skills
- having the skills to gain access to relevant research and evidence
- having a critical understanding of research processes
- being able to read and critically appraise research and other types of evidence
- having an awareness of ethical issues related to research.

By possessing these skills and being 'research literate', nurses should be able to assess the appropriateness of using specific types of evidence in their daily practice. It should be a natural activity for nurses to keep up to date and use research findings and evidence in their work, and being 'research literate' is one of the basic skills.

In this chapter we consider the historical context of nursing research, the nature of nursing research, including different definitions and the development of evidence-based practice.

Learning outcomes

This chapter is designed to enable the reader to:

- **Understand the nature and historical context of nursing research**
- **Define research in nursing**
- **Identify the three elements of evidence-based practice**
- **Identify the five stages of evidence-based practice**

KEY TERMS

Capability building, Capacity building, Evidence-based practice, Hierarchy of evidence, Nursing research, Research literate

---

The historical context of nursing research

Florence Nightingale is often seen as the very first nurse researcher. Her research in the 1850s focused on soldiers' morbidity and mortality during the Crimean War. Nightingale identified 'research' questions in practice and undertook a systematic collection of data to try to find answers to the problems. Her 'research' eventually led to changes in the environment for sick people, including cleanliness, ventilation, clean water and adequate diet. However, Nightingale's contribution is seen as atypical with Kirby (2004) pointing out that the development of **nursing research** in the United Kingdom really only started with the inception of the National Health Service (NHS) – now the world's largest publicly funded health service – in the late 1940s. Prior to this, the development of nursing research had relied on a few highly determined individuals and was bound up with the professionalisation of nursing, the demands for suitable nurses, and the raising of educational standards for nurses (Kirby, 2004). Furthermore, in the 1950s, sociologists and psychologists were more likely to be undertaking research into nursing and nurses; only a small number of pioneering nurses were researching nursing and nurses themselves, one being Marjorie Simpson, who started the first self-help group for nurse researchers in 1959 called the Research Discussion Group (Hopps, 1994). This went on to become the Research Society of the Royal College of Nursing, which continues today. The Royal College of Nursing is the body in the UK that represents nurses and nursing, promotes excellence in practice and shapes health policies.

Tierney (1998) presented a picture of the development of nursing research across Europe. She identified the UK, Finland and Denmark as having developed in a similar way over the past 30 years, with Estonia, Lithuania and Slovenia only developing in the last 10 years. Growth was particularly evident in the 1980s and 1990s. It can be seen that though overall growth has been slow, it has been more rapid in developed European countries. Many factors have affected this growth, such as the lack of resources and funding to support research, slow development of research training, **capacity** and **capability building**, and the low status of nurses relative to other health professions, particularly medicine. Tierney pointed out that there are four elements that support development: 'bottom-up' initiatives by forward looking individuals; 'top-down' initiatives through government support; growth of a research infrastructure as seen through universities; and a strategic approach rather than ad hoc initiatives.

In the 1970s, serious consideration of nursing research in the UK came with the publication of the Briggs report (DoHSS, 1972) that recommended nursing should become a 'research-based' profession. This is often seen as a turning point in the historical context of nursing research, and as something that was badly needed for professional status. However, in the decades following the publication of the Briggs report, many suggested that nursing had not become 'research-based', nor had research made an impact on the daily practice of nurses (Hunt, 1981; Thomas, 1985; Webb and Mackenzie, 1993). Specifically, the arguments were that nurses did not read or understand research, nurses did not know how to use research in practice, nurses did not believe research, nurses were not able to use research to change practice, and nurse researchers did not communicate well. It is interesting to think about the current position: Do nurses read research? Do they understand research? Is research impacting on practice?

In 1993 the *Report of the Taskforce on the Strategy for Research in Nursing, Midwifery and Health Visiting* (DoH, 1993) was published. It sought to address many of the deficiencies noted earlier about nursing becoming a 'research-based' profession. It was suggested that nurse education, support and research infrastructure needed to be developed to support progress. The report did not suggest that all nurses should be undertaking research, rather it recommended that all nurses should become **research literate**, an essential skill for knowledge-led nursing practice. It became much clearer that all nurses needed to become equipped with the skills of understanding the research process, and an ability to retrieve and critically assess research findings, increasing capacity, with only a few nurses needing to be prepared to undertake research, increasing capability.

Changes in research preparation and training have been seen at all levels of nurse education. Research is now fully integrated into the pre-registration curricula (UKCC, 1986) and there are changes to post-registration provision that include research education (UKCC, 1994). The move of nurse education into higher education institutions in the 1990s has supported ongoing academic development at Masters and Doctoral levels, with 900 nurses registered on PhD programmes in 2005 (Higher Education Statistics Agency, 2005). Despite these developments there remains a shortfall of research-capable nurses (Rafferty et al., 2003), recognised by the Higher Education Funding Council, a body that promotes and funds high-quality, cost-effective teaching and research in higher education in England (HEFCE, 2001). The under-funding of research for nurses and allied health professions led to the HEFCE supporting capability building for both professional groups following the 2001 Research Assessment Exercise (RAE). The RAE is an audit of research volume and quality, soon to be superseded by the Research Excellence Framework, which allocates research funding to Higher Education Institutions based on the quality of research activity. Nursing departments scoring 3a and 3b in the 2001 RAE received funding through the Research Capability Fund. The results of the 2008 RAE and subsequent funding allocations are yet to be announced (at the time of going to press). Attention has also been given to developing the clinical research workforce. The UK Clinical Research Collaboration (UKCRC) reported in 2007 on 'Developing the best research professionals. Qualified graduate nurses: recommendations for preparing and supporting clinical academic nurses of the future'. This report was part of the agenda to modernise nursing careers, developing and preparing nurses to lead in a modernised healthcare system (DoH, 2006). The report recommends the establishment of a range of research training opportunities including Masters and Doctoral studies and fellowships, career flexibility that allows the combination of research and clinical practice and information provision to promote career opportunities for nursing. Programme work related to the implementation of these recommendations is planned for 2008.

The development of nursing research has also been aided by nursing organisations both nationally and internationally. This is acknowledged by Tierney (1997), who suggests that national nursing associations across Europe have been instrumental in strengthening the support for nursing research. In the UK the Royal College of Nursing has a well-established Research and Development support resource that can be accessed via the World Wide Web as well as the Research Society, an institute, and occasional funding for research projects. In the UK the Foundation of Nursing Studies and the Queen's Nursing Institute are just a couple of the organisations that support nursing research. The Department of Health has occasional streams of funding specifically for nursing research as well as multi-disciplinary health research funding opportunities. Nurses now compete on a national basis with other disciplines for research funding, and European research funding is becoming easier to access.

Rafferty (1997), however, argues that we cannot ignore the 'politics' of nursing research, particularly the economic and organisational factors that influence research priorities. In nursing, these influences are powerful and there is no doubt that they affect the direction and development of nursing research in the UK.

Economic, political and organisation factors influence the types of research that nurses undertake and can influence where the research funding is allocated.

The nature of nursing research

Though the growth of nursing research has been slow it continues to develop and is broad ranging, relating to practice, policy, education and management. It encompasses, for example, research about the effectiveness of nursing care, the development and evaluation of new types of care delivery, the expansion of nursing theories and concepts, the impact of policy on practice, new roles, and new ways of educating the nursing workforce. Nursing research is interested in what patients and clients feel and experience, how nurses learn and develop through-out their careers, how multi-disciplinary working and learning contributes to the care of patients, and the outcomes of nursing practice. The nursing profession is continually striving to develop its own body of research, and to contribute to health services research and the social sciences.

The nature of nursing research is complex. We have already suggested that nursing research is broad and wide ranging, capturing research into practice, care outcomes, education and management issues. Additionally, it should be remem-bered that nurses work as part of interprofessional teams and in different health-care settings. A number of research issues and questions might therefore arise that relate to interprofessional working. These factors impact on how nursing research is defined. Definitions of nursing research reflect the perspective of those researching nursing.

Bowling, in describing research on health and health services, defines research as '… the systematic and rigorous process of enquiry which aims to describe phe-nomena and to develop explanatory concepts and theories. Ultimately it aims to contribute to a scientific body of knowledge' (2002: 1). She then goes on to acknowledge the importance of multi-disciplinary health services research, which includes anthropologists, epidemiologists, health economists, medical sociologists and statisticians amongst those who conduct such research. They would each come with their own perspective on what defines research and how it should be conducted. Thus in defining nursing research there must be recognition of the potential multi-disciplinary nature of research teams and the consequential wide range of 'qualitative' and 'quantitative' research methods that will be employed to address the broad range of research issues.

Before moving on to consider definitions of research it is important to understand the main research approaches used, qualitative and quantitative, and to appreciate that often to address the complexity of nursing research both approaches can be combined within one study. The research approach is the whole design, which includes the researcher position and assumptions, the process of enquiry and the way data is collected and analysed. Qualitative research is part of an interpretivist or constructivist position that has long been part of social and behavioural sciences (Guba and Lincoln, 1982). The approach is used to describe and understand individual perspectives and experiences. For example, qualitative research may be used to answer questions about the patient experience or staff perceptions of new ways of working or new roles in nursing. Qualitative research can explore questions such as: What are patient's experiences of NHS Direct? How do patient's feel about the development of local NHS services? To gather information about personal views and experiences, research methods such as interviewing and observation are used, collecting textual or visual data for analysis.

Quantitative research has its origins in a scientific paradigm and roots in positivism, which believes human phenomena can be subjected to measurement and objective study. In nursing research quantitative approaches can be used to measure whether one treatment has a better effect than another. For example, quantitative designs might answer research questions such as 'Is treatment A better than treatment B?' The researcher may be guided by a hypothesis, a statement for testing (see Chapter 6), for example, 'Adults classed as clinically obese receiving an exercise programme of 30 minutes per day will have greater weight loss within two months of starting the programme than those undertaking a 10 minute exercise programme for two months.' Quantitative research takes a formal approach to the collection and analysis of numerical data.

In this book we discuss the different types of research in detail, identifying the strengths and limitations of each (see Chapters 11 to 18, 20 and 21). In doing this we introduce the readers to the range of research methods that might be used either independently or as part of a mixed-methods approach.

Given the complex nature of nursing research, finding one definition that achieves consensus is difficult. However, in most definitions of research there are some core elements:

- a systematic process
- a search for new knowledge or deepening understanding
- activities that are planned and logical
- a search for an answer to a question.

We use the following basic definition for the purposes of this book:

A systematic approach to gathering information for the purposes of answering questions and solving problems in the pursuit of creating new knowledge about nursing practice, education and policy. (Hek and Moule, 2006: 10)

Who does research in nursing?

As mentioned previously, researchers from other disciplines carried out much of the early nursing research in the 1950s, 1960s and early 1970s, including sociology, psychology, social and welfare policy, and history. Research was undertaken from a discipline perspective and nurse researchers at the time learnt about a wide range of research approaches and methods. Nurse researchers developed their research skills from social scientists and health researchers who included them on research teams. Historians, economists, statisticians, epidemiologists, geographers and anthropologists also brought their own approaches and techniques to nursing research.

This position has changed in the last 30 years or so, with many nurses now leading and undertaking their own research as well as being involved in multi-disciplinary research teams. Increasingly, health services research involves multi-disciplinary teams including health professionals, statisticians and health economists. Nurses can be part of these teams, directly employed on a specific project; for example, a clinical trial examining the effectiveness of a nurse-led service, or an evaluation looking at what works in family support or child protection. Nurse researchers are more likely to have a larger input into studies than in the past, when nurses may have been employed as data collectors. Nurses can undertake project design and management, as well as data collection and analysis. We could think about local examples of research that might provide further evidence of this change, for example: Are there research projects in practice that involve nurses? What are the roles of nurses in these projects?

As mentioned at the beginning of this chapter, all nurses need to become 'research literate'. Nurses studying at diploma level are most likely to undertake activities such as designing a questionnaire or interviewing colleagues as exercises to help them understand research methods and the research process. Most commonly, nursing students will practise skills to enable them to find and critically appraise research literature. All nursing students are likely to write essays using research findings and evidence, and all these activities are important and necessary in helping nurses to become 'research literate'. Some nurses, particularly at degree level, may undertake their own literature-based review or research study. This may be a small individual research project as part of a pre- or post-qualifying degree course or can involve being a member of a project team, exploring an aspect of practice.

An increasing number of nurses are educated to Master's level, with the number aspiring to Doctoral level education increasing (Higher Education Statistics Agency, 2005) both in Higher Education Institutions and clinical practice settings. This is a major change from 30 years ago when Doctorates and Master's level nurses were less common. This means that nurses have undertaken major pieces of research to a high level, and as nurses improve their capabilities as researchers they are more likely to lead research projects and teams and secure external funding through competitive tendering for major sources such as the Department of Health and Research Councils. There are many more Chairs in Nursing (Professors) than ever before and nurses are holding senior board level positions in higher education, the NHS, and other healthcare organisations. This all signals a healthy situation for nursing research with nurses becoming more deeply involved in research, though with still some way to go (UKCRC, 2007). We can probably find evidence to support these changes in the local setting, for example: Are there nurses studying for Masters degrees and Doctorates in the locality? Are Professors of nursing employed in the hospitals or local universities? Is nursing literature published by Professors and those completing Doctorates and higher studies?

What is evidence-based practice?

Making decisions about the type of nursing care to give to patients and clients is not easy. It may mean making choices between a number of alternative actions that involve treatment choices, provision of services or efficiency.

One definition of **evidence-based practice** suggests it is the use of best evidence in making decisions about patient care (Sackett et al., 2000).

From this definition we can see that the decision should be based on the current best evidence, as well as using the practitioner's own expertise, and that the decision should be made explicit.

These days, the view of the patient or client is seen as paramount to any decision that is made about the provision of healthcare for an individual. Therefore, it is reasonable to say that there are three clear key components to evidence-based practice. When making an 'evidence-based' decision about the care of a particular patient, the nurse should:

- use the best available current evidence
- consider the preferences of the individual client/patient
- use their own expertise and experience to make decisions.

In making decisions about how to care for a patient, the nurse should search for and use the best available evidence in their practice, they should consider the requirements, values, circumstances and preferences of the patient and they should integrate their own professional experience, expertise and judgement when making a decision. All three elements need to be used together, although the importance of each may vary in different situations. The overriding principle is that of giving the most effective care to maximise the quality of life for an individual.

How do you 'do' evidence-based practice?

Evidence-based practice is seen as comprising five explicit steps:

1   Identify a problem from practice and turn it into a specific question. This might be about the most effective intervention for a particular patient, or about the most appropriate test, or about the best method for delivering nursing care.
2   Find the best available evidence that relates to the specific question, usually through a thorough and systematic search of the literature.
3   Critically appraise the evidence for its validity (closeness to the truth), usefulness (practical application) and methodological rigour.
4   Identify and use the current best evidence, and together with the patient or client's preferences and the practitioner's expertise and experience, apply it to the situation.
5   Evaluate the effect on the patient or client, and reflect on the nurse's own performance.

Current pre-qualifying nurse education helps students address all these stages, but specifically practitioners need to learn how to search effectively for appropriate evidence and research through a range of literature sources (see Chapters 7 and 8) and how to critically appraise research (Chapters 7, 8 and 9).

Origins and development of evidence-based practice

Evidence-based practice rapidly emerged in the space of 10 years since the early 1990s and has had a significant impact on the health services including nursing. Evidence-based medicine was the starting point of the movement (Reynolds, 2000), and this was swiftly adopted in other professional groups including nursing (Trinder, 2000a).

The successful emergence of evidence-based practice has been argued by those within the movement as being due to the obvious, simple, sensible and rational idea 'that practice should be based on the most up-to-date, valid and reliable research' (Melnyk and Fineout-Overholt, 2005). The context in which it has developed may go some way to explain why the movement has been flourishing in many areas of healthcare practice. Within recent years there has been a cultural shift within the healthcare professions from one of trusted professional judgement-based practice to that of evidence-based practice.

Glicken (2005) suggests that there are a number of contributing factors including: growth in an increasingly well-educated and well-informed public; increasing awareness of the limitations of science; growth in consumer and self-help groups; intensive media scrutiny; explosion of the availability of different types of information and data; developments in information technology; increasing emphasis on productivity and competitiveness; emphasis on 'value-for-money' and audit; increase in scrutiny, accountability and regulation of professional groups; lawsuits and compensation; and major adverse events within the health services.

This cultural shift has resulted in an explosion of evidence-based initiatives and new terminology within the health services since the mid-1990s. These include initiatives such as Evidence-based Child Health and Evidence-based Mental Health; specialist 'evidence-based' journals; websites and web-based discussion lists. It also includes the NHS Centre for Reviews and Dissemination at York (2001) that undertakes the review and dissemination of research results to the NHS, and the UK Cochrane Centre that collaborates with others to build, maintain and disseminate a database of systematic, up-to-date reviews of randomised controlled trials of healthcare. This has had an effect on how research and evidence is considered and used by nurses and how evidence and practice drives (and is driven by) practice and policy more than ever before.

Criticisms of evidence-based practice

The growth of evidence-based practice has critics across all areas of healthcare, and there is limited consensus on the merits of evidence-based practice. Critics point out that there is no evidence that evidence-based practice actually works; that it constrains professional decision-making and autonomy; that it is too simple and is 'cook-book' practice; that it is a covert method of rationing resources; that it exalts certain types of research evidence over other types of knowledge and evidence and that research trials are usually not directly transferable (Jenicek, 2006). There are also concerns that the effective implementation of evidence-based practice has been hindered by the **hierarchy of evidence** that promotes randomised controlled trials as the highest form of evidence and neglects to recognise the value of reflection in developing best practice (Mantzoukas, 2008). Nurses need to be aware of the debates surrounding evidence-based practice both within their own professional group and more generally in the health and social services (see Trinder, 2000b for a useful critique).

There are limitations with evidence-based practice in all aspects of healthcare but particularly with nursing. First, there is a shortage of research in some areas of nursing, that is useful in identifying the 'effectiveness' of nursing care. In other words, whether a particular nursing activity 'works' or not, or is effective. There are many reasons for this, including time and resources to undertake the type of research needed such as controlled trials, the skills and training of nurse researchers to conduct this type of research, and the cultural barriers in health organisations and the organisation of nursing education. Second, nurses may not be appropriately trained in the skills of evidence-based practice, such as literature searching and reviewing, critical appraisal, audit and change-management. Third, nurses in practice may be hampered in their search for evidence as limited access to literature-searching facilities in some clinical settings remain.

It is possible to overcome some of these barriers, particularly through education and training. Also, there is research examining the barriers to evidence-based practice, and ways to overcome them. Finally, there are ways of finding evidence that has already been reviewed and appraised. These include evidence-based clinical guidelines from: Cochrane Reviews (systematic reviews of healthcare interventions and promotes the search for evidence in the form of clinical trials and other studies of interventions), Effective Healthcare Bulletins (based on a systematic review and synthesis of research on the clinical effect, cost-effectiveness and acceptability of health service interventions), and National Institute for Clinical Excellence (NICE) (an independent organisation responsible for providing national guidance on promoting good health and preventing and treating ill health).

Hierarchy of evidence and research

The idea of a hierarchy of evidence has evolved as a response to the notion that some research designs, particularly those using quantitative methods, are more able than others to provide robust evidence of effectiveness, that is, what works. The most common type of hierarchy therefore places evidence gathered through research at the top, with a systematic review of evidence from multiple randomised controlled trials being the pinnacle:

1 Evidence from a systematic review of multiple well-designed randomised controlled trials.
2 Evidence from one or more well-designed randomised trials.
3 Evidence from experiments without randomisation or from single before-and-after studies, cohort, time series or matched case-controlled studies or observational studies.
4 Evidence from well-designed descriptive studies or qualitative research.
5 Opinions from expert committees or respected authorities based on practice-based evidence.
6 Personal, professional and peer expertise and experience.
   (See Gray, 1997; Khan et al., 2003; and www.york.ac.uk/inst/crd/ NHS Centre for Clinical Reviews and Dissemination, for more detailed types of hierarchy.)

This hierarchy of evidence is only appropriate for research questions that are seeking an answer about what works. For example, if a nurse wanted to know the best way to dress a particular type of wound, say a burn, then the above would help in making decisions about the best type of evidence. This would be well-designed randomised controlled trials, or even better, a systematic review of randomised controlled trials. However, if nurses wanted to develop understanding about what it feels like have severe burns, so that they could develop their communication and empathetic skills, then qualitative research would be more informative.

Chapter summary

- Nursing research today has been shaped by its historical roots, and political, economic and organisation influences.
- Defining 'what is research' is not easy, and debates surround the nature of nursing and health services research.
- The recent development of evidence-based practice has been rapid and influential.
- All nurses must become 'research literate' and learn the essentials of evidence-based practice.
- Some nurses will become researchers as part of their role in practice, or through a career in teaching, policy development or leadership.

References

Bowling, A. (2002) *Research Methods in Health: Investigating Health and Health Services*, 2nd edition. Buckingham: Open University Press.

Department of Health (1993) *Report of the Taskforce on the Strategy for Research in Nursing, Midwifery and Health Visiting*. London: Department of Health.

Department of Health (2006) *Modernising Nursing Careers: Setting the Direction*. London: Department of Health.

Department of Health and Social Security (1972) *Report of the Committee on Nursing*. London: HMSO.

Glicken, M. (2005) *Improving the Effectiveness of the Helping Professions: An Evidence-based Approach to Practice*. Thousand Oaks, CA: Sage.

Gray, J. (1997) *Evidence-based Healthcare: How to Make Health Policy and Management Decisions*. London: Churchill Livingstone.

Guba, E. and Lincoln, Y. (1982) 'Epistemological and methodological bases of naturalistic enquiry', *Educational Communication and Technology*, 30 (4): 233–52.

Hek, G. and Moule, P. (2006) *Making Sense of Research: An Introduction for Health and Social Care Practitioners*, 3rd edition. London: Sage.

Higher Education Funding Council for England (HEFCE) (2001) *Promoting Research in Nursing and the Allied Health Professions*. Bristol: HEFCE.

Higher Education Statistics Agency (2005) cited in UK Clinical Research Collaboration (UKCRC) (2007) *Developing the Best Research Professionals. Qualified Graduate Nurses: Recommendations for Preparing and Supporting Clinical Academic Nurses of the Future*. London: UKCRC. p. 17.

Hopps, L.C. (1994) 'The development of research in nursing in the United Kingdom', *Journal of Clinical Nursing*, 3: 199–204.

Hunt, J. (1981) 'Indicators for nursing practice: the use of research findings', *Journal of Advanced Nursing*, 6 (3): 189–94.

Jenicek, M. (2006) 'The art of soft science: evidence-based medicine, reasoned medicine or both?', *Journal of Education in Clinical Practice*, 12: 410–19.

Khan, K., Kunz, R., Kleijnen, J. and Antes, G. (2003) *Systematic Reviews to Support Evidence-based Medicine*. London: The Royal Society of Medicine Press.

Kirby, S. (2004) 'A historical perspective on the contrasting experiences of nurses as research subjects and research activists', *International Journal of Nursing Practice*, 10: 272–9.

Mantzoukas, S. (2008) 'A review of evidence-based practice, nursing research and reflection: levelling the hierarchy', *Journal of Clinical Nursing*, 17: 214–23.

Melnyk, B. and Fineout-Overholt, E. (2005) *Evidence-based Practice in Nursing and Healthcare: A Guide to Best Practice*. Philadelphia, PA: Lippincott Williams & Wilkins.

National Health Service Centre for Reviews and Dissemination (2001) *Undertaking Systematic Reviews of Research on Effectiveness: CRD Report Number 4*, 2nd edition. York: University of York, NHS CRD.

Rafferty, A. (1997) 'Writing, researching and reflexivity in nursing history', *Nurse Researcher*, 5 (2): 5–16.

Rafferty, A., Bond, S. and Traynor, M. (2003) 'Does nursing, midwifery and health visiting need a research council?', *Nursing Times Research*, 5 (5): 325–35.

Reynolds, S. (2000) 'The anatomy of evidence-based practice: principles and methods', in L. Trinder (ed.), *Evidence-based Practice: A Critical Appraisal*. Oxford: Blackwell Science.

Sackett, D.L., Straus, S.E., Richardson, W.S., Rosenberg, W. and Haynes, R.B. (2000) *Evidence-based Medicine: How to Practice and Teach EBM*, 2nd edition. Edinburgh: Churchill Livingstone.

Thomas, E. (1985) 'Attitudes towards nursing research among trained nurses', *Nurse Education Today*, 5 (1): 18–21.

Tierney, A. (1997) 'Organization report: the development of nursing research in Europe', *European Nurse*, 2 (2): 73–84.

Tierney, A. (1998) 'Nursing research in Europe', *International Nursing Review*, 45 (1): 15–19.

Trinder, L. (2000a) 'The context of evidence-based practice', in L. Trinder (ed.), *Evidence-based Practice: A Critical Appraisal*. Oxford: Blackwell Science. pp. 1–16.

Trinder, L. (2000b) 'A critical appraisal of evidence-based practice', in L. Trinder (ed.), *Evidence-based Practice: A Critical Appraisal*. Oxford: Blackwell Science. pp. 212–41.

United Kingdom Central Council (UKCC) (1986) *Project 2000: A New Preparation for Practice*. London: United Kingdom Central Council for Nursing, Midwifery and Health Visiting.

United Kingdom Central Council (UKCC) (1994) *The Future of Professional Practice: The Council's Standards for Education and Practice Following Registration*. London: United Kingdom Central Council for Nursing, Midwifery and Health Visiting.

UK Clinical Research Collaboration (UKCRC) (2007) *Developing the Best Research Professionals. Qualified Graduate Nurses: Recommendations for Preparing and Supporting Clinical Academic Nurses of the Future*. London: UKCRC.

Webb, C. and MacKenzie, J. (1993) 'Where are we now? Research-mindedness in the 1990's', *Journal of Clinical Nursing*, 2 (3): 129–33.

Suggested further reading

Brown, B., Crawford, P. and Hicks, C. (2003) *Evidence-Based Research: Dilemmas and Debates in Health Care*. Maidenhead: Open University Press.

Freshwater, D. and Bishop, V. (2004) *Nursing Research in Context*. Basingstoke: Palgrave Macmillan.

Glasby, J. and Beresford, P. (2006) 'Commentary and issues: who knows best? Evidence-based practice and the service user contribution', *Critical Social Policy*, 26 (1): 268–84.

Gray, J.A.M. (1997) *Evidence-based Healthcare: How to Make Health Policy and Management Decisions*. London: Churchill Livingstone.

McCormack, B. (2006) 'Evidence-based practice and the potential for transformation', *Journal of Research in Nursing*, 11: 89–94.

Sackett, D.L., Straus, S.E., Richardson, W.S., Rosenberg, W. and Haynes, R.B. (2000) *Evidence-based Medicine: How to Practice and Teach EBM*, 2nd edition. Edinburgh: Churchill Livingstone.

Trinder, L. (ed.) (2000) *Evidence-based Practice: A Critical Appraisal*. Oxford: Blackwell Science.

Websites

Cochrane Reviews: www.cochrane.org/
Effective Health Care Bulletins: www.york.ac.uk/inst/crd/ehcb.htm
Evidence-based Medicine: www.openclinical.org/ebm.html
Foundation of Nursing Studies: www.fons.org/
National Institute for Clinical Excellence (NICE): www.nice.org.uk/
NHS Centre for Clinical Reviews and Dissemination: www.york.ac.uk/inst/crd/
Queen's Nursing Institute: www.qni.org.uk/
UK Clinical Research Collaboration: www.ukcrc.org/

2

SOURCES OF NURSING KNOWLEDGE

Nursing knowledge is drawn from a multifaceted base and includes evidence that comes from science (research and evaluation), experience and personally derived understanding. Scientific knowledge is developed through enquiry and can use the research approaches discussed throughout this book. It is, however, not the only form of evidence used by nurses in their practice. Nurses also use experience gained from practice itself and their own personal learning. The relationship between research and the generation of scientific knowledge is understood and accepted by many. In contrast, a number of writers have proposed frameworks that describe knowledge as being generated through experience and personal understanding. Carper (1975, 1978) discusses the four fundamental patterns of knowing: empirics (know what), aesthetic (know-how), personal knowledge (do I know myself and others?) and ethics (know why I should). This work draws together a range of essential knowledge that can be used to inform nursing practice, acknowledging the importance not just of scientific knowledge, but of knowledge developed through experience, personal understanding and interpretation and of moral and ethical reasoning. Schon (1987) developed the concept knowing how as part of 'knowing-in-action'. This supports the generation of personal and tacit knowledge that Rolfe (1998) suggests we all possess but are unable to articulate.

This chapter considers the range of knowledge available to inform practice decisions. First, we review scientific knowledge and consider how it is generated. Second, we consider other sources of knowledge developed through experience that include tradition, intuition and tacit understanding. Third, personal knowledge is presented as individual knowledge used to support care delivery on an individual basis. Liaschenko and Fisher (1999) describe this as person knowledge, that of knowing the patient as an individual person.

It should be noted that, in making decisions to deliver care and using evidence to support practice delivery, nurses may draw on a range of sources of knowledge. None exists exclusively and nurses may use scientific, personal knowledge and experience in making judgements. Having considered the complexities of nursing knowledge, we will review the development of policy to support nursing research. The chapter will end in conceptualising nursing research, defining it and considering how it informs nursing practice as part of a range of evidence that supports care development and delivery.

Learning outcomes

This chapter is designed to enable the reader to:

- **Identify the sources of knowledge available to inform nursing and health-care practice**
- **Understand the complex nature of nursing research**
- **Appreciate the importance of research and evidence-based knowledge in informing practice, theory and policy**

KEY TERMS

Intuition, Personal knowledge, Scientific knowledge, Tacit knowledge, Tradition

---

Scientific knowledge

Scientific knowledge is positioned at levels one through to four of the hierarchy of evidence (see Chapter 1) and makes a significant contribution to the development and application of nursing practice. Scientific evidence also informs nursing education, policy and management. This form of knowledge is generated through research activity, where a rigorous approach is followed to obtain findings that will be used to inform nursing practice. We discuss the process that researchers use to generate scientific knowledge in Chapter 3, and within the book we explore a number of approaches that can be used to support scientific knowledge generation (see Chapters 13 to 17). Whereas many forms of knowledge can be based on individual experience, gained through trial and error and based on **traditions**, scientific knowledge results from a methodological process that is laid open for scrutiny and critical review.

Research activity can be classified as being part of inductive and deductive approaches. Generally, a deductive approach implies that there is a theory or knowledge in existence which will be tested through the research process, whereas an inductive approach suggests that research will try to develop theory (Hek and Moule, 2006). Deductive and inductive positions in research are often described as being part of positivist and interpretivist research. Postivists emphasise the positive sciences, developing knowledge through testing and systematic experience. They employ quantitative methods to answer research questions and use scientific methods to test theory in a rigorous and controlled way. They aim to establish 'truth' that will allow the generalisation or wider use of the results (Pearson et al., 2007).

The 'gold standard' randomised controlled trial is often employed in quantitative research to evaluate the effectiveness of interventions (Centre for Reviews and Dissemination, 2001), such as to see whether one approach to hip replacement works better than another. Elements of randomisation (selecting patients for either the control or research groups randomly), control (having the control group receiving the usual hip to compare with the research group) and manipulation (the research and control groups having different hips) are used (Polit and Beck, 2006) (see Chapter 13). Evidence from randomised controlled trials contributes to levels one and two of the hierarchy of evidence (see Chapter 1), whilst evidence at level three would come from experimental designs without randomisation (see Chapters 13 and 21). There are likely to be examples of care delivery based on scientific knowledge in practice settings. Consider examples of these: Where has a randomised controlled trial or experimental design led to changes in practice?

Whilst positivist scientific approaches to knowledge generation have been important to the development of healthcare practice, especially medical practice, it is recognised that not all research questions can be addressed through such designs. Nursing and healthcare have a number of research questions related to the social aspects of life, wanting to explore the lived experience of patients, carers and staff. Research conducted in the interpretivist paradigm through qualitative approaches is employed to answer such questions and forms level four of the hierarchy of evidence (see Chapter 1). Interpretivists believe that in order to understand and make sense of the world, researchers must interpret human behaviour in natural settings. Qualitative researchers are therefore interested in gaining understanding of complex phenomena, rather than testing for cause and effect relationships seen in positivist approaches (Burns and Grove, 2005). Qualitative methods involve listening to and observing people's interactions and patterns of behaviour. The types of designs used include ethnography, phenomenology, grounded theory, but may also encompass feminist and action research (see Chapters 13 and 17). Data collection is likely to include interviews, focus groups, diary recording and observations. This research approach, rather than seeking to control and measure, avoids exerting any influence on data collection and aims to describe reality and draw understanding from this.

Many studies use a mixed method approach that includes both qualitative and quantitative research (Bryman, 1988) (see Chapter 20). The use of mixed methods in social research allows the researcher to employ a number of methods to investigate research problems (Denzin, 1989). For example, when exploring the effectiveness of pain control, quantitative measures might include recording of physiological signs, with qualitative approaches gaining the patient's views on pain control. Measuring pain relief outcomes would draw on both qualitative and quantitative methods to provide a picture of patient experience and effectiveness of pain control.

Scientific evidence is not the only form of knowledge employed to support decision making in practice. It should be remembered that a range of sources informs nursing decision making and care delivery.

Other sources of knowledge

Tradition

Knowledge passed down through generations of nurses forms the basis of traditional understanding. Traditional practices can be conveyed through observed practice, role modelling, written documents, books, journal articles, and often from 'experienced' practitioners. These practices can be imposed: 'This is the way it should be done because this is the way it has always been done.' Such an approach can lead to the development of a nursing culture that accepts practices as being right, without questioning their foundation and evidence base. Examples from current practice can include the daily washing or bathing of patients before mid-morning, recording observations of temperature, respirations, blood pressure and pulse on a regular basis. Some traditional practices can have a useful place in today's nursing. Team handovers serve a useful purpose in ensuring the transfer of patient and other ward-related information from the out-going to the in-coming nursing team. The practice can also facilitate learning for student nurses and new staff members and offers an opportunity for socialisation of the team. We can see evidence of tradition informing other areas of practice. Consider, for example: Which practices are informed by tradition? Why might this be the case?

As new evidence emerges there is often a need to challenge and change traditional and ritualistic practices. The need to practise using current evidence is expressed as part of the Nurses Code of Professional Conduct (Nursing and Midwifery Council, 2008; www.nmc-uk.org) requires all practitioners to

Keep your knowledge and skills up-to-date throughout your working life. (NMC, 2008: 7)

One major example of such challenge to traditional knowledge through the development of new evidence came in the 1990s. Manual handling practices underwent change, using risk assessment and equipment to encourage patients to move themselves. These guidelines, presented by the National Back Pain Association and the Royal College of Nursing (1997), replaced traditional lifting practices and improved the safety of staff and patients.

Intuition and tacit knowledge

Any experienced practising nurse would probably be able to provide examples of employing **intuition** and **tacit knowledge** in practice situations. The use of intuition and tacit knowledge can include anticipating cardiac arrest, the need for pain relief or belief that a patient's life is near its end. Burnard (1989) has described intuition as an acute sensitivity or 'sixth sense', drawing on experience and knowledge to make a care judgement. Tacit knowledge is also developed through experience gained by engagement in practice. Gunilla et al. (2002) propose that tacit practice can be role modelled and displayed in practice delivery to future generations of nurses.

Benner (1984) has suggested that nurses evolve into expert practitioners, using experience to develop aesthetic knowledge (know-how). Expert nurses will use know-how to identify patients' needs, engaging in the delivery of holistic care as intuitive doers (Benner, 1984). Whilst Benner also acknowledges that the expert nurse will draw on scientific or 'know what' knowledge, the idea that nurses' practice can be informed by intuition, a knowledge base that Walsh (1997) suggests is not explicit, has led to debates around accountability.

It is suggested that a lack of objectivity and ability to identify a rationale behind decisions taken using intuitive and tacit knowledge prevents it being viewed as a phenomenon for scientific study and adversely affects its recognition and standing as a knowledge base for practice (Hek and Moule, 2006). There are occasions however, when such knowledge is effectively employed to support decision making. Rew and Sparrow (1987) cite the use of intuition and tacit knowledge in situations where there may be limited information with which to interpret a possible behavioural response or in cases where ethical dilemmas are presented. Try to identify some examples of the use of intuition and tacit knowledge in practice: When is this type of knowledge used?

Dreyfus and Dreyfus (1985) offer a model of intuitive practice, described by Benner and Tanner (1987), which includes six elements of intuitive practice (See Table 2.1)

The model provides a framework for the analysis of intuitive practice that includes know-how.

As debates surrounding the value and role of intuitive and tacit knowledge in nursing practice continue (Gunilla et al., 2002; Whitehead, 2005), it should be acknowledged that intuition and tacit knowledge can inform the development of **personal knowledge**. Such knowledge may ultimately, therefore, form part of the understanding that informs professional practice.

Table 2.1 Elements of intuition

Element	Form of intuition
Pattern recognition	The ability to recognise patterns of responses and changes of behaviour; for example, to recognise a rise in patient temperature through behaviour patterns.
Similarity recognition	Recognising patient characteristics seen previously and using these as part of interpreting a situation.
Commonsense understanding	Recognising and using commonly accepted practice.
Skilled know-how	Making judgements about what seems to be the appropriate care for a patient.
Sense of salience	Recognising the importance of a particular information source, even though this may be contradicted by another.
Deliberative rationality	Maintaining a broad view of the situation.

Source: Adapted from Benner and Tanner, 1987

Personal knowledge

Personal knowledge is individual knowledge shaped through being personally involved in situations and events in practice. Liaschenko and Fisher (1999) refer to 'person knowledge', to knowing a person as an individual, understanding personal experience of illness and care delivery. Benner (1984) describes five levels of experience (see Table 2.2).

Often experience is developed through observing role models in practice, and as such can be developed to include traditional and tacit knowledge. Trial and error can also play a part in the development of knowledge gained through experience, trying a different

Table 2.2 Five levels of experience

Level	Type of experience
Novice	No personal experience of the activity. Preconceived ideas and expectations of practice that are refined and developed through experience.
Advanced beginner	Some experience to guide interpretation and intervention in recurrent situations.
Competent	Use personal knowledge gained through experience to undertake care that is deliberate and organised.
Proficient	Works with the individual patient and family, recognising the need to treat holistically and individually.
Expert	Extensive experience to analyse situations and deliver skilful care.

Source: Adapted from Benner, 1984

approach with unknown outcomes (Burns and Grove, 2005). Knowledge gained through this method becomes personal, often without formal documentation, sharing or research of the practice to confirm effectiveness for more general use. There are probably examples of drawing on trial and error to develop personal knowledge that we can identify. Consider an aspect of practice that may have been developed in this way.

Personal knowledge can be developed through the student reflecting on practice experiences. Personal expertise is therefore developed through a range of experiences and can be based on a number of sources of knowledge. Its status as a form of evidence on which to base practice is, however, subject to question. Closs (2003) suggests we should question expert knowledge that may be formed on limited experience and personal bias, without reliable foundation.

Nursing research policy in the UK

Nursing research has the potential to make a significant contribution to evidence-based practice and the development of cost and clinically effective care. At the time of publication, a number of key documents have highlighted the importance of developing nursing research (see Table 2.3). Additionally, there are publications relating to nursing research development within Wales, Scotland and Ireland (National Assembly for Wales, 1999; Scottish Executive Health Department, 2001; Department of Health and Children, 2003).

Table 2.3 Key strategy documents

Document	Development issues
Making a Difference: Strengthening the Nursing, Midwifery and Health Visiting Contribution to Health and Healthcare (DoH, 1999)	• Need for nurses to develop critical research appraisal skills. • Need for nurses to influence the government's research and development policies.
Towards a Strategy for Nursing Research and Development (DoH, 2000)	• Need for monies to support research programmes. • Need for capability building through collaborative partnerships.
Promoting Research in Nursing and the Allied Health Professions (HEFCE, 2001)	• Need for capability building to support evidence-based practice and RAE.
Best Research for Best Health: A National Health Service Research Strategy (DoH, 2006)	• Need to develop a world-class environment for health research, development and innovation.
Developing the Best Research Professionals (UKCRC, 2006) (Consultation exercise in place during the writing of this text)	• Need to develop clinical research career structures for nurses – suggested models based on clinical academic career model.

It should be noted that policy changes rapidly, and readers may find it useful to keep updated by accessing the Department of Health website (www.dh.gov.uk).

For some time there has been concern that nursing needs to influence the Department of Health (DoH) research and development (R&D) agenda and help build its research capacity (an ability to appreciate and use research) and capability (an ability to undertake research). Presenting at an R&D workshop on the contribution of nursing research in R&D, Rafferty (2000) suggested that nurses are the largest part of the NHS workforce, accounting for 70 per cent of the wage bill and 40 per cent of the overall budget. It was postulated that perhaps 40 per cent of the R&D budget should be invested in research that impacts on the work undertaken by such a majority workforce. Additionally, the need to build research capacity and capability in nursing has been acknowledged and upheld through achievements in the Research Assessment Exercise (RAE). Unit of Assessment 10 (UoA) relates to nursing and midwifery. The data are entered by university departments and include research income, publications and doctoral studies completions. Esteem indicators are scored and achievements are related to research funding allocations. Following the last RAE in 2001, the Higher Education Funding Council for England suggested that nursing is starting from a low baseline, though it did acknowledge a funding increase from 3 million in 1996–7 to 9.7 million in 1999–2000 from the DoH, NHS regional offices and trusts (HEFCE, 2001). Despite this increase it is still recognised that nursing research is not only competing against a range of health professionals well established in research, but is also affected by the lack of research monies available for nursing research, as highlighted above (Rafferty 2000). To help address this the HEFCE has provided additional capability, building monies to nursing linked to the RAE 2001 achievement (HEFCE, 2001), and nursing is being encouraged to influence the R&D agenda.

The Department of Health aims to see the UK as a world-class environment for health research, development and innovation, employing a strategy set out in *Best Research for Best Health: A National Health Service Research Strategy* (DoH, 2006). It outlines a five-year development plan that aims to see more patients and healthcare professionals engaged in health research that will increase the evidence-base and improve health and healthcare. To support this, the development of research policy and commissioning of research through the NHS R&D programme has been recast into three key programmes:

- Health Technology Assessment – devices, equipment, drugs and procedures across all healthcare sectors.
- Service Delivery and Organisation R&D programme – how organisation and delivery of services can promote quality care.
- New and Emerging Applications of Technology Programme (NEAT) – use of new and emerging technologies to develop healthcare products and interventions.

The UK Clinical Research Collaboration (UKCRC) established in 2004 has an aim to increase research capacity in the NHS, developing an expert workforce. It is currently engaged in developing a research career structure for nurses, building on the model of development for clinical academic careers. Presented as a consultation document, *Developing the Best Research Professionals* (UKCRC, 2006), a final report is due in 2008 (www.ukcrc.org.uk). The possible career structures include integrated pathways supporting education and practice development in research that require collaborations between universities and the NHS. There is no doubt that all parties involved will welcome the move to recognise and develop nurse researchers, though we must wait and see how this is operationalised. There are many issues requiring clarification, such as the funding of the initiative, the need for collaboration and agreement on knowledge and skills required, and there is still a need to support nursing-led research.

Conceptualising nursing research

In thinking about nursing research, a broad view of professional practice needs to be taken. Nursing research encompasses the practice of nursing, which is in itself complex. Practice-based research questions may try to test new practice or support care development. Additionally, they can measure the effectiveness of care, explore carer and family issues, or consider the interprofessional nature of care delivery.

Nurses do not work in isolation, but with a range of professionals in different healthcare environments. The research agenda needs to reflect this and consider questions where a multi-disciplinary approach to care is required.

Nursing research also explores the educational preparation of nurses, reviewing the pedagogy of nursing, and how best to support learning and teaching of nurses and other healthcare professionals. Research will additionally review the management of nursing services, such as the development and effectiveness of new roles.

Nursing is an emerging profession and one that often draws on other disciplines in its execution of research. The social sciences, psychology, physical sciences, environment sciences and epidemiology can inform nursing research. Indeed, research teams may often reflect a number of disciplines in their make-up, utilising a range of professions and taking on board different discipline perspectives in the research design. For example, researching aspects of mental healthcare can take a pharmaceutical, psychological or sociological perspective. In Chapter 1 we discussed the developing research roles of nurses, engaging in nursing research within universities and practice settings. Attempts to increase the research capacity (number of nurses able to understand research) and capability of nurses (nurses able to research) through career mapping are under development (UKCRC, 2006) and formally recognise the need for nurses to engage in researching their own professional practice, as highlighted in previous reports (HEFCE, 2001). Such drivers acknowledge the need to link practice, education and research within nursing in order to secure an evidence-based future (HEFCE, 2001).

Nurses should be involved not only in researching their practice but also in identifying the research agendas. In 2000 the Department of Health (DoH, 2000) emphasised the need to identify research priorities within nursing to ensure that appropriate aspects of nursing delivery are considered. This aimed to engage nurses in developing the research priorities for practice and to ensure the focus of research activity.

In undertaking such research, a multitude of research methods will be employed, in both positivist and interpretivist paradigms. Depending on the research question(s), those exploring nursing issues will draw on qualitative and quantitative approaches and a range of methods of data collection. The social sciences play a key role in much nursing research activity as they are employed to consider issues related to the patient, carer and family that can be physiological, psychological or socially derived. These are not the limits of nursing research, however, which may need to test theory and practice developments through more rigorous positivist approaches. Given the scope and nature of nursing research, our definition offered in Chapter 1 reflects its complexity and recognises the need to employ a range of methods and methodologies to address the broad range of questions and create new knowledge for practice education and policy. As a reminder, our definition based on that within Hek and Moule (2006) is:

> A systematic approach to gathering information for the purposes of answering questions and solving problems in the pursuit of creating new knowledge about nursing practice, education and policy. (2006: 10)

The remaining chapters of the book consider more fully the complexities of developing, undertaking and implementing nursing research to support decision making and practice. Whilst we should acknowledge that a range of evidence can inform practice, that derived through scientific approaches is significant to the support of evidence-based practice.

Chapter summary

- Nursing knowledge is multifaceted and is developed through science and experience.
- Nurses can draw on a range of sources of knowledge to support decision making and care delivery.
- Scientific knowledge is constructed through methodological processes and is open to scrutiny.
- Scientific knowledge can be developed through deductive and inductive research approaches.
- Tradition, intuition and tacit understanding can underpin nursing care delivery.
- Personal knowledge is knowing the patient as an individual.
- The knowledge base for practice should be questioned.
- Nurses need to be involved in developing research agendas and in researching practice.
- Nurses are still developing research skills and expertise.

References

Benner, P. (1984) *From Novice to Expert: Excellence and Power in Clinical Nursing Practice*. Menlo Park, CA: Addison-Wesley.

Benner, P. and Tanner, C. (1987) 'How expert nurses use intuition', *American Journal of Nursing*, 87 (1): 23–31.

Bryman, A. (1988) *Quantity and Quality in Social Research*. London: Routledge.

Burnard, P. (1989) 'The sixth sense', *Nursing Times*, 85 (50): 52–3.

Burns, N. and Grove, S. (2005) *The Practice of Nursing Research: Conduct, Critique and Utilization*, 5th edition. St Louis, MO: Elsevier/Saunders.

Carper, B. (1975) *Fundamental Patterns of Knowing in Nursing*. Dissertation for Degree of Doctor in Education. Columbia University, USA.

Carper, B. (1978) 'Fundamental patterns of knowing in nursing', *Advances in Nursing Science*, 1 (1): 13–23.

Centre for Reviews and Dissemination (2001) *Undertaking Systematic Reviews of Research on Effectiveness*, 2nd edition. University of York: CRD.

Closs, S.J. (2003) 'Evidence and community-based nursing practice', in R. Bryer and J. Griffiths (eds), *Practice Development in Community Nursing*. London: Arnold. pp. 33–56.

Denzin, N. (1989) *The Research Act: A Theoretical Introduction to Sociological Methods*, 3rd edition. Englewoods Cliffs, NJ: Prentice-Hall.

Department of Health (1999) *Making a Difference: Strengthening the Nursing, Midwifery and Health Visiting Contribution to Health and Healthcare*. London: Department of Health.

Department of Health (2000) *Towards a Strategy for Nursing Research and Development: Proposals for Action*. London: Department of Health.

Department of Health (2006) *Best Research for Best Health: A National Health Service Research Strategy*. London: Department of Health.

Department of Health and Children (2003) *Research Strategy for Nursing and Midwifery in Ireland*. Dublin: Department of Health and Children.

Dreyfus, H. and Dreyfus, S. (1985) *Mind over Machine: The Power of Human Intuition and Expertise in the Era of the Computer*. New York: Free Press.

Gunilla, C., Drew, N., Dahlberg, K. and Lutzen, K. (2002) 'Uncovering tacit caring knowledge', *Nursing Philosophy*, 3 (20): 144–51.

Hek, G. and Moule, P. (2006) *Making Sense of Research: An Introduction for Health and Social Care Practitioners*, 3rd edition. London: Sage.

Higher Education Funding Council for England (HEFCE) (2001) *Promoting Research in Nursing and the Allied Health Professions*. Research Report 01/64. Bristol: Higher Education Funding Council for England. Available at www.hefce.ac.uk/Pubs/hefce/2001/01_64.htm.

Liaschenko, J. and Fisher, A. (1999) 'Theorising the knowledge that nurses use in the conduct of their work', *Scholarly Inquiry for Nursing Practice: An International Journal*, 13: 29–40.

National Assembly for Wales (1999) *Realising the Potential: A Strategic Framework for Nursing, Midwifery and Health Visiting in Wales into the 21st Century.* Cardiff: National Assembly for Wales.

National Back Pain Association and the Royal College of Nursing (1997) *The Guide to the Handling of Patients.* Teddington: National Back Pain Association.

Nursing and Midwifery Council (2008) *The Code: Standards of Conduct, Performance and Ethics for Nurses and Midwives.* London: NMC.

Pearson, A., Field, J. and Jordan, Z. (2007) *Evidence-based Clinical Practice in Nursing and Health Care: Simulating Research, Experience and Expertise.* Oxford: Blackwell.

Polit, D. and Beck, C. (2006) *Essentials of Nursing Research: Methods, Appraisal and Utilization*, 6th edition. Philadelphia, PA: Lippincott Williams & Wilkins.

Rafferty, A.M. (2000) 'Influencing the research and development agenda'. Paper presented to a Department of Health Research and Development Workshop. York, March 2000.

Rew, L. and Sparrow, E. (1987) 'Intuition: a neglected hallmark of nursing knowledge', *Advances in Nursing Science*, 10 (10): 49–62.

Rolfe, G. (1998) *Expanding Nursing Knowledge.* Oxford: Butterworth Heinemann.

Schon, D.A. (1987) *Educating the Reflective Practitioner.* San Francisco, CA: Jossey-Bass.

Scottish Executive Health Department (2001) *Caring for Scotland: The Strategy for Research and Development in Nursing and Midwifery in Scotland.* Edinburgh: Scottish Executive Health Department.

United Kingdom Clinical Research Collaboration (2006) *Developing the Best Research Professionals.* London: UKCRC. Available at www.ukcrc.org/activities/ researchworkforce.aspx.

Walsh, M. (1997) 'Accountability and intuition: justifying nursing practice', *Nursing Standard*, 11 (23): 39–41.

Whitehead, D. (2005) 'Empirical or tacit knowledge as a basis for theory development?', *Journal of Clinical Nursing*, 14 (2): 299–305.

Suggested further reading

Estabrooks, C., Rutakumura, W., O'Leary, K., Profetto-McGrath, J., Milner, M., Leavers, M.-J. and Scott-Findlay, S. (2005) 'Sources of practice knowledge among nurses', *Qualitative Health Research*, 15 (4): 460–76. http://qhr.sagepub.com/cgi/ reprint/15/4/460.

Glasby, J. and Beresford, P. (2006) 'Commentary and issues: who knows best? Evidence-based practice and the service user contribution', *Critical Social Policy*, 26 (1): 268–84. http://csp.sagepub.com/cgi/reprint/26/1/268.

Pearson, A., Field, J. and Jordan, Z. (2007) *Evidence-based Clinical Practice in Nursing and Health Care: Simulating Research, Experience and Expertise*. Oxford: Blackwell.

Rice, M. (2008) 'Psychiatric mental health evidence-based practice', *Journal of the American Psychiatric Nurses Association*, 14 (2): 107–11. http.//jap.sagepub.com/cgi/reprint/14/2/107.

Rolfe, G. (1998) *Expanding Nursing Knowledge*. Oxford: Butterworth Heinemann.

Websites

Department of Health: www.dh.gov.uk
Higher Education Funding Council for Higher Education: www.hefce.ac.uk
Nursing and Midwifery Council: www.nmc-uk.org
UK Clinical Research Collaboration: www.ukcrc.org.uk

3

THE RESEARCH PROCESS

The research process guides research activity. It is a series of steps or stages undertaken by researchers in order to address research questions. In this chapter we discuss the main steps guiding nursing research, which are not unique to the profession but can be mirrored in other disciplines. Nursing employs the research process to consider questions arising from practice and education, providing a 'scientific' approach to generating evidence on which to base practice. In adopting such an approach, the process taken to answer practice questions is founded in an objective framework that is open to scrutiny and critical review. Thus, judgements can be made about the quality of the research process and its outcomes.

The process, though presented in a linear framework in Figure 3.1, is not necessarily implemented in this way. Researchers can be engaged in moving backwards and forwards between the stages and may not be involved in them consecutively or sequentially. An understanding of the research process is needed to identify published research, with knowledge of the processes involved in each stage being required to support critical appraisal and evaluation of research papers.

The publishers of nursing research assist identification of the stages of the process through providing authors with templates for the presentation of research papers (see Figure 3.2). A comparison of the two Figures shows distinct overlap and a cognisance between the process of research and its presentation to readers. It should be acknowledged that within this book our aim is to provide readers with the knowledge and skills to critically read research. We also provide insight into the stages and processes of research activity that might support the development of a research proposal. Additionally, theoretical guidance in the text will support those engaged in the activity of research, where the skills of research will be developed under supervision.

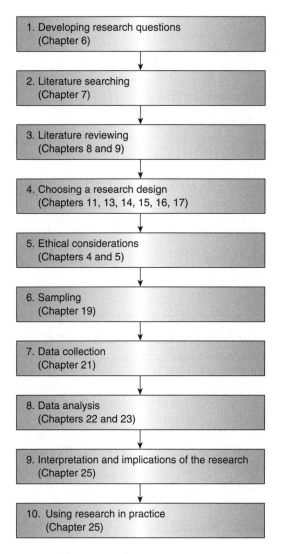

Figure 3.1   The stages of the research process

Learning outcomes

This chapter is designed to enable the reader to:

- Identify the stages of the research process
- Understand how the research process guides research activity

Introduction

Background (literature review)

The study

    Aims (research questions/hypothesis)

    Design/methodology

    Sample/participants

    Data collection

    Validity and reliability/rigour of the study

    Ethical considerations

    Data analysis

Results/findings

Discussion

Conclusions

Figure 3.2 *Journal of Advanced Nursing*: **research paper headings**
Source: www.journalofadvancednursing.com, accessed 23 November 2007

KEY TERMS

Deductive reasoning, Inductive reasoning, Research design, Research process

---

Stages of the research process

Developing research questions

Research questions are often derived from nursing practice, emerging from issues or problems in care delivery, or a desire to enhance practice. They can be key questions proposed at government through to individual level, sometimes with funding being offered to support the **research process**. Government research agendas are often linked to changes in policy; for example, recent commissions have considered the use of information technology by nurses in decision making, linked to the publication of the initial National Health Service Plan (DoH, 2000). Individual professionals in the workplace might identify local research questions. This can result from experiences of immediate practice delivery, and could include questions about patient information provision or user perspectives. Examples might include: 'What are patients' experiences of cancer care treatment?' or 'Is the new process of patient handover more effect for the nurse?'

Further details on problem identification and the formulation of research aims, questions or the development of research hypotheses are reviewed in Chapter 6. Chapter 6 also considers the importance of developing research questions based on establishing the current evidence base through literature searching and review. This will ensure that the initial thinking about the research problem area is well founded and should provide evidence of the research base that already exists, confirming whether further research is needed. The literature review can also provide some ideas on how the research should be designed and conducted to answer the research problem. Thus, the stage of finalising the research question will overlap with the steps of literature searching and literature reviewing, with the formulation of a question being guided by practice experience and critical review of the existing literature.

Literature searching

This stage of the research process is not only important in developing the research question, but also potentially links to all other stages of the research process. Successful searching is the key to identifying the existing literature in the field of study and will determine the current knowledge base. It should be ongoing throughout the period of research study, enabling the researcher to draw on any new thinking in the field that might impact on the study.

The literature search can inform the development of the **research design,** sample, data collection and data analysis and is drawn on in identifying the research interpretations and implications for practice. These relationships and the process of literature searching are discussed in Chapter 7, which suggests the need for a systematic approach to ensure that all relevant literature is accessed. Given the importance of adopting a rigorous approach to searching, the chapter includes a number of strategies that can be employed, including the identification of key terms, sources and development of inclusion and exclusion criteria. It also highlights a number of organisations and key personnel with advanced searching skills, whose expertise can be drawn on.

Researchers undertaking literature-based studies complete a systematic critical appraisal of existing research-making literature searching (see Chapter 18), a crucial component of the research methodology.

Literature reviewing

A review of the literature follows the literature search, though in practice the researcher is likely to begin this process whilst still obtaining papers and can use the review to identify further literature that should be sourced. Reviewing can be guided by a critical review framework and conducted following an appraisal process, as discussed in Chapters 8 and 9. The critical review framework (see Chapter 9) is based on the stages of the research process and is developed to include a number of questions that allow the user to interrogate the published research paper. The questions will relate to presentation and content, and when applied through an appraisal process will enable the reviewer to analyse the strengths and weaknesses of the paper. The process of review aims to support evaluation of the quality of the published literature identified in the search.

The advent of the Internet has facilitated access to a wider range of literature than previously available. Not all papers found on the Internet have been subjected to a formal peer review process and postings can present personal opinion. Those reviewing material will therefore need to appreciate the different levels of evidence available. To assist readers in this, Chapter 1 provides an introduction to the sorts of information and evidence accessible to support research, whilst Chapter 2 reviews the different sources of nursing knowledge.

Choosing a research design

There is a range of research designs available for use in addressing research questions. Their function is to ensure that the evidence collected is able to answer the research questions. In other words, the design chosen should enable the researcher to collect the evidence needed to answer the research problems or questions. The design is the plan of how the research will answer the research question and should include the overall research approach taken, ethical considerations, sampling, methods of data collection and analysis. Chapter 11 presents further discussions on selecting a research design. Often research designs and approaches can be presented as being either part of qualitative or quantitative research, as a dichotomy, that polarises the approaches. This position isn't necessarily helpful as the designs, such as case study methods (see Chapter 17), can include data collection methods that might be viewed as qualitative (participant observation) or those seen as more quantitative (surveys).

Quantitative research, in the crudest sense, is research that tends to be driven by a positivist or scientific approach, but more latterly by a post-positivist approach. It is often described as being part of deduction or **deductive reasoning** that starts with a general theory about something and moves to test the theory through undertaking further observations or by developing tests. Quantitative research is seen as attempting to answer questions and hypothesis through generating research data, often involving numerical data collection that can be analysed through statistical techniques. There is often an aim to generalise results to a wider population, applying the results to a broader group of people.

Qualitative research is most commonly seen as inductivist, where the aim is to develop concepts and themes from the interpretation of observations and interviews. **Inductive reasoning** is a process of starting with the details of an experience or our observations of something and using these to develop a general understanding of phenomena. Specific observations and descriptions are made and used to develop a hypothesis and theory of a more general situation that can be tested.

In its simplest form, qualitative research aims to generate data that comprises words and pictures. Qualitative researchers often focus on language, perceptions and experiences in order to understand and explain behaviour. They believe that the social world needs to be interpreted to be understood. Qualitative research may be used to explore beliefs and experiences. Evidence is analysed to identify key themes and issues. The results often describe the local context and can be open to transferability to other contexts.

Chapters 11, and 13 to 17, include more in-depth discussions on a range of research designs, including those that might be employed in quantitative research such as experimental and survey design and those that can be drawn on within qualitative approaches, phenomenology, ethnography and grounded theory.

Crucially, the researcher needs to adopt the most suitable research approach to answer the research question. The selection of approach should take account of the existing literature base and subject of the study. In some cases adopting a qualitative approach might be reasonable and in others a combined approach might afford better answers. For example, if research aimed to review nurse's learning and skill development, a combined approach would offer scope to test knowledge and skill attainment measuring specific criteria and elicit experiences of learning. Data collection in this case would include a range of methods such as pre- and post-tests of knowledge, testing skill attainment against proved criteria and interviewing individuals about their learning experiences.

The selection of a research design will also be influenced by a number of practical issues. In designing a study the researcher will think about their own research skills and the expertise of the research team and preferred working methods. Designing a study with methods of data collection the researchers prefer not to engage with, or are not skilled in, wouldn't be sensible. The team also needs to consider the amount of time for the study and the resources to support it. For example, it may be that there is a limited amount of time and resources available, in which case selecting a longitudinal study with the need for participant observations would not be sustainable. It may be more practical to arrange to collect some key interviews for analysis, though obviously the design selected must enable the researcher to collect the evidence needed to address the research question, so must be valid.

Rigour and trustworthiness must also be apparent in the application of the research design. Chapter 12 reviews issues of rigour, validity and reliability in quantitative research, and considers how these key characteristics reflect the quality in research design. Though measures of rigour in qualitative research are less developed, it must establish trustworthiness through being auditable, checking that the interpretations of data are credible, transferable, dependable and confirmable.

Ethical considerations

Often the ethical issues of research are given less credence than is afforded within this book. Ethical considerations are placed here, as we believe ethical issues should be considered prior to undertaking sampling and data collection. In fact, one could argue that ethical issues should be placed at the top of the research process, being reviewed prior to developing the research question, rather than being referred to at the end of the research process, as is often the case.

Within healthcare research there are clear guidelines for researchers to work with that are not necessarily afforded in all professions where researchers might be working with vulnerable subjects, such as within the field of education. The British Educational Research Association (BERA) provides guidelines (BERA, 2004) to support ethical practice, encouraging researchers to reflect on their practice, but this operates at an individual level. Formal mechanisms rarely exist to review research proposals, as, with the exception of universities, education structures don't tend to encompass an ethics committee of any kind. *Research Governance* (DoH, 2005) guides the practice of anyone researching with patients, clients or health and social care staff, and applies to all those undertaking research, whether it is part of professional development or a large-scale project. Currently healthcare is leading the way in the approach to researching ethically, though other professions are set to follow.

Sampling

Data is collected from a sample, drawn from a population that the researcher is interested in. Such populations may be composed of subjects or incidents. The size and scope of the selected sample will depend on the research design that is being used to answer the research question and the methods of data collection employed. For example, an experimental design might employ a statistician to compute a power calculation to estimate the sample size needed for the study. The research would then aim to recruit that number to support rigour and confidence in the data analysis. In general, qualitative approaches can include smaller samples based on the characteristics of the population. Where phenomenological approaches are taken to explore the lived experience of a particular group, sampling will be purposive and sample selection will aim to include members of that population in the study.

Sampling theory includes two main strategies or techniques. These are commonly referred to as probability and non-probability sampling. Probability sampling techniques involve the use of random selection, where in theory every member of the population has a chance of being included in the final sample. In contrast, non-probability sampling does not attempt to include random selection processes and selection can be determined at researcher level. Within each technique there are a number of approaches to sampling. These are discussed in further detail as part of Chapter 19.

Data collection

Each research design can employ a number of data collection techniques or methods. A case study design, for example, might encompass documentary analysis, observations, interviews and diary collection. Each data collection tool affords the researcher access to different types of data relevant to addressing the research question. Interviews will allow the researcher to explore experiences of providing patient care, whereas observations facilitate insight into actual practice delivery, and documentation provides written accounts of practice provision. A number of data collection techniques are presented in Chapter 21, spanning those that might be employed within the range of research designs. Commonly used techniques include interviews, questionnaires, tests and measurement scales. These are discussed in Chapter 21, and reference is made to the use of life history, critical incident technique and emerging Internet and web-based approaches. The discussion will cover the main approaches to data collection, identifying the potential strengths and weaknesses of each.

Data analysis

The approach to data analysis will depend on the type of data that has been collected. Quantitative data analysis techniques are presented in Chapter 22. The chapter discusses the analysis of numerical data, using descriptive and inferential statistics. The management of data is considered, including working with data sets, understanding levels of measurement, the application of statistical tests and generation of probability figures. There is also discussion of the types of computer packages available to assist those analysing numerical data. The chapter will guide those interested to resources that cover the mechanics of calculation, as it does not aim to equip readers with the skill to compute tests, but rather to appreciate how researchers work with data and present it.

A further chapter presents the key issues of qualitative data analysis, which involves the researcher describing and presenting findings through developing interpretations of text or observational data. Chapter 23 considers the preparation of qualitative data and processes of analysis, including the use of computer software to support analysis and the presentation of findings.

Interpretation and implications of the research

Health care research often addresses research questions that are specifically related to issues in practice. There is an expectation, therefore, that research findings will have direct relevance to practice and possibly to policy development. Research may also identify the need for ongoing study in a particular field and make recommendations regarding the need for further research, identifying questions and possible designs. Chapter 25 reviews the implications, arising from research activity, for practice, policy and further research. In doing so it considers the importance of recognising any limitations in the research design that might affect the strength of the findings and quality of the research.

Using research in practice

Historically, nursing has reported difficulties in applying research findings to practice, identifying key obstacles to its use. Chapter 25 considers potential barriers to research implementation, though also comments on the use of research in developing clinical guidelines, practice protocols and in developing standards of care as part of clinical audit. Effective strategies used to increase research implementation are reviewed, including the dissemination of research through the provision of research reports, journal papers and conference presentations. These activities should be a mandatory part of the research process for any researcher. Research proposals, whether developed as part of an application for funding, for professional development, private study or as part of a review for ethical approval, should include a strategy for the dissemination of research findings.

Chapter summary

- The research process is a series of steps or stages undertaken by researchers in order to address research questions.
- The research process includes the following stages: Developing the research question; Literature searching; Literature reviewing; Choosing a research design; Ethical considerations; Sampling; Data collection; Data analysis; Interpretation and implications of the research; Using research in practice.

- The stages can be inter-related as research activity does not always follow the process sequentially.
- Appreciation of the stages of the research process enables professionals to identify and critically appraise research.

References

British Educational Research Association (2004) *Revised Ethical Guidelines for Educational Research*. Macclesfield: BERA. Available at www.bera.ac.uk/publications/guides.php, accessed 11 February 2008.

Department of Health (2000) *The NHS Plan*. London: Stationery Office.

Department of Health (2005) *Research Governance Framework for Health and Social Care*. London: DoH. Available at www.dh.gov.uk/en/Publicationsandstatistics/Publications/PublicationsPolicyAndGuidance/DH_4108962, accessed 11 February 2008.

Suggested further reading

Bowling, A. (2002) *Research Methods in Health: Investigating Health and Health Services*, 2nd edition. Buckingham: Open University Press.

Department of Health (2005) *Research Governance Framework for Health and Social Care, Department of Health*, 2nd edition. London: Department of Health. Available at www.dh.gov.uk/en/Publicationsandstatistics/Publications/PublicationsPolicyAndGuidance/DH_4108962.

LoBiondo-Wood, G. and Haber, J. (2006) *Nursing Research: Methods and Critical Appraisal for Evidence-based Practice*, 6th edition. St Louis, MO: Elsevier Mosby.

Polit, D. and Beck, C. (2006) *Essentials of Nursing Research: Methods, Appraisal and Utilization*, 6th edition. Philadelphia, PA: Lippincott Williams & Wilkins.

Welch, A. (2004) 'The researcher's reflections on the research process', *Nursing Science Quarterly*, 17 (3): 201–7.

Websites

BERA guidelines: www.bera.ac.uk/publications/guides.php

Department of Health Publications, Policy and Guidance: www.dh.gov.uk/en/Publicationsandstatistics/Publications/PublicationsPolicyAndGuidance/DH_4108962

4

RESEARCH ETHICS AND GOVERNANCE

Ethical issues arise at all stages in the research process. They start at the very beginning with decisions about whether or not the research should be conducted at all. For example, there may be some research that is so offensive that it would be unethical for it to be conducted. On the other hand, there may be some research that it would be unethical to not do, such as evaluations of new services or acceptability of new treatments to patients. There is also a strong argument that supports the idea that research should only be undertaken when it is apparent (usually based on findings from a comprehensive literature review) that there is no clear answer to a question or problem and that research will help to provide an answer.

For most research the intention should be to improve knowledge, whether it is about treatment and care, diagnosis and prophylactic procedures or gaining an understanding of people's experiences, perspectives and behaviours. Certainly, anyone funding research or giving permission for research to be conducted, such as a Research Ethics Committee (REC), research and development department of a healthcare institution or grant-giving body, will want evidence and a justification for carrying out the research before giving funding or approval for a specific research project. This includes researchers having their proposals subjected to independent scrutiny through Research Ethics Committees established by, for example, universities, healthcare institutions and social care providers, to ensure that the research is ethical.

This chapter concentrates on the significance of ethics committees and governance when conducting nursing research, including multi-disciplinary and interdisciplinary studies. The next chapter (Chapter 5) discusses the principles that determine whether research is ethical, with particular emphasis on the responsibilities that a researcher must consider in relation to any potential and actual participants.

Learning outcomes

This chapter is designed to enable the reader to:

- Recognise the specific guidance and ethical codes for nurse researchers
- Recognise the important legislation that nurse researchers need to consider
- Have an understanding of Research Governance
- Have an understanding of research ethics committees and their role
- Have an appreciation of the principles of Good Clinical Practice in research.

KEY TERMS

Anonymity, Confidentiality, Data Protection Act 1998, Ethical principles, Good Clinical Practice in research, Human Tissue Act 2004, Mental Capacity Act 2005, Research ethics, Research ethics committees, Research Governance Framework, Storage

---

Regulations and legislation

The imperative of healthcare research is to balance the advancement of knowledge with the need to respect human integrity and the right to self-determination. The ethical approach should always err on the side of caution: participants should be exposed to minimum risk of harm whilst benefiting directly or indirectly from the outcome of research.

There is no doubt that research has produced benefits in the past and continues to do so. However, in response to some major blunders in research history, a need for guidance and regulation has been recognised as being necessary, as virtually all research is potentially harmful. Probably the most well-known abuse of research participants was the use of human subjects in biomedical experiments in the Second World War. The subsequent Nuremberg War Crimes Trials resulted in the creation of the Nuremberg Code in the late 1940s.

The Nuremberg Code set out the standards for judging physicians and scientists who had conducted biomedical experiments on concentration camp prisoners. This code became a prototype for many later regulations, particularly those relating to human experimentation, with voluntary consent being the central tenet.

The Nuremberg Code was superseded in 1964 by the Declaration of Helsinki when the World Medical Association adopted the code. It is regularly amended to take into account changing perspectives and is currently being updated. The Declaration of Helsinki sets out principles to safeguard research participants, has voluntary consent fundamental to the principles and clearly states that the interests of society should never take precedence over the well-being of participants.

More recently, in Europe and the UK there has been a steady increase in the regulations, requirements and governance relating to conduct of research in health and social services. These have been driven by highly publicised scandals such as: research without consent using the organs of children who had died; malpractice and misconduct by health researchers which have been reported in the press; increased public interest in health and research issues; an increasingly litigious society and increased public expectation for accountability, transparency and fairness within health and social services. Furthermore, in the past many health and social care organisations have not always had a comprehensive record of all the research being undertaken in their organisations, on their premises or involving their staff and patients/clients. All of these factors, together with legislation that relates to the protection of the rights of individuals, have contributed to new policies and practices that are designed to protect research participants and give greater confidence to the general public who are potential research participants.

This means that there are a number of regulations and legislation that have to be complied with when undertaking research, and it is incumbent on individual researchers to ensure compliance. Legislation that has an impact on research includes:

- *Data Protection Act 1998*

  This is a very important Act for researchers, who must consider how they handle and process personal information and data. The **Data Protection Act** lays down the legal requirements for handling personal data to protect the confidentiality of the individual and the interests of those who have legitimate reasons for using personal information. Personal information includes both facts and opinions about the individual, including images, recordings and samples. It places obligations on those who process information (controllers), and rights of those, living or dead, who are the subject of the information (subjects). There are eight principles of good practice and anyone processing (controllers) personal information (written or electronic) must comply with them. The Act require that personal data must:

  1 be fairly and lawfully processed
  2 be processed for limited purposes; these must be specified and lawful and must not be further processed in any way incompatible with the purpose
  3 be adequate, relevant and not excessive for the purpose
  4 be accurate and kept up to date
  5 not be kept longer than is necessary for the purpose; for research purposes this can be an unspecified period providing it can be justified
  6 be processed in accordance with the individual's rights (see below)
  7 be kept secure
  8 not be transferred to countries outside the European Economic Area (EEA) unless the country has adequate protection for the individual.

Some data is particularly sensitive and there are extra provisions for information about ethnic or racial origin, political opinions and religious beliefs, trade union membership, physical or mental health condition, sex life, criminal proceedings and convictions. These conditions include having the explicit consent of the individual concerned or there are legal requirements or protection issues associated with the data.

The subjects of the information also have rights under the Data Protection Act. There is a right to find out what information is held about them on computer and some manual records. A data controller can be asked by an individual not to process information relating to him or her that causes substantial unwarranted damage or distress to them or anyone else and not to process information for direct marketing purposes. Subjects of the information also have the right to compensation for damage or distress caused by breach of the Act and to apply for a court to order get rectification, blocking or destruction of data if it is inaccurate or based on opinions formed from inaccurate information.

In addition, all National Health Service (NHS) providers of healthcare have someone appointed as a 'Caldicott Guardian' (named after the *Caldicott Report* of 1997). This is usually a senior manager who has the responsibility for the safekeeping of patients' records and for ensuring that patient information is used appropriately by staff. Caldicott Guardians also ensure that patients' rights are respected in relation to records, and may need to give approval for researchers to have access to patients' records.

- *Freedom of Information Act 2000*

This Act allows access to information regardless of when it was created or how long the public authority has held it. There are, however, a number of exemptions, for example, information relating to national security and confidential information. Other exemptions also require a public authority to consider whether it is in the public interest to withhold information. If an individual wants to gain access to information about themself, they should use their rights under the Data Protection Act. However, personal data about other individuals cannot be released, as it would breach the Data Protection Act.

For researchers, knowledge about what is available from public authorities under the Freedom of Information Act can be useful if background information is required. Furthermore, in some types of research, access to such public information may be an important stage in the research process and researchers should familiarise themselves with the guidelines available.

- *Human Rights Act 1998*

In terms of research, the Human Rights Act has no specific conditions other than requiring that researchers respect the basic human rights of participants and anyone connected with the research at all times.

- *Mental Capacity Act 2005*

The **Mental Capacity Act** (MCA) is a particularly important Act for researchers in the field of health and social care. Many nurse researchers want to undertake research with vulnerable participants or those who lack capacity to give consent, this is possible provided that the requirements of the MCA are fulfilled. Any nurse wanting to involve participants who lack capacity to consent must be fully conversant with the requirements under the MCA.

Of specific interest to researchers are sections 30 to 34 of the MCA. These go into detail about undertaking research with individuals who lack capacity to consent, and what is required by law. This includes approval of a research project involving people who lack capacity to consent by an appropriate body when it is satisfied that the research is connected to the impairing condition affecting the individual or its treatment. There must be justification that the research cannot be carried out on individuals who have the capacity to consent and the study must have the potential to benefit participants without imposing a burden disproportionate to the benefit, or an intention to provide knowledge of the causes or care and treatment of people affected by the same or similar condition.

Researchers who involve individuals who lack capacity to consent must have reasonable grounds for believing that participating carries negligible risk to the individual, is not unduly invasive or restrictive and does not interfere with the participants' freedom of action or privacy. They must also do nothing to participants that the participant appears to object to (unless this is to protect the individual from harm or reduce or prevent pain and discomfort). Researchers must also withdraw such individuals from the study if the participant indicates in *any way* that they wish to be withdrawn, or withdraw them from the study if the researcher believes there is a risk to the participant and, at all times, the interests of the participants must be assumed to outweigh those of science and society.

As well as establishing whether an individual has mental capacity to make a decision, such as whether to participate in a study or not, researchers must consider the likelihood of whether an individual will at some other time have capacity and, as far as is reasonably practical, encourage them to participate in any decision affecting them. This might also include considering the person's past and present wishes and feelings, their beliefs and values, and the views of anyone who has been named by the individual, cares for them or has a lasting power of attorney and would consider what was in the person's best interests.

The MCA provides a legal framework to protect people with impaired capacity and support them so that they are given every opportunity to make decisions for themselves. It sets out a number of principles that should be used when determining whether a person has mental capacity. A person is defined as lacking capacity if *at the time* of the decision, or act, they are unable to make a decision for themselves because of impairment or disturbance of brain function. This disturbance can be temporary or permanent and assessment of capacity should not be referenced to their age, appearance or aspect of behaviour that might lead to unjustified assumptions about their mental capacity.

A person is deemed to be unable to make a decision for themselves if they are unable to understand the information relevant to the decisions (the information must be given in a way appropriate to the individual's circumstances, for example, simple language, visual aids); retain the information (even if it is only for a short period it does not prevent them from making a decision); weigh up information and reasonably foresee the consequences of deciding one way or another as part of the decision-making process; communicate the decision by talking, sign language or other means.

The MCA also contains a duty to consult, where practicable and appropriate, the next of kin of a person with impaired capacity and has introduced new forms for proxy decision making and advocacy.

- *Public Interest Disclosure Act 1998*

Decisions about breaking confidentiality 'in the public interest' are complex. Each case is considered on its merits as to whether the duty of confidentiality to the research participant should prevail over the disclosure of information. In terms of research, if **confidentiality** or **anonymity** cannot be guaranteed, participants must be warned in advance before they agree to participate. If information needs to be disclosed in the public interest without a participant's consent, there must be a benefit to the individual or society that outweighs the individual's right to confidentiality, for example, if the health and safety of anyone has been, is being or is likely to be endangered.

The Public Interest Disclosure Act is particularly important for nurse researchers who want to include work colleagues as participants.

- *Human Tissue Act 2004*

For anyone involved in research with organs or tissue, the full legislation of the **Human Tissue Act** must be consulted and particular reference made to the consenting process. The National Research Ethics Service gives specific guidance on this. The Human Tissues Authority (HTA) has a specific role in informing the public about **storage** and use of human bodies and tissues and the disposal of human tissue. They also license and inspect some activities, including research activities, and produce good practice guidelines.

The Human Tissue Act has come about as a direct result of a number of enquiries into the retention and use of organs and tissues. The public enquiries showed that storage and use of organs and tissue without proper consent after people had died were commonplace. A legal review also found that the law on tissue retention was inadequate and, following public consultation, the Human Tissue Act (2004) replaced the 1989 Human Organ Transplant Act. This Act introduced a new offence of DNA theft and also includes a change that allows museums to move human remains out of their collections.

Human tissue is defined in the Act as material that has come from human body cells. Hair and nail from living people are excluded, as are live gametes and embryos, which are covered under the 1990 Human Fertilization and Embryology Act.

The fundamental principle of the Human Tissue Act is consent. It lists the purposes for which consent is required and these include research, clinical audit and training including training for research purposes. There are a few exceptions, for example, where 'residual' tissue from the living that cannot be identified and can be used provided certain conditions apply, existing holdings of tissue, and where there is a case of extreme public health emergency.

Understandably, these recent developments have resulted in more formalised ethics procedures and additional bureaucracy for researchers in the fields of health and social care. Social science research, which often spans health and nursing research, has now also become more bureaucratised and moved it away from its former reliance on self-regulation and professional codes. However, it must be recognised that protection of participants, and researchers, is the prime reason for these procedures being put into place.

Research Governance Framework

Research governance has developed in order to promote high standards in the conduct of research. In the UK this governance developed out of existing guidance, acts as a reference for all human research, and recognises that research participants have the right to have their physical and mental integrity respected and safeguarded. These rights are set out on the basis of a commitment to, and acceptance of, the need for research to enhance an effective health and social care service provision.

Specifically, the *Research Governance Framework for Health and Social Care* (DoH, 2005) was developed with the overall aim of setting standards; defining mechanisms to deliver standards; describing the monitoring and assessment arrangements; improving research quality; and safeguarding the public. The expectation is that there are high ethical, scientific and financial standards; clear allocation of responsibilities; transparent decision making; risk management and robust monitoring arrangements in healthcare organisations that are research-active. Ensuring proper governance of research undertaken in the NHS and its close partners should help the public have confidence in, and benefit from, good quality research. Research governance is one of the core standards of all organisations delivering NHS care.

All research-active healthcare organisations must comply with the **Research Governance Framework**. This means having systems in place to ensure that the principles and requirements of the framework are consistently applied. It applies to all types of research and research methods and to all health contexts including hospitals, the community and primary care, public health and prison healthcare. Research in this context is described as

the attempt to generate generalisable new knowledge by addressing clearly defined research questions with systematic and rigorous new methods. (DoH, 2005: 3)

It means that studies that both test and generate hypotheses come under the remit of the Framework.

There are five areas of responsibility in the Research Governance Framework, and different legislation and guidance applies to the different areas: science, information, health and safety, finance and intellectual property, ethics.

Science

It is expected that existing sources of evidence, for example, literature reviews, should be carefully considered before new research is undertaken. Proposals for research should be subjected to peer review that gives independent advice on quality, though this should be proportionate to the scale of the research and the risks involved. For example, a small-scale student project should not be subjected to the same level of review as a multi-centre randomised controlled trial. All research involving patients should apply the principles of **Good Clinical Practice** (MRC, 1998), and the Medicines and Healthcare products Regulatory Agency (MHRA) must authorise any trials on people of medicines/devices. Finally, any data collected must be retained for an appropriate period to allow for further analysis, subject to consent, and to support monitoring by appropriate bodies.

Information

The Framework states that there should be free access to information on the research and the findings after appropriate critical scientific review. This information should be presented in a format understandable and accessible to those who have participated, those who have the potential to benefit and the general public. Opportunities to develop commercial medicines, devices and aids should be taken, subject to the protection of intellectual property and commercial confidentiality.

Health and safety

The safety of participants and researcher should be given priority at all times, and health and safety regulations must be strictly observed.

Finance and intellectual property

There must be financial probity and compliance with the law and rules of HM Treasury for the use of public funds. This includes employers having in place arrangements for compensation if any of their staff harm anyone through negligence. Consideration for the exploitation of intellectual property should be part of the governance framework for any research study.

Ethics

The dignity, rights, safety and well-being of participants are paramount in any research project. For research involving patients, service users, healthcare professionals or volunteers or their organs, tissues or data, there must be independent review to ensure that ethical standards are met. There must be appropriate arrangements for obtaining informed consent. This includes the provision of suitable material, such as written or pictorial information, so that participants, caregivers, parents or supporters have clear explanations that they can understand. When tissues and organs are to be used, the special arrangements specified under the Human Tissues Act (2004) must be applied.

It is expected that researchers be aware of their ethical and legal responsibilities in relation to the confidentiality, protection and storage of participant information. Wherever possible, service users, caregivers and representative groups should be involved in the design, conduct, analysis and reporting of the research. The research design, methods and techniques should reflect the diversity of society where relevant, and take account of age, disability, gender, sexual orientation, race, culture and religion of participants and users of research. Risks in research must be in proportion to the potential benefit and should be kept to a minimum. Risks, pain and discomfort must be explained to potential participants, and there should be arrangements for compensation in the event of non-negligent harm.

Within the Research Governance Framework there are different responsibilities for different groups of people, that is: researchers, participants, the care organisation and responsible health care professionals, the organisation employing the researchers, the research funders and the sponsor of the research.

Responsibilities of sponsors

The sponsor of the research is usually, but not always, the employer of the researcher or the supervisor of the student. They could also be the funder or the care organisation, or there could be joint sponsor arrangements between a university and a care organisation, for example.

Essentially, sponsors are responsible for ensuring that the research proposal respects the dignity, rights, safety and well-being of participants, and that the relationship with care professionals and arrangement are consistent with the Research Governance Framework. This will include confirming that an independent expert review and appropriate **research ethics committee** or independent ethics reviewer have given favourable opinions about the proposal. If the study involves medicine sponsors, or someone acting on their behalf, a clinical trial authorisation must be obtained and checks made that the arrangements for the trial comply with the law.

It is also the responsibility of sponsors to ensure that the chief investigator and other key researchers, including those at collaborating sites, have the necessary expertise and experience and have access to the resources needed to conduct the proposed research successfully. This includes confirming that the arrangements and resources proposed will allow the collection of high-quality, accurate data, that the systems and resources proposed are those required to allow appropriate data analysis and data protection. Arrangements about compensation in the event of harm to research participants are the responsibility of sponsors (DoH, 2005). Finally, throughout the study sponsors are expected to assist with any enquiry, investigation or audit related to each research project.

Responsibilities of researchers

Researchers also have detailed and specific responsibilities under the Research Governance Framework. They must follow the agreed research proposal or protocol; select a means of communication which ensures that potential participants are fully informed before deciding whether to participate or not; help healthcare professionals to ensure that participants receive appropriate care whilst involved in the research; report adverse events and protect the confidentiality of records and data. In addition, a senior individual with suitable experience and expertise must be designated as the chief investigator. The chief investigator has additional responsibilities, such as: undertaking the design, conduct, analysis, reporting, gaining ethical approval and ensuring that the study adheres to the standards required in the Research Governance Framework. Responsibilities for the financial management and other resources, including intellectual property, dissemination of findings and feeding back appropriately to participants, are also the responsibility of the chief investigator, though it is acknowledged that many of these responsibilities will often be delegated to appropriate other members of the research team.

Nurse researchers, particularly those leading projects, must thoroughly familiarise themselves with the requirements of the Research Governance Framework if they are conducting research in health services.

Research ethics approval

There are essentially two processes for gaining approval to carry our research in health and (in some) social services:

- NHS Trust Research and Development department approval.
- Research Ethics Committee approval.

However, if you are doing research as part of an educational qualification, you will also need to gain approval from your university.

The focus for gaining ethical approval is on 'risk'. It does, however, recognise that risk can be complex and not necessarily physical; for example, it might relate to a person's personal values and beliefs, social standing, family or community circumstances.

NHS Trust Research and Development approval processes

There is a requirement, in the NHS, for any care provider Research and Development (R&D) department to be satisfied that a number of research governance requirements as set out in the Research Governance Framework have been fulfilled. This means that all research undertaken within each organisation is notified to, and monitored by, the R&D department. It is now also expected that users of the research outcomes will be involved at as many stages of the research process as possible.

A *research passport* system has recently been introduced that provides a mechanism for pre-engagement information about a researcher to be shared with relevant NHS organisations in which the applicant will be conducting research. It means that a researcher who is not employed by an NHS organisation or does not have a contractual relationship with the NHS *may* need a research passport. Students undertaking research and who will be supervised within clinical settings by an NHS employee, or university staff member with an honorary clinical or research contract, do not ordinarily need a research passport. A research passport may be project-specific or may be valid for a period of three years for a number of projects.

What is a research passport?

A research passport is a way of consolidating the checks on a researcher conducting research in the NHS, so there is just one standard form for each researcher that is completed by the researcher and her/his employer, and validated by an NHS organisation. The completed research passport is presented to all the relevant NHS organisations and obviates the need for checks to be repeated by all collaborating NHS organisations. This should allow faster study start-ups.

Exactly what checks are needed depends on the type of passport and nature of the research. Essentially the passport provides information that the holder has satisfied the NHS requirements about his or her character and suitability that are commensurate with the role of the researcher, the type of research and the duty of care. The checks are akin to those that would be undertaken for anyone applying for employment with the NHS and are likely to include a criminal record check and an occupational health clearance. Most NHS R&D departments now also require anyone conducting research in their organisation to have undertaken Good Clinical Practice training (this is described later).

NHS R&D departments will also monitor and audit research that is within their sphere of responsibility as well as giving approval for the research to begin once they are sure that the above conditions have been satisfied. Researchers are responsible for ensuring that the requirements of NHS R&D departments are met.

Research Ethics Committees

Before a research project can start, any researcher has to seek an independent ethical review of their proposed research. There are a number of different types of Research

Ethics Committees, and which committee(s) needs to give approval depends on the nature of the research proposed. For NHS research which involves patients and/or clients, access to notes and records, access to staff within health and social services and access to health or social care premises, a researcher must apply to a Local NHS Research Ethics Committee (REC). If the research is to be undertaken at more than five different NHS or social service premises, then the application for ethical approval needs to be made to an REC that can give approval for a multi-centre research study. For research by a student or member of staff of a university, a University Research Ethics Committee (UREC) will need to be approached to approve the research and this will usually be required in addition to the NHS REC approval. In the social services there may be a Social Services Ethics Committee or, more likely, a UREC or REC will provide this function. Similarly, research that falls outside the NHS and social services but is social science research will also require independent ethics scrutiny and approval. Again, this will usually be gained through a UREC or REC or a Social Services Ethics Committee.

Ethics committees are multi-professional, with members having experience across all types of research design. Lay people are included on these committees to provide an ordinary person's perspective. Ethical review involves completing an application form, providing a research proposal that gives details of the proposed research, providing copies of research instruments (for example, questionnaires, interview schedules) and, most importantly, production of participant information sheets and consent forms. Some committees require the researcher(s) to attend a committee meeting to answer questions about the proposed research. Research may not start until a favourable ethical opinion has been given.

NHS Research Ethics Committees

In the case of health research, members of an REC will scrutinise research applications and give opinions as to whether the proposed research has considered and responded to all ethical issues. The arrangements for applying to an REC are now standardised and the application form is completed and submitted online via the National Research Ethics Service (NRES) (www.nres.npsa.nhs.uk/).

Codes for nursing research

Nursing research is no different from any other health research. The ethical and governance requirements for nurses are the same as those for doctors, radiographers, physiotherapists and other healthcare professionals who want to conduct research in the NHS, and any other healthcare partners in the independent, private and charitable sectors. For nurses working in the social care sector, the structures and support for research are, as yet, not so well developed. However, the principles still apply and the NHS ethics review procedures are often seen as 'gold standard'.

Most professional bodies have their own codes of conduct, which usually include research, and in nursing there is specific guidance produced by the Royal College of Nursing (RCN, 2004). The RCN guidance makes clear the responsibilities of any nurse involved in research. There is particular focus on vulnerable participants, consent and confidentiality: these issues are discussed in detail in the next chapter (Chapter 5), which addresses ethical issues of research.

Good Clinical Practice

All of the issues that have been discussed so far are designed to promote the principles of Good Clinical Practice (GCP) in research. The International Conference on Harmonisation of Technical Requirements for Registration of Pharmaceuticals for Human Use (ICH) produced a consolidated document setting out a standard for the conduct of clinical trials in 1996. This is an international ethical and scientific quality standard established to provide a unified standard for the European Union (EU), Japan, the USA, Australia, Canada and the Nordic Countries, as well as the World Health Organization (WHO). Compliance with the standard should provide public assurance that the rights, safety and well-being of research participants are protected and that the clinical research data are credible (ICR, 1997). Although the principles were designed primarily for the conduct of drug trials, there is an expectation that all research studies comply with them to give assurance of the quality and safety of research.

The main principle of the ICH Good Clinical Practice is that clinical trials should be conducted in accordance with the **ethical principles** that have their origin in the Declaration of Helsinki, and that are consistent with GCP and the applicable regulatory requirement(s). It is expected that, before a trial is initiated, foreseeable risks and inconveniences should be weighed against the anticipated benefits for the individual trial participant and society. A trial should be initiated and continued only if the anticipated benefits justify the risks, as well as being scientifically sound and described in a clear, detailed protocol. The rights, safety and well-being of the trial participants are the most important considerations and should prevail over interests of sciences and society. Available non-clinical and clinical information on an investigational product should be adequate to support the proposed clinical trial, and GCP expects that any trial be conducted in compliance with a protocol that has received prior institutional review and independent ethics committee approval. This will include a clear account of how freely given informed consent is to be obtained from every participant prior to participation and how data collected will be recorded and stored in a way that allows its accurate reporting, interpretation and verification. It is also expected that each individual involved in conducting a trial should be qualified by education, training and experience to perform his or her respective task(s) and, where necessary, be supervised by an appropriately experienced researcher.

However, the medical care given to, and medical decisions made on behalf of, participants should always be the responsibility of a qualified physician, or when appropriate, a qualified dentist.

Chapter summary

There is an expectation that any health and social service research is ethical, of good quality, safe, and that data are credible.

- Ethical and governance issues must be considered at all stages of the research process.
- Individual researchers have a responsibility to abide by the regulations and legislation as they apply to research and their professional practice.
- All NHS research is subject to the Research Governance Framework (DoH, 2005).
- Researchers are expected to follow the Good Clinical Practice principles (ICR, 1997).
- Any health and (some) social service research has to be approved by:

    - NHS Trust R&D department(s)
    - REC.

- The approval processes, research governance, regulations and legislation are all designed to ensure that the integrity and safety of any research participant are respected and safeguarded.

References

Department of Health (2005) *Research Governance Framework for Health and Social Care*, 2nd edition. London: DoH.

Institute of Clinical Research (1997) *ICH Guidelines for Good Clinical Practice*. Bourne End: The Institute of Clinical Research.

MRC (1998) *Guidelines for Good Clinical Paractice in Clinical Trials*. London: Medical Research Council. Available at: www.mrc.ac.uk/Utilities/Documentrecord/index. htm?d=MRC002416.

Royal College of Nursing (2004) *Research Ethics: RCN Guidance for Nurses*. London: Royal College of Nursing.

Suggested further reading

General Medical Council (2002) *Research: The Role and Responsibilities of Doctors*. Available at www.gmc-uk.org/guidance/library/index.

Institute of Clinical Research (1997) *ICH Guidelines for Good Clinical Practice.* Bourne End: The Institute of Clinical Research.

Lowrance, W. (2003) 'Learning from experience: privacy and the secondary use of data in health research', *Journal of Health Service Research and Policy*, 8 (suppl.): 2–7.

Mason, J.K. and Laurie, G.T. (2006) *Law and Medical Ethics*, 7th edition. Oxford: Oxford University Press.

Pattinson, S. (2006) *Medical Law & Ethics.* London: Sweet & Maxwell.

Royal College of Nursing Research Society (2004) *Research Ethics: RCN Guidance for Nurses.* London: Royal College of Nursing.

Royal College of Nursing Research Society (2005) *Informed Consent in Health and Social Care Research.* Available at www.rcn.org.uk/publications.

Soteriou, T. and Hek, G. (2003) 'Research governance and students: what are NHS Trusts looking for?', *Nurse Researcher*, 1 (1): 22–31.

Website

National Research Ethics Service: www.nres.npsa.nhs.uk/

5

RESEARCHING ETHICALLY

Evaluating research involving human beings is difficult and puzzling as this research is both necessary and problematic. The need for such research can be justified because of the potential benefits. Regrettably, research has also been associated with unethical conduct. The imperative, however, for anyone undertaking a research project has to be the maintenance of ethical standards.

The aim for this chapter is to explain the principles that underpin ethical conduct in research and how these can be put into practice in developing a project and when actually carrying out a research study.

Learning outcomes

This chapter is designed to enable the reader to:

- **Appreciate ethical principles and how they relate to research practice**
- **Understand the needs of vulnerable research participants**
- **Understand the nature of informed consent**
- **Recognise what needs to be included when giving information to a participant**
- **Understand how anonymity and confidentiality can be preserved in a research project**
- **Appreciate and understand the need for data storage**
- **Be able to identify the risks to researcher safety**
- **Appreciate the issues raised when in a role of researcher and nurse**

KEY TERMS

Anonymity, Beneficence, Confidentiality, Dual role of researcher and nurse, Informed consent, Justice, Non-maleficence, Participant information, Research ethics committees, Respect for autonomy, Safety of researchers, Vulnerable participants

---

Brief history of the ethics of research involving humans

The justification given for undertaking research on humans is that we lack the knowledge to be able to predict, with confidence, the outcome of an intervention. The aim, therefore, is to eliminate uncertainty as far as is possible by testing different options. This will often take the form of an experiment. There is, however, a need for a systematic and co-ordinated approach in order to reduce the risks associated with ad hoc research of tragedies, such as the cases of blindness in premature babies resulting from supplemental oxygen therapy that occurred between 1942 and 1952 (Silverman, 1985).

There is a long history of and association between medicine and experimentation, with Brieger (1978) and Ibn Sina,[1] for example, suggesting that experiments must be done on man because animal testing proved nothing about the effects of drugs on humans. As medical science progressed, experiments continued to be performed on humans, including trials with smallpox variolation and cowpox inoculations in attempts to prevent smallpox infections (Bazin, 2001). Early in the 19th century, experimenters tended to use themselves as their own 'guinea pigs' (Howard-Jones, 1982). Although there were rapid developments in medicine in the second half of the 19th century and early 20th century, which led to an increasing realisation of the need for research to rationalise and improve the safety of drug therapies in particular (Howard-Jones 1982). This also resulted in an institutionalisation of research and demands for more accountability of researchers.

Although there were no international or UK codes/guidelines relating to the ethical conduct of researchers experimenting on humans prior to the Nuremberg Code of 1947, it was expected that medical researchers would be guided by their personal or professional values. For medicine, the Hippocratic Oath underpins

---

1 Ibn Sina (980–1037), also known as Avicenna, was an Iranian physician, the most famous and influential of the philosopher-scientists of Islam. He wrote *The Canon of Medicine*, which is one of the most famous books in the history of medicine (*Encyclopaedia Britannica*).

professional conduct. The Oath has no specific reference to research but does includes reference to the following:

> ... system of regimen which according to my ability and judgment, I consider for the benefit of my patients, and abstain from whatever is (to their harm or injustice) deleterious and mischievous. (Hippocratic Oath as translated by Francis Adams in 1891; the section in brackets is from the 1996 translation by Heinrich von Staden)

Unethical research is often epitomised by the concentration camp experiments that took place in Germany during the Second World War. The irony is that in the early 20th century Germany had been one of the first countries to develop a code of ethics for research experiments (Capron, 1997). There are, however, examples of what is regarded as unethical research in other countries that demonstrated a need for specific codes to guide the conduct of research. The natural history of syphilis study in Tuskegee, Alabama, USA, was developed in 1943 to investigate the effects of syphilis on a group of African-American men. However, the men who agreed to participate in the study were not told that a treatment for syphilis (penicillin) was being withheld from them for the purpose of studying the long-term effects of the disease. This study not only contradicted the ethical guidance then in place in the USA, but continued until the 1970s.

In the UK, the death of Ronald Madison at the Chemical Defence Establishment, Porton Down, in 1953 after unknowingly being exposed to the nerve agent Sarin also highlighted the need for more rigorous monitoring of research involving humans. A recent review of the Porton Down Volunteer Programme included an independent Ethical Assessment of the trials conducted between 1939 and 1989. This Ethical Assessment, undertaken by Sir Ian Kennedy, came to the conclusion:

> ... that research was carried out at Porton in a thorough, painstaking, careful and often ingenious manner ... there is no evidence to justify a conclusion that the conduct of a trial at any point went beyond the limits of what should ever be contemplated, far less tolerated, in a civilized society.

> ... however, I am persuaded that there were trials, albeit a few out of the many thousands of trials ... when it may be said that the research may not have met the ethical standards required of researchers and, where relevant, those who approved the trials. (Kennedy, 2006: 432–3)

Unfortunately, despite the introduction of codes of ethics for the conduct of research there have continued to be examples, albeit rare, of unethical research. It appears that this is associated with a lack of attention to detail and failure to follow the codes for research conduct. The TeGenero TGN1412 drugs trial is a recent example in the UK, where it appears that there was a failure to follow the approved research protocol and that the independent critical review was not as rigorous as it should have been (Kenter and Cohen, 2006). This episode serves as a reminder that it is important for all researchers to adhere to research protocols once they have been approved, and to ensure that they are aware of, and apply, ethical principles when conducting any research involving humans.

Ethical principles

Before embarking on a discussion of ethical principles it is important to understand the term *ethics*. Ethics is a generic term for various ways of understanding and examining the moral life. There are two types of ethical enquiry: normative and non-normative:

- Normative ethics attempt to answer the question *'Which general moral norms for the guidance and evaluation of conduct should we accept and why?'* (Beauchamp and Childress, 2001). Practical or *applied* ethics is the attempt to implement general norms and theories for practical problems and contexts.
- Non-normative ethics fall into two categories: descriptive and meta-ethics. Descriptive ethics refer to the factual investigation of moral conduct and beliefs, and meta-ethics analyse language, concepts and methods of reasoning.

Morality refers to 'norms about right and wrong human conduct that are so widely shared that they form a stable (although usually incomplete) social consensus' (Beauchamp and Childress, 2001). For example, not lying, stealing or killing, keeping promises, respecting rights of others. Because most of us are comfortable with these 'rules' there is no debate about them and they are accepted as *common morality*. *Professional morality* again refers to commonly accepted norms of conduct, but specifically about moral responsibilities applicable to a specific profession. From a healthcare professional perspective, it refers to things like ensuring **informed consent** and patient **confidentiality**.

There is a long history in the field of biomedical ethics, with many putting forward theories, definitions and principles based on moral theory and 'common morality'. The most influential theorists have probably been Beauchamp and Childress who, in 1983, set out four clusters of moral principles: **respect for autonomy**, **non-maleficence**, **beneficence** and **justice**. Fundamental to most is the notion that with good moral reasoning it is possible to make ethical decisions with which all 'reasonable' people will agree. In terms of medical research, as previously mentioned, the Nuremberg Code and the Declaration of Helsinki in 1964 were hugely influential, with protection of the individual and informed consent as essential for the conduct of medical research (see National Institutes of Health, 2006 and World Medical Association, 2000).

The ethical principles that should guide nurse researchers, particularly in relation to protecting potential research participants, are essentially the same as those that guide nursing practice. These principles are set out in codes of conduct nationally and internationally, for example, the International Council of Nurses *Code of Ethics for Nurses* (2006). In the UK the Royal College of Nursing (RCN) provides specific guidance for research as it may relate to nurses involved in research in any way. The ethical principles that are usually associated with research include: veracity, justice, non-maleficence, beneficence and confidentiality.

- **Veracity:** Veracity is the ethical principle of 'telling the truth'. Researchers must be honest with participants and inform them of potential risks and benefits, as well as of the right to decide whether to participate or not, without any coercion, and to withdraw at any time. The principle of veracity also links to the need for researchers to consider how they will establish a trusting relationship, and how they will respect the rights of participants. This includes a duty to respect the rights, autonomy and dignity of participants.
- **Justice:** The principle of justice is about being 'fair' to participants and not giving preference to, or being discriminatory with, some participants over others. Being fair also means that the interests of the participants must come before those of the researcher(s) and before the objectives of the study. Justice also requires that there is no abuse or exploitation of participants on the grounds of race, religion, sex, age, class or sexual orientation.
- **Non-maleficence:** Non-maleficence is the principle of 'doing no harm' to research participants. Essentially, it is a duty wherever possible to prevent physical, psychological, emotional, social and economic harms. Though it is recognised that it will not always be possible to avoid harms and that some harms may be necessary to avoid other harms and promote an eventual good, the trauma associated with an operation, for example, is acceptable provided that the outcome is recovery of health. There is also a duty to protect the weak, vulnerable and incompetent by adapting procedures and processes to take into account their vulnerabilities.
- **Beneficence:** This is the principle of 'doing good' to both research participants and society. The expectation is that research should benefit both the individual participants and society in general. The imperative of beneficence is to do good and prevent harm. Harm is defined as being whatever is bad for someone is harmful, and nothing is harmful, unless it is bad for the one harmed. In healthcare, consideration must be given to patients' evaluation of the harmfulness of a proposed or actual intervention irrespective of what is perceived to be the outcome of the intervention.
- **Confidentiality:** Confidentiality is the ethical principle of 'safeguarding' the personal information which has been gathered in a study. This means that researchers should never report data about an individual without that individual's explicit permission. It requires that researchers explain to participants who will have access to their data and that sharing of data with others is only permissible with participants' permission. Contained within this principle is also a duty to store data safely.

These principles can be used as a framework to critically appraise research and to examine the effects of research on the participants. It must be noted, however, that some research designs, as will be seen later, will need to have ethical issues considered in certain and more specific ways. For example, in some ethnographic studies, such as observation of crowd behaviour, the participants may not know they are being observed and therefore have no choice about participating or not; in disseminating the research findings of **action research**, issues of confidentiality may be compromised; in experimental research a random selection might result in a voluntary group which is not representative of the target population, such as being better educated, of a higher social class or more socially involved.

In addition to the methods and procedures used in research, the topic being considered may also raise ethical concerns. For example, research in the area of abuse or criminal activity, or with particularly vulnerable groups such as the very old, or people with a severe learning disability or severe mental illness. The challenge for readers of research or nurses undertaking research is to ensure that research evidence is produced ethically whilst employing good research practices.

Vulnerable participants

Some people who may participate in research may be considered to be vulnerable for a variety of reasons. Some individuals may feel obligated to take part in a study because a researcher has power or perceived power, such as when the researcher is a member of the healthcare team. Others may have the capacity to give consent to participate, but might find it difficult to withhold consent if they are put under implicit or explicit pressure. Individuals with learning disabilities, or who have a mental health problem, or are frail and elderly, or are living in an institution such as a residential home or prison, may all be considered vulnerable, as may children and young people, and women who are pregnant. Furthermore, in theory at least, any individual can be considered to be vulnerable if they are in any way debilitated, and this means that any patient can be considered as being vulnerable in some respect.

Other potential participants may be vulnerable because they have limited ability to decide whether or not to participate in research due to difficulties in making a reasoned decision because they do not understand what is involved. For example, potential participants who do not speak the same language as the researcher, or have special language needs due to visual, hearing or learning impairments, or they may conceal particular needs such as limited reading and writing ability. Some potential participants may be temporarily vulnerable, for example, if they have just received bad news or are just about to receive treatment. Researchers must be sensitive to these issues and, when necessary, make specific arrangements when seeking to recruit such participants to ensure that they can have appropriate and timely information, and in a medium that helps them understand what might be involved when deciding whether or not to participate.

Some adults may not have the capacity to give consent. There must be clear justification for researchers including such groups of participants in research, and they should never be asked to participate if the research could be equally undertaken with other adults. However, if a researcher wants to involve adults who lack the capacity to give consent, it should be limited to the areas of research related to their incapacity (see Chapter 4, Mental Capacity Act). A researcher will also need to demonstrate that the research could be of direct benefit to, or improve knowledge of, their health or that of people with the same state of health or same incapacity. Furthermore, the researcher must establish that the individual has not expressed any objection either verbally or physically, and that participation will not cause the participant emotional, physical or psychological harm. The risks to participants must be negligible and not interfere with their freedom of action or privacy.

Researchers may want to involve children and young people in research; however, as a potentially vulnerable group they must not be exploited. It must be remembered that they will not always be able to express their own needs or protect themselves from harm, or make informed choices about being involved in research. However, children are capable of giving consent if they are deemed as 'Gillick' competent (also known as the principle of 'Fraser'). This means that children who are felt to be competent to understand the proposed research and make decisions on their own behalf can consent on their own behalf. They may need extra time to understand what is involved and be given suitable media for explaining the research, such as pictures or drama. If children and young people are not competent to give consent independently to participate in research, the consent of someone with parental responsibility must be obtained and, in addition, the child must not object to participation. Researchers wanting to include children in their study must be familiar with the Children Act 1989, which sets out the legislation related to consent and the responsibilities of parents.

Other areas where there may be issues of vulnerability are particularly related to when the researcher is in a position of power over potential participants. For example, lecturers wanting to study their students, or managers wanting to undertake research with their staff, will need to carefully consider whether their participants are in a potentially vulnerable position. Vulnerability may be in terms of their relationship with participants and issues of power and authority, or it may be because participants feel themselves to be in an obligatory position and, therefore, unable to make a fully autonomous decision whether to participate. There is also potential for coercion and, in some instances, peer pressure to participate. This can be especially so when students want to research other students, or colleagues undertaking a course want to research their work colleagues.

Including vulnerable individuals in research requires careful consideration, as excluding them from research may be a form of discrimination or may mean that some groups are not researched adequately. This may be because of difficulties relating to consent or perceptions that specific groups should not be approached to participate because of their vulnerability, such as palliative care patients. Therefore, researchers need to justify why certain groups of people should be included in research. Consideration should be given to an individual's ability to comprehend the information given, but just as important is the form and nature of the explanation given, and the way that consent is obtained, particularly if participants are only intermittently competent to consent or have difficulty retaining information, such as individuals with dementia.

Nurse researchers must be fully aware of the issues of involving **vulnerable participants** and recognise that it is up to individual participants to decide whether or not to participate in research. The next section on informed consent considers how vulnerable participants can be included in research with due regard to their vulnerability.

Informed consent

Informed consent is a concept familiar to all nurses, particularly with reference to treatment and care. The principles of informed consent are also applied to potential research participants and are fundamental to the conduct of ethical research. The consent of participants is accepted both legally and professionally *only* when a participant has been properly informed, has agreed without any coercion and is deemed competent to give consent.

Communicating clearly with potential participants in a form they can understand, and that is prepared in a manner that meets their individual needs, is key to the consent process. The information given to potential participants should be written, or given in another appropriate format, such as an audio or video recording. Potential participants should be given the opportunity to ask questions, allowed adequate time to consider taking part, and given the opportunity to discuss with others if they wish. Only after this process should participants be asked to give written consent or other form of consent, such as video or audio consent if written consent is not possible. For some participants, ongoing consent is required, this applies particularly in longer studies, in research that has a number of stages or research that involves participants who may have difficulty retaining information. Figure 5.1 gives an indication of what research participants need to know before deciding to take part in a research project.

Preparing information that will enable potential participants make an informed decision about whether to participate takes time and effort and should be built into the research process. Potential participants should be given information in the most suitable format to meet their individual needs, for example, written, audio/video recorded, using pictures or artwork, read aloud, using an interpreter and so on. The person discussing the information with the potential participant should not be in a position of power or authority where there could be coercion; if this is the case, then someone else should be responsible for the information giving and consent process. Wherever possible, an appropriate period of time, such as three to four days, should be allowed between giving the information and seeking written consent. Written information sheets should be non-technical and written in a language that is easily understood by a layperson. Short sentences and words should be used with clear sub-headings and a font size that is easy to read. Bullet-point lists should be used when appropriate. The language should be appropriate to the intended audience, for example, patient, work colleague, student or manager. Where necessary, the information should be on appropriately headed

Participants should:

- know that they are being invited to take part in a research study
- have time to consider being involved and consult with family and friends if they want to
- be assured that they can decline to participate or withdraw at any time without giving a reason
- understand that their care, treatment, education or support will be unaffected whether they decide or not to participate, or if they withdraw at any point
- understand the purpose of the research
- know why they have been chosen
- understand what will happen to them if they agree to take part; for example, how long they will be involved, whether they need to do anything such as have an interview, keep a diary, give blood, complete a questionnaire, visit a clinic, take some medication, have a telephone interview etc.
- understand any risks, costs, disadvantages and benefits
- know whether there will be any discomfort or psychological or emotional distress
- understand how their confidentiality will be safeguarded, how their data will be collected and stored, e.g. anonymously, who will have access to the data, and how long it will be retained
- understand arrangements for any payments, expenses or benefits
- understand what will happen at the end of the study
- know who is organising and funding the study
- know who to contact for queries and for any complaints
- know the name of the Research Ethics Committee who reviewed the study
- have the opportunity to ask questions and have full and honest answers.

Figure 5.1   What research participants need to know before deciding to take part in a research project

paper such as that of the university or NHS Trust, and have a short self-explanatory title appropriate for a layperson. The tone of the information should be invitational and not overly persuasive or coercive. It should be clear that potential participants have free choice whether to accept or decline the invitation without any impact on their current or future care. The information sheet should be dated. An example of a participation information sheet for a nursing research study is given in Figure 5.2.

For any researcher undertaking research with NHS patients, there is clear guidance for preparing information sheets on the National Research Ethics Service (NRES) website (www.nres.npsa.nhs.uk), and the latest guidance should always be used.

Written consent should be obtained whenever possible, and if it is not possible there should be a justifiable reason. **Participant information** sheets and consent forms need to be prepared on separate sheets of paper, and participants should keep the information sheet and be given a copy of the consent form they signed.

Consent forms should record specific information on headed paper entitled 'Consent Form'; researchers are advised to use the format suggested by the NRES, which includes the title of the project, name and signature of researcher

1. **Study title:** Patient self-monitoring of bowel habits study.

2. **Invitation paragraph**

You are being invited to take part in a research study being conducted by the Practice Development Team at XXXX NHS Trust. Before you decide it is important for you to understand why the research is being done and what it will involve. Please take time to read the following information carefully and discuss it with others if you wish. Ask us if there is anything that is not clear or if you would like further information. Take time to decide whether or not you wish to take part. Thank you for reading this.

3. **What is the purpose of the study?**

Constipation is a problem that can affect any individual at any time of life and ill health is likely to increase the risks of developing constipation.

Although constipation is rarely life threatening it can cause a variety of physical discomforts and have psychological and social consequences which may contribute to a reduction in a person's quality of life. The development of constipation and associated discomforts may also delay a patient's recovery, leading to an increase in the associated risks, and for in-patients may result in longer hospitalisation.

It is, however, known that there is often reluctance by some patients, and even some health care professionals, to discuss bowel function until it has become a significant problem. It has been suggested that an effective way of assessing patients' bowel function is by asking patients to self-record frequency, type of stool and whether there is any defecation discomfort. The idea is that self-recording is more likely to result in a more realistic record of bowel function and avoids patients have to discuss bowel function with a healthcare professional when there are no problems. It should also increase patients' understanding about what is considered 'normal' bowel function and act as a prompt for seeking advice when their bowel function is not normal.

The aim of this study is to determine whether a patient-held bowel monitoring card is an effective way of monitoring bowel function for patients who are at risk of becoming constipated. We are doing this by asking some patients to use a Bowel Monitoring Card (BMC) to record their bowel movements for themselves. We will then compare the information on the BMC with that of the records of those patients who have not used the BMC.

The study is being undertaken on a few wards at XXXX NHS Trust and with District Nursing Teams in XPCT.

4. **Why have I been chosen?**

You have been chosen because you are either a patient on one of the wards at XXXX NHS Trust or a patient of a District Nursing Team in XPCT taking part in the study.

5. **Do I have to take part in the research?**

It is up to you to decide whether or not to take part in the research. If you do decide to take part you will be given this information sheet to keep and be asked to sign a consent form. Even if you decide to take part you are free to withdraw at any time without giving a reason. A decision to withdraw at any time, or a decision not to take part, will not affect you in any way.

6. **What do I have to do?**

Complete and return a signed copy of the consent form. Then you just need to complete our questionnaire, put it in the addressed envelope provided, seal the envelope and give it back to a

Ward Nurse or your District Nurse. Your Ward or District Nurse will then return your questionnaire with a copy of your bowel function record – this will be a bowel monitoring card or a copy of the part of your notes where your bowel function has been recorded. No other details will be taken from your healthcare records.

7. What are the possible benefits of taking part?

It is unlikely that you will gain any immediate benefit from taking part in this study; however, the information we get from this study may help us to improve the way patients' bowel function is recorded. This in turn should help to improve the way patients' bowel function is monitored, and help to highlight those patients who are at risk of developing constipation.

8. Will my taking part in this study be kept confidential?

All information received will be treated as confidential. Your name will not appear on the questionnaire; instead, a code number will identify you. Questionnaire data will be input on to a datasheet that can be accessed via a password known only to the research team.

9. What will happen to the results of the research study?

The results of the study will be presented as a report to XPCT and XXXX NHS Trust and used to inform the development of effective bowel function monitoring. The findings will also be disseminated at conferences and in academic publications. As already mentioned, results will be reported in such a way that preserves confidentiality. It will be the responsibility of the research team to collect and analyse all data.

10. What if I have any concerns?

If you have any concerns or other questions about this study or the way it has been carried out, you should contact the principal researchers.
MLG and EF Tel: ………………….. or Email………………

Contact for further information:
M L G and E F
Governance Office, East Wing,
XXXX Hospital,

Thank you
M L G and E F

Figure 5.2   Example of a participant information sheet

and of participant, and the date that consent is given. There should be tick boxes for the participant to initial the following statements where appropriate:

☐ I have read the information sheet dated … and have had opportunity to consider the information, ask questions and have had these answered satisfactorily.

☐ I understand that my participation is voluntary and that I am free to withdraw at any time without giving any reason, without my healthcare/education/work circumstances or legal rights being affected.

☐ I give permission for my medical records/work records/exam marks to be examined.

- ☐ I agree to my interview being audio-taped/video-taped.
- ☐ I understand that direct quotes may be used when the project is written up, although they will be anonymised.
- ☐ I agree to my GP being informed of my participation.
- ☐ I agree to take part in the above study.

There are a few situations when implied consent can be used. The most likely is when a participant implies their consent by returning a questionnaire. In such cases, a letter of invitation to complete the questionnaire will be sent together with an information sheet to potential participants. It should be clear from the letter and the information sheet that returning the questionnaire implies consent and that a separate consent form is not required. The information sheet should contain all the information previously outlined. However, some ethics committees require researchers to obtain informed written consent prior to administration of the questionnaire.

Anonymity

Not using the names and addresses of participants and assigning each of them a unique identity number can achieve **anonymity**. This process should be undertaken as close as possible to when the data is collected. A list of the unique identity numbers together with the individual's name should be kept separately and securely and not referred to, unless there is specific need, such as a medical emergency, in order to ensure that the researcher cannot link data with a particular participant. This is mainly for insurance purposes or in the case of a complaint where there may be a need to find out the identity number of a particular participant. An ethics committee will expect an explanation about how data will be anonymised.

A common understanding in the NHS is that NHS-anonymised data is basically a 'free good'. For 'routine' uses of data, for example, when conducting an audit, consent need not be 'explicit' under the Data Protection Act but can be 'implied'. However, obtaining data for research purposes is not usually considered a routine use and informed and explicit consent is nearly always required before researchers can access patient-identifiable records or data. Introducing anonymisation techniques before data is passed to a third-party researcher may be an option for some researchers, and this is allowable under the Data Protection Act. However, advice will be needed from an NHS Trust data protection officer and permission obtained from the Research and Development (R&D) office.

In the UK, under section 60 of the Health and Social Care Act (2001), the Secretary of State for Health is authorized to allow the processing of personal medical data for specific purposes without consent. This includes surveillance of communicable diseases, diagnosis and treatment of cancer and some limited research activity; however, support will be required from the Patient Information Advisory Group (PIAG), under Section 60 of the Health and Social Care Act, and researchers will need to discuss their project with them.

If a researcher wants direct access to patients' records to get names and addresses of patients to invite them to participate in a study, this can be a problem. Section 60 guidance makes it clear that either explicit informed consent is required to gain access or the researcher must apply to PIAG for section 60 support. Alternatively, a clinician such as a doctor or nurse who is directly responsible for the patients could approach them to invite them to participate, thus avoiding the need for the researcher to have access to the patients' confidential records.

Personal fully non-reversible anonymised data should be used whenever possible by researchers, and it should be processed and stored appropriately for the purposes of a research project. In all other circumstances, explicit informed consent should be obtained at the very first stage, including consent to access the names and addresses of potential participants.

Confidentiality

Participants in research have a right to expect that any information that they provide will be treated confidentially and that any disclosure of information about them will only be done with their consent. There must be a clear understanding between the researcher and participant concerning the use to be made of the data provided and how personal information will be stored. Participants must be given details, usually on the participant information sheet, of who will have access to their data other than the researcher, for example a supervisor or other research team members. Research participants should not be discussed beyond the needs of the project team and the data must be kept secure at all times. This is particularly important with data stored on a computer, and an ethics committee will normally expect electronic data to be password protected. Access to the data should be restricted to only those people who have a legitimate reason to see it.

If confidentiality or anonymity cannot be guaranteed, participants must be told in advance before they agree to participate. For example, when interviewing nurses, a participant may reveal that they have made a drug error, or that they have a heavy drinking problem, or that they have witnessed another member of staff dealing in drugs, or have cheated in an exam. The researcher needs to make it clear on the information sheet that if, for example, criminal activity or issues of misconduct are revealed, then they will need to take some action. The action needs to be appropriate to the situation and risk and could be, for example, encouraging them to speak to their line manager; encouraging them to phone a help line; offering a counsellor; or reporting them to their line manager. This all needs to be made clear on the information sheet – although, of course, not everything a participant may reveal or be observed doing can be anticipated. If information needs to be disclosed in the public interest without a participant's consent (see Chapter 4), there must be a benefit to the individual or society that outweighs the individual's right to confidentiality.

Data storage, retention and security

Data collected during the process of research needs to be kept safely and with due regard to issues of confidentiality and anonymity as outlined above. Information on paper, audio-tape, video-tape, and portable data such as memory sticks, CDs and DVDs should be stored in locked, fireproof cabinets. Data kept electronically should be password protected, and have firewall, virus and spyware protection. Researchers need to consider how this will be achieved and if there are any cost implications for their project. Transporting data in cars and trains, for example, needs careful consideration not just to protect the confidentiality of participants' information, but also to protect the data collected in the research project and avoid the risk of having to repeat data collections.

The Data Protection Act (see Chapter 4) makes it clear that data must be fairly and lawfully processed, accurate and up to date, kept secure, and should be adequate, relevant and not excessive. All this applies to research data; however, some types of data are exempt, such as data which has been anonymised and where the link between the data and the individual has been irreversibly broken so that the individual can never be identified, for example data that has been supplied by another organisation which has the code.

Data should be retained for the most appropriate time in which to facilitate realistic completion of a project, dissemination, any future analysis, and any potential claims for insurance purposes. Not all data needs to be retained; for example, once transcripts of audio-tapes are made, the original recording could be destroyed. Clinical research data used during clinical trials has to be kept for a specific length of time depending on the trial agreements. This is usually 15 years but can be longer. Other types of data should be stored from between five and ten years, but this is dependent on what data is to be kept, and is likely to be shorter for students on short courses such as Masters' degrees, where the requirement may be to keep the data for only three years. Some forms of historical research may need to be kept much longer for justifiable reasons. The advice of the **Research Ethics Committee** where the research is being reviewed is necessary to ensure that data is retained for an appropriate length of time, and how it should be destroyed at the end of the project.

Safety for researchers

Nurse researchers may be undertaking their research in unfamiliar environments or in private dwellings. This may put them in potentially risky situations, and requires some preparation to be done to reduce and control risks and minimise any anxieties that the researcher may have. Research managers may need to budget for the **safety of researchers** on a project, such as providing taxis, special training, counselling for staff researching on difficult topics, providing mobile phones, or budgeting for extra time to allow researchers to work in pairs, or have overnight accommodation.

There may be potential risks in a research project that are more than the risks encountered in daily life. Clearly, each research project is different, but researchers need to consider whether there is a possibility, and the potential consequences, of causing physical or psychological harm to participants. For the researcher, risks of physical or psychological threats, abuse or trauma, increased risk of exposure to infections, accidents or harm and the possibility of researcher or participant being in a compromising position with a risk of accusation of inappropriate behaviour to either person must all be considered.

Many of the potential risks can be avoided or reduced by careful planning at early stages in the project, and careful preparation before setting up and undertaking research in unfamiliar environments or private dwellings. This should be done within project teams, or with supervisors. There is an expectation, as part of insurance agreements and research governance procedures, that researchers have considered safety for both their participants and themselves. All research projects in the NHS must have appropriate insurance and indemnity arrangements, usually arranged through employers or sponsors of the researcher, and are detailed in NHS Research Ethics Committee applications, with similar requirements for non-NHS research ethics committees.

Early planning for fieldwork stages in a research project, such as interviewing or observation, should, where appropriate, consider and prepare for the sensitive nature and possible consequences of any topics being discussed. Any cultural and social issues such as age, gender and ethnicity of interviewers/participants, venue for interviews, observation studies and so on should be considered, as well as how these can be resolved. Issues related to use of body language, physical contact and cultural norms such as social distance to establish and maintain an appropriate professional relationship with participants must be resolved before the research starts. When interviews are to be conducted, then decisions about the site should reflect the need for the participant to feel comfortable and safe or whether a neutral area might be possible and safer for the researcher. For example, carrying a mobile phone and having an arrangement whereby a colleague/office knows where researchers are and to confirm safety. When appropriate, researchers should also work out how to not look 'out of place' and how best to keep valuables and equipment out of sight. It may also be worthwhile visiting unfamiliar environments before starting fieldwork to identify any specific risks. Researchers should not forget the tiring and emotional effects of interviewing and observing. Carrying identification related to the research and an employer which can be checked by participants may be necessary, and it is also worth considering whether local police should be informed if cold calling is involved.

During an interview, in particular, participants may become distressed or angry and researchers need to be able to spot the signs and be prepared to terminate an interview or take some other action; the health of the participants must come before the needs of the research. After interviewing, researchers, particularly inexperienced ones, may need a period of debriefing and, in some situations, counselling. There should certainly be a discussion and review of the fieldwork with a supervisor or other team member as to whether there were any safety issues or difficult situations to deal with, or things that needed to be done differently.

Dual role of researcher and nurse

Nurses must always uphold the principles of their own code of conduct, as well as research-related codes and guidance. Nurses undertaking research should possess the relevant research skills and knowledge compatible with the demands of the proposed research as with any other professional role, and this includes acknowledging any limitations of their ability.

As can be seen from the previous sections in this chapter, there are a number of ethical issues that can arise and need to be prepared for by nurses undertaking research either as part of their job or as course work. All research is potentially exploitative and researchers' motives can be mixed with a blurring of roles. This is particularly so when the researcher is a healthcare professional such as a nurse, or is undertaking the research as part of career development. Nurses undertaking research may also feel that some of the tasks they perform, such as seeking consent and inter-viewing patients, are the same as in their normal nursing role and this can lead to lack of thought and proper preparation for a research role.

Nurses must always make it clear to participants that they are undertaking a research project and that they are acting as a researcher rather than a nurse. This is particularly important when seeking consent, as patients could be easily coerced or misled into taking part in a research project by mistakenly thinking that it is all part of their nursing care. Furthermore, participants who see researchers as nurses may disclose too much, and this can create difficult situations for both the participant and researcher, particularly if the researcher is the 'normal' carer for the participant. Similarly, managers researching their own staff can get into difficult situations if the participants are not fully aware of the role the manager is playing – researcher or manager – hence the importance of fully comprehensive participant information before seeking informed consent.

Finally, nurses must be satisfied that any 'funded' research is ethically and scientifically sound and that, as an individual, they are not associated with any promotion of a particular product. Many research projects are externally funded by a wide range of funding agencies, including commercial sponsors; nurse researchers need to be wary of being inappropriately influenced by funders and how the research can be independently conducted, including dissemination, so that there is no inappropriate promotion of products or organisations. Most employers, including NHS Trusts and universities, have people who can advise about commercial sponsorship, copyright and intellectual property.

What are members of a research ethics committee looking for?

This final section considers what an ethics committee will be looking for in an ethics application. All these points have been covered by earlier sections in this chapter and the list below could be used as an aide-memoire.

The application forms and associated papers such as research protocols, information sheets, consent forms, interview schedules and questionnaires should:

- be written in language suitable for an intelligent layperson
- be free of grammatical and typographical errors
- provide clear explanation about how the physical, psychological and emotional well-being of participants will be protected
- give clear descriptions of the potential health and safety issues for both participants and researchers, and what will be done about them
- give clear descriptions of how consent will be gained and how it will be recorded.

There should also be clear descriptions in the application and the participant information sheet of:

- how potential participants will be identified, approached and recruited
- any inclusion/exclusion criteria for participation
- any special groups that need justifying, which should include:

  - real and direct benefit to participants
  - foreseeable risks
  - foreseeable discomforts
  - others giving consent

- whether there will be any withholding of treatment or care from participants
- any procedures additional to normal care
- the length of time each individual will participate in the study
- any sensitive, embarrassing or upsetting questions
- any possibility of disclosures by participants and what will be done about this

- any risks and hazards, pain and discomfort to participants
- any benefit to participants
- any risks and hazards to researchers
- the length of time participants have to decide whether to take part
- what will happen if any information becomes available during the course of a project that may have an impact on the study
- whether a participant's general practitioner is being informed of their participation
- any payments or expenses due to participants and how they will claim them
- how results will be given to participants
- how data will be protected and stored, and for how long
- how the study is being funded
- who is sponsoring the study.

The information for participants should be provided in the most appropriate format, particularly for those who might not understand written or verbal explanations or have special communication needs. This might be written, audio-taped or video-taped, for example, and for those participants unable to retain information it may need to be repeated. There may need to be accompanying letters of permission for access to organisations, and all information and interview schedules, questionnaires and research tools must be produced on headed notepaper.

Chapter summary

- All research should be undertaken ethically.
- Nurse researchers should be guided by ethical principles.
- Conducting research with vulnerable participants is ethically acceptable provided care and attention is given to their specific needs, particularly in respect of ensuring effective communication with them.
- Informed consent is a prerequisite for undertaking any research with human beings.
- Consent can only be informed if potential participants are given information in a form that they can understand and is prepared in a manner that meets their individual needs.
- NHS researchers should follow the guidelines from NRES in the content and format of information sheets and consent forms.
- Information/data given by participants to researchers should be anonymised as close as possible to when the data is collected.
- Participants have a right to expect that any information they give to researchers will be treated confidentially and only disclosed with their full consent.
- Data must be stored safely and with due regard to issues of confidentiality and anonymity.
- Researchers and participants have an equal right to be protected from harm.
- Nurses must maintain awareness of the potential conflicts of interests associated with the dual role of practitioner and researcher.
- Ethics committees are looking for evidence to confirm that any proposed research will be conducted ethically and have 'rules' about the information that researcher need to provide to them.

References

Adams, F. (1891) *The Genuine Works of Hippocrates*. New York: William Wood.

Bazin, H. (2001) 'The ethics of vaccine usage in society: lesson from the past', *Current Opinion in Immunology*, 13: 505–10.

Beauchamp, T.L. and Childress, J.F. (2001) *Principles of Biomedical Ethics*, 5th edition. Oxford: Oxford University Press.

Brieger, G. (1978) *History: Human Experimentation*. New York: Free Press.

Capron, A. (1997) 'Human experimentation', in R. Veatch (ed.), *Medical Ethics*. Boston: Jones & Bartlett. pp. 135–84.

Howard-Jones, N. (1982) 'Human experimentation in historical and ethical perpectives', *Social Science and Medicine*, 16: 1429–48.

International Council of Nurses (2006) *Code of Ethics for Nurses*. Geneva: ICN. Available at www.icn.ch.

Kennedy, I. (2006) 'An ethical assessment', in *Historical Survey of the Porton Down Service Volunteer Programme 1939–1989*. London: Ministry of Defence. Chapter 23.

Kenter, M. and Cohen, A. (2006) 'Establishing risk of human experimentation with drugs: lessons from TGN1412', *The Lancet*, 368: 1387–91.

National Institutes of Health (2006) *Directives for Human Experimentation*: Nuremberg Code. Bethesda, MD: NIH. Available at www.nihtraining.com/ohsrsite/guidelines/nuremberg.html, accessed 4 May 2006.

Silverman, W. (1985) *Human Experimentation: A Guided Step into the Unknown*, Oxford: Oxford University Press.

von Staden, H. (1996) '"In a pure and holy way:" personal and professional Conduct in the Hippocratic Oath', *Journal of the History of Medicine and Allied Sciences*, 51: 406–8.

World Medical Association (2000) *Declaration of Helsinki: Ethical Principles for Medical Research Involving Human Subjects*. Available at www.nihtraining.com/ohsrsite/guidelines/helsinki.html.

Suggested further reading

Beauchamp, T.L. and Childress, J.F. (2001) *Principles of Biomedical Ethics*. Oxford: Oxford University Press.

Department of Health (2003) *Research Governance Framework for Health and Social Care*, 2nd edition. London: Department of Health.

General Medical Council (2002) *Research: The Role and Responsibilities of Doctors*. London: GMC. Available at www.gmc-uk.org/guidance/library/index.

Gillon, R. (1994) *Philosophical Medical Ethics*. Chichester: Wiley.

Medical Research Council (2001) *Human Tissue and Biological Samples for Use in Research: Operational and Ethical Guidelines*. London: MRC.

Randall, F. and Downie, R.S. (2001) *Palliative Care Ethics: A Companion for All Specialities,* 2nd edition. Oxford: Oxford Medical Publications.

Royal College of Nursing (2007) *Research Ethics: RCN Guidance for Nurses*. London: RCN.

Royal College of Nursing Research Society (2005) *Informed Consent in Health and Social Care Research*. London: RCN. Available at www.rcn.org.uk/publications.

Soteriou, T. and Hek, G. (2003) 'Research governance and students: what are NHS Trusts looking for?', *Nurse Researcher*, 11 (1): 22–31.

ten Have, H. and Clark, D. (eds) (2002) *The Ethics of Palliative Care*. Buckingham: Open University Press.

Available on the HMSO website www.hmso.gov.uk/acts

Children Act 1989
Data Protection Act 1998
Health and Social Care Act 2001
Human Rights Act 1998
Mental Capacity Act 2005
Public Interest Disclosure Act 1998

Websites

British Educational Research Association: www.bera.ac.uk
British Psychological Association: www.bps.org.uk
British Sociological Association: www.brtisoc.co.uk
Economic and Social Research Council: www.esrcsocietytoday.ac.uk
International Council of Nurses: www.icn.ch
Medical Research Council: www.mrc.ac.uk
National Research Ethics Service: www.nres.npsa.nhs.uk
Royal College of Nursing: www.rcn.org.uk

6

DEVELOPING RESEARCH QUESTIONS

Every research project begins with an idea or set of ideas. At a very general level these ideas can be seen as situations or experiences which we would like to know more about or better understand. They may prompt questions such as:

- Why does this happen?
- Is it possible to stop or prevent this from happening?
- Does this happen anywhere else?

When reflecting on nursing practice, situations or experiences the following types of question may be prompted:

- Is it possible to improve the way I/we do this?
- Is there a way of doing this more quickly/less expensively/less painfully?
- Are our patients satisfied with the care we give?

Turning these broad ideas into a researchable question is the first stage of the research process. It is, however, easy for novice researchers to conceive the idea that the breadth of their research project equates with its value. This misconception coupled with an initial enthusiasm often results in broad and unfocused research questions and, hence, over-ambitious research proposals. The purpose of this chapter is to give guidance on how to translate a broad query into a question that can be answered by undertaking a research study.

Learning outcomes

This chapter is designed to enable the reader to:

- **Understand the importance of having a research question**
- **Have a understanding of where research questions come from**

- **Recognise the processes involved in developing a research question**
- **Understand the differences between research questions, aims and objectives**

KEY TERMS

Hypothesis, Replication studies, Research aims, Research objectives, Research problems, Research questions, Secondary research

---

Generating research problems and research questions

Research is about finding answers to questions, but where do these questions come from? The terms 'research problem' and 'research question' can be confusing:

- A **research problem** is identified as a broad topic area of interest that has perplexing or troubling aspects which can be 'solved' by the accumulation of relevant information or evidence.
- A **research question** is more concise and is a description of exactly what issues the research intends to acquire information about.

For example, if a nurse is concerned about the healing of wounds in patients with burns, then this is the research problem. This is a very broad topic and needs to be narrowed down to a manageable focus. The following research questions could be developed from this research problem: 'Does patient mobility have an effect on the rate of healing in patients with lower limb burns?' or 'To what extent does mobility affect the rate of wound healing in patients with lower limb burns?'

Alternatively, research around this topic could be expressed as a problem statement: 'The purpose of this study is to examine the effect of patient mobility on the rate of wound healing in patients with lower limb burns.'

A good research question is one that is clearly expressed and focused on a researchable problem. A research question or problem statement may be further amplified through an aim that serves to focus more directly on the significant and relevant issue which is to be researched. This may be necessary because a research question is expected to be short, precise and direct. In some types of research a **hypothesis** is used, instead of a research question, to attempt to answer a question and predict an outcome. These terms will be discussed in more detail later in this chapter.

A **research aim** is, in effect, a description of exactly what issues the research intends to address. A research aim is a broad statement that often uses words such as

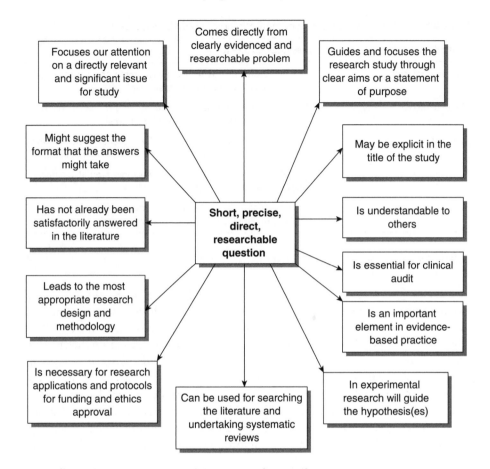

Figure 6.1   Key components of the research question

examine, describe, explore, and so on. Using the earlier example of wound healing, the aim might be: 'To investigate whether mobility promotes healing in patients with lower limb burns.'

Research objectives are a way of breaking down and detailing a research aim into more manageable sections. It is likely that a research study will have an overall aim and a number of objectives which explain how the research question will be answered.

In addition, for some types of research, the research question can be expressed in a particular way so that it indicates the methodological approach being used. Table 6.1 shows how use of the different methodologies might be expressed for research on the wound healing topic:

Table 6.1 Examples of how different methodologies might be expressed

Methodology	Research question
Experimental study	Wound healing in patients with lower limb burns: a randomised controlled trial of mobilisation strategies.
Phenomenological study	What is the lived experience of patients who are beginning to mobilise after suffering from lower limb burns?
Systematic review	To determine the effectiveness of different types of mobilisation techniques on wound healing in patients with lower limb burns.
Observational study	How do patients with lower limb burns move around and how does this affect the rate of wound healing?
Ethnographic study	How do community nurses help patients mobilise after burns injuries? An ethnographic study of family and nurse interactions.

Sources of research questions

Ideas or topics for research come from a number of sources. However, it is important to remember from the outset that doing research usually requires a commitment in addition to other continuing demands on time (Edwards and Talbot, 1999). Therefore, it is a good idea, particularly when just starting out as a researcher, to focus on topics that create a real interest and that can help with personal professional development. Even when the general topic for research is being determined by an employer, educational institution or funder, it is likely that there will be an opportunity to link the project with specific interests or focus on part of a project that does create interest (Blaxter et al., 2006). Having an interest in a topic is important for a researcher to be able to retain motivation throughout the research process and make completion of a study more likely.

The actual source or inspiration for a research project can come from a number of areas. Occasionally a research question may arise from simple curiosity: 'a desire to satisfy an intellectual query that comes out of the blue' (Sim and Wright, 2000: 17).

More commonly, for nurses, ideas or inspiration for research are influenced by factors from both professional practice and their own thoughts on life. The most likely sources of topics or interest are those that arise from problems and questions identified through clinical experience (see Table 6.2).

Clinical experience

Clinical experience could be problems faced in clinical practice, such as: why particular patients are reluctant to take their medication; concerns about how best to break bad

Table 6.2 Sources of research questions

Subject	Related questions	Examples
Clinical experience	Patient problems Carer problems Clinical problems Patterns and trends Frequently occurring problems Effectiveness Outcomes New roles High incidence Prevalence Costly procedures	Some patients seem reluctant to take their medication; some wards appear to have more patients with MRSA than others; more patients appear to be discharged on Fridays than any other day.
Professional development	New approaches, e.g., inter- professional learning Behavioural change Preparation for new roles Student problems Evaluation of courses Conferences and literature identifying new areas for research Programmes of research identified by NHS Trusts	What is the best way of retaining student nurses? What are the educational needs of modern matrons? Are short intense full-time cardiac care courses better than longer part-time courses? What are the benefits of nurses learning together with doctors and social workers?
Theoretical frameworks	Theory testing Theory development Replication studies Validation of tools Methodological testing	Validation of a post-operative pain assessment tool for young children; testing a Finnish care dependency scale in British nursing homes; evaluating the validity, reliability and readability of a critical care family needs assessment tool.
Other sources	Unusual or unanticipated events, e.g. BSE crises; new phenomena; radiation leak; violent event; natural disasters such as floods and storms	The long-term health needs of survivors of an earthquake; the impact of contaminated food products on mothers' attitudes to breastfeeding; post-traumatic stress disorder in older victims of crime.
Policy imperatives	National initiatives Consensus activities National priorities Local service delivery National Service Frameworks Clinical guidelines Nursing policies Health and social care policies Public health policies	The effect of policy changes on the health needs of asylum seekers; the impact of a National Service Framework on staff training needs; the nature of school nursing following the new public health policies.

news to carers; an observation that male surgical patients seem to mobilise more quickly than female patients even though they have the same type of surgery; concern that patients who complain appear to receive less attention from nurses than patients who don't complain; an interest in the difference between a specialist nurse and an advanced nurse practitioner; an observation that MRSA appears to be increasing in a particular area; wondering what happens to patients who are discharged early. Clinical experience is a key source of research questions that interest nurses because it is based on everyday work experience.

Professional development

Professional development issues may also be a rich source of topics for nursing research, and these could lead to questions such as:

- Does inter-professional learning result in enhanced patient care?
- Is e-learning as effective as traditional lectures in terms of student knowledge?
- To what extent does a nursing degree influence career opportunity?
- Do small tutorial groups reduce attrition rates more than large lecture groups?
- Is clinical skills laboratory learning as effective as learning in the clinical environment?

Attending a conference on a particular topic, such as cancer nursing, exposes nurses to cutting-edge research. Some presentations will conclude with new research questions that need to be answered, or areas/topics that need further research may become apparent in the course of the presentation. Likewise, many published research studies will identify further research questions that need to be addressed. This can be a very useful way of generating research questions as they come directly from research that is topical and has a good evidence foundation.

Most local NHS Trusts support particular programmes of research that relate to their specific provision of care. For example, an acute NHS Trust with a Regional Oncology Centre is likely to support a programme of research related to the care of people with cancer. Local Research and Development Departments may also be able to identify specific questions that need researching to help build up expertise in a particular area as well as support the research remit of the Trust.

Theoretical frameworks

Some researchers are interested in developing theory in a particular area. The research questions they seek to answer might be about testing an existing theory or developing a new theory. The theories may have arisen from the work of other disciplines such as sociology or psychology, but may need to be tested in practice. Part of this might be about validating a particular data collection tool to ensure that it measures the phenomena accurately, reliably and without bias. Or it may be about testing a previously validated tool such as the BARRIERS to research implementation scale (Funk et al., 1991) using a different sample and in different settings. The BARRIERS scale has been tested in different groups of nurses in various countries such as the USA, Sweden, Australia and the UK. The research questions in these types of research studies will thus focus on what group is to be used in testing the tool. They may also be referred to as **replication studies** and use the same research questions and the same or a similar sample at different times.

Other sources

Research questions might also be developed from events that are unpredicted or accidental. The BSE crises might have led to nurses in rural areas exploring the impact of such an event on the mental health of farmers, or the effects of a salmonella outbreak in a small community might interest school nurses and public health nurses.

Policy imperatives

Another rich source of research questions may come from policy imperatives. These might be associated with, for example, health policy, health and social care policy, nursing policy or even international policy. In these cases, an organisation such as the Department of Health or the Royal College of Nursing may advertise that they want research in particular areas, and they often identify problems or concerns that need to be answered through research. This is sometimes called 'an invitation to tender' and can be highly competitive. For example, the Department of Health Research Programmes that are driven by policy imperatives have recently wanted research undertaken in the areas of: inpatient discharge procedures; information needs of patients; urban community hospitals; the relationship between A&E and Primary Care; the outcomes and effectiveness of rehabilitation programmes for patients being looked after at home; and patients' and carers' social needs. The Research for Patient Benefit (RfPB) programme is intended to provide a real opportunity for projects to emerge out of healthcare practice and to be designed to improve that practice. While it deliberately does not specify topics to be covered, applicants need to ensure that a clear case is made for the potential for patient and/or public benefit arising from the study. Alongside rigorous research designs and methodologies, they also look for dissemination strategies that will enhance the likelihood that the results can be rolled out within the NHS.

In many cases, such as those cited above, there is just an indication of the area where research is needed. However, the Social Care Workforce Research Initiative identified indicative research questions that it wanted answering through robust research studies. These included: How effective in recruiting or retaining staff are schemes that attempt to offer improved work/life balance? Are managers equipped to understand and use workforce information for planning? What do staff identify as areas in which they would most like training? What is the impact of user involvement in training and education? Does the use of agency staff make a difference to user experiences and outcomes?

The questions identified are developed as a result of changes in policy where the government wants to consider what effect these policies may have had. These could be related to issues such as modernising services; changes in the workforce; expansion and diversity in the workforce; turnover of staff, and so on, all of which are the focus of new policies that could affect nurses and nursing practice. They are usually posted on relevant websites (see Websites).

National Service Frameworks and Clinical Guidelines

National Service Frameworks (NSFs) might also highlight questions that need researching. Recent NSFs have identified new roles for nurses that need evaluating and key priorities that require actions that will have to be tested or assessed to see if they are effective. For example, the NSF for children has a priority of reducing teenage pregnancy and may prompt research questions such as:

- Does a dedicated teenage sexual health service provided by school nurses reduce pregnancy?
- What do teenage boys think about love and relationships?
- Would easy access to free condoms in secondary schools have an effect on teenage pregnancy rates?
- What is the role of mothers and fathers in reducing teenage pregnancy?

Similarly, clinical guidelines such as those produced by the National Institute of Clinical Excellence (NICE) are likely to identify areas where further research is needed because they have found minimal evidence. For example, the pressure ulcer prevention guideline (NICE, 2003), which focuses on how to prevent pressure ulcers in both primary and secondary care settings, made the following recommendations for further research:

- The effectiveness of re-positioning patients.
- A need for data on patient comfort in different positions.

- A comparison of different positions such as 30 degree/lateral tilt with other positions.
- The perceptions of individuals vulnerable to pressure ulcers (and their carers).

For novice researchers looking for a topic to research, clinical guidelines produce a rich source of ideas that are topical. Such guidelines are based on a systematic literature review of previous research on the topic and will identify where there are shortfalls in the evidence base and suggest where further research is needed.

Consensus activities can also lead to new areas that need researching. A recent Delphi study about career pathways in nursing and midwifery (Beattie et al., 2004) found that there is still uncertainty about whether nursing should become an all-graduate profession. Outcomes from this study include recommendations for further research to identify exactly what level of education is required for a nurse today.

Published studies

Despite the fact that all research studies have a research question, it is often really difficult to find the question clearly expressed in published literature. In the literature, it is more common to find aims and objectives specified, or a hypothesis may be presented. This may be because the publisher has word limits for articles and the authors try to be succinct in their writing. Research studies, however, need a research question to guide the whole research process – it is the starting point. Furthermore, the research question will be one of the first things that needs to be formulated in a research proposal, an application proposal for funding and an application to a Research Ethics Committee.

A simple examination of recently published studies in high-quality research journals can indicate how authors describe their research problem and specify the focus of their research. In Table 6.3, ten published studies have been identified to demonstrate the ways in which authors use research questions, research aims, problem statements, research objectives and hypotheses. For all cases the authors' exact words are used. In addition to the aims and research questions (when provided), the title of the article is given to demonstrate how they link together.

It can be seen from these examples that the range is enormous and that some studies clearly express what the research is trying to find, whilst in others it is not so obvious. Furthermore, some titles of published articles are nearly the same as the research questions, whereas in others they differ. In some cases there is also an indication of the research methodology adopted, such as Reilley et al. (2004) and Lloyd-Williams et al. (2007), which include 'a controlled trial' and 'a qualitative study' in their respective titles.

Table 6.3   Examples of research questions in recent published literature

Research question, aim or hypothesis	Title of published article	Authors
Aim: To investigate Swedish undergraduate nursing students' attitudes and awareness of research and development within nursing, and to illuminate factors that may have an impact on their attitudes and awareness.	'Swedish nursing students' attitudes to and awareness of research and development in nursing'	Björkström et al. (2003)
Aim: To evaluate the Breast Care Nursing Service from the patients' perspective. **Question 1**: How do patients with breast cancer experience the Breast Care Nursing Service? **Question 2**: What are the strengths and weaknesses of the Breast Care Nursing Service from the patients' perspective?	'A patient-focused evaluation of breast care nursing specialist services in North Wales'	Carnwell and Baker (2003)
Aim: To determine if occupational orientation, educational level, experience, area of practice, level of appointment and age are related to clinical decision-making in a sample of Australian nurses. **Question 1**: To what extent do nurses participate in clinical decision making and to what extent do they want to participate? **Question 2**: What occupational orientations (role values) do nurses working in an Australian acute care context hold? **Question 3**: Are there any significant relationships between occupational orientation (role value), educational level, experience, age, level of appointment and area of clinical practice and frequency of clinical decision making? **Question 4**: Which variables are the strongest predictors of clinical decision making?	'Decision-making in clinical nursing: investigating contributing factors'	Hoffman et al. (2004)
Overall aim: To describe the views and experiences regarding end of life, as described by a group of older people in their eighties.	'The end of life: a qualitative study of the perceptions of people over the age of 80 on issues surrounding death and dying'	Lloyd-Williams et al. (2007)
Objective: To determine whether provision of health advocacy for homeless patients would reduce the burden of care for a primary healthcare team. **Hypothesis**: That a dedicated health advocacy service for homeless patients can reduce the workload of GPs and other health workers.	'Can a health advocate for homeless families reduce workload for the primary healthcare team? A controlled trial'	Reilley et al. (2004)

(Continued)

Table 6.3 *(Continued)*

Research question, aim or hypothesis	Title of published article	Authors
The **aim** of the evaluation was to provide case studies of families and their key supporting agency members' perceptions and experiences of the PATCH service.	'Evaluation of the PATCH nursing service: partnership and training supporting children with complex needs at home'	Runciman and McIntosh (2003)
A study that was undertaken **to investigate** newly recruited student nurses' attitudes to gender and nursing stereotypes and pinpoint any change of attitude from 1992–2002.	'Angel, handmaiden, battleaxe or whore? A study which examines changes in newly recruited student nurses' attitudes to gender and nursing stereotypes'	Jinks and Bradley (2004)
Aim: To determine whether cognitive behaviour therapy would promote behavioural change on fluid consumption due to increased awareness and acknowledgement of the impact. **Question:** Can cognitive behavioural therapy reduce interdialactic weight gain?	'Can cognitive behaviour therapy assist adherence to fluid restriction with dialysis patients: a case series'	Ekers and Kingdon (2003)
Aim 1: To elicit the views of consultants, GPs and patients on the idea of copying GP referral letters to patients. **Aim 2:** To describe the experiences of a smaller group of GPs and patients actually involved in copying and receiving copies of referral letters.	'Copying GP referral letters to patients: the benefits and practical implications'	Jelley et al. (2003)
Aim: To understand how general practitioners conceptualise binge-eating disorder.	'Binge eating disorder: general practitioners' constructs of an ambiguous pathology'	Henderson et al. (2003)

Research questions

As we have just seen, it can be difficult to find research questions clearly stated within published literature. However, researchers need to be able to clearly express the research question(s) and, usually, they will also identify aims and objectives.

A good research question is clear and focused and is based on a researchable problem. Background information, brief details of previous research that identifies the problem and an underlying rationale as to why it is an important question to answer, will all support the research question. However, actually formulating a question can be troublesome, and it can be quite difficult to get the length of the

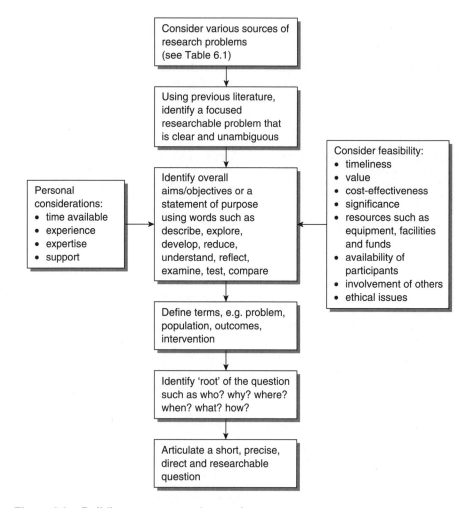

Figure 6.2   Building up a research question

question right. There is a need to find a balance between being succinct and trying to get everything fully detailed in the question. Identifying the key elements and then moving them around so that they make sense can help the development of a research question. The earlier example given in this chapter includes 'rate of wound healing', 'mobility' and 'patients with lower limb burns'. Focusing on these elements will assist in determining exactly what question the research is attempting to answer.

Figure 6.2 suggests a number of stages in developing both research questions and research aims and objectives. At this stage it is also worth remembering that the research question and the title of the research will not necessarily be the same, and it is not unusual to have a short working title for headings on information sheets and so on, reserving the use of the full research question for the full research proposal.

Having identified what problem(s) the research will address, or focus on, the problem needs to be clearly articulated. When asked by an interested colleague, a researcher needs to be able to succinctly answer the question 'What is the research problem?' If the researcher cannot do this, then further background work needs to be undertaken by looking at the literature and other research.

When preparing research questions, and ultimately research aims, it helps to consider personal constraints, such as how much time is available, how much experience and expertise is needed and what support is available. At this stage a researcher should also think about:

- the feasibility of undertaking the study, that is, will it actually be possible to conduct this research study?
- the availability of participants
- what resources will be required
- the availability of necessary equipment and facilities
- how others will be involved, including service users; Smith et al.'s (2008) review of the evidence and practice of user involvement gives an indication of the different roles of users in research
- ethical issues.

Remember that the significance of a research study may have an impact on the responses of others to the proposed research and may even determine whether it will be possible to get the necessary co-operation and resources required. It is also worth seeking advice from more experienced researchers at this early stage on any of the above aspects, as well as enlisting their help in devising the research question.

Research questions that are about intervention studies may use a PICO framework: **P**roblem, **I**ntervention, **C**omparison, **O**utcomes (Sackett et al., 1997). This framework is mostly used to frame questions when searching for evidence on effectiveness, as in systematic literature reviews. However, it can be useful in intervention studies to help identify key concepts and terms. If PICO were applied to the earlier example, we might end up with a question such as: 'For young people aged 12–16 with lower limb burns (*problem*), does a supported walking programme of 30 minutes a day (*intervention*) when compared to bed rest (*comparison*) increase the rate of wound healing and reduce rates of infection (two *outcomes*)?' The use of PICO is not appropriate for every research study, but it may help to tease out the key issues in certain types of experimental studies.

Another activity that can help with framing research questions is to consider words such as: who, why, where, when, how and what. These can be extended to phrases such as: To what extent ...? How do ...? What are ...? This is particularly useful in qualitative research, which by its nature has a more open and 'holistic' approach in its methods.

Prioritising research questions

Sometimes research questions need to be prioritised. This can help in determining what is the most important thing to study and can be of benefit, particularly for the novice researcher, when undertaking a time-limited project. One way to prioritise is to consider the following:

1 Level or degree of importance to patients', clients' or participants' well-being.
2 Most feasible to answer in the time available.
3 Most interesting question.
4 Most likely to be a recurring problem in own practice.
5 Level or degree of importance to nursing.
6 Most likely to produce recommendations that can be implemented.

There may be other aspects such as cost, ethical considerations, accessibility to facilities and/or participants or policy imperatives that need to be taken into consideration.

Research aims and objectives

Once the research question is explicit, it is possible to begin to specify research aims and objectives. Research aims describe the overall purpose of a project and research objectives describe the individual tasks that need to be carried out in order to meet the aims.

The clearly articulated problem can then be used to identify the aims of the research. A common difficulty when trying to explain what problem is to be addressed is to think 'too big' and try to do too much in a single research study. Research aims are usually quite broad and will summarise the overall goal of the research and maybe identify key variables (see later in this chapter). The research question, however, is very narrow and 'small'. Consider the difference between the question 'Does mobility influence wound healing in patients with lower limb burns?' compared with 'In 12- to 16-year-old young people what is the effect of a "supported walking" programme, of 30 minutes per day, on the rate of wound infection of lower limb burns?'

Specifying overall aims can be aided by using words such as describe, explore, reduce, and so on. It is also useful to define specific terms such as the type of problem (lower limb burns and healing), population or sample (young people 12–16 years of age), and outcome (rate of wound infection or increased healing rate). If the study is looking at a particular intervention, then this too will need to be defined (supported walking programme of 30 minutes per day).

Although objectives are usually a way of giving detail based on a research aim, the term 'objective' is sometimes used interchangeably with 'aim'. In Table 6.3, the study by Reilley et al. (2004) had an objective 'To determine whether provision of health advocacy for homeless patients would reduce the burden of care for a primary healthcare team', and many readers would see this as an aim rather than an objective. In reality, a research study will usually have something quite broad called an aim or a 'statement of purpose' and then some statements that are more specific and broken down into smaller researchable chunks. These might be called objectives or be worded as research questions. Looking at the examples in Table 6.3, the variability amongst aims, questions and objectives can be seen. Rather than debate the difference between aims, objectives and questions, it is important to recognise that each research study should have a clear research question(s) that is short, precise, direct, researchable and that drives the study. The three boxed examples below show more detail about how research aims, research questions and hypotheses are used in specific studies.

Box 6.1 Example of a study with a research aim and specific research questions

This Australian study describes the results of a study that investigated the contextual factors that influence clinical decision making. The **aim** of the study was to determine if occupational orientation, educational level, experience, area of practice, level of appointment and age are related to clinical decision making in a sample of Australian nurses. Four specific research questions were asked:

1   To what extent do nurses participate in clinical decision making and to what extent do they want to participate?
2   What occupational orientations (role values) do nurses working in an Australian acute care context hold?
3   Are there any significant relationships between occupational orientation (role value), educational level, experience, age, level of appointment and area of clinical practice and frequency of clinical decision making?
4   Which variables are the strongest predictors of clinical decision making?

The design of the study was a one-group prospective correlational postal survey of a convenience sample of registered nurses' perceptions of their participation in clinical

(Continued)

(Continued)

decision making. Multiple regression was used to model and weigh the relative influence of a number of factors on decision making. A response rate of 58 per cent was achieved, with 96 questionnaires out of 174 being returned.

Results indicated that education and experience were not significantly related to decision making. The most important factor that accounted for the greatest variability of clinical decision making was holding a professional occupational orientation. Other important factors were level of appointment, area of clinical speciality and age. Experience had no influence on decision making. The authors concluded that holding a professional orientation to work is important, and it is important to develop a professional outlook in all practising nurses, including students.

Source: Hoffman et al., 2004

Box 6.2　Example of a study with specific research aims

This study describes the quality of life and related factors in clients with schizophrenia in the Hong Kong Chinese population. The study had an overall aim and three specific aims:

Overall aim: To investigate the quality of life (QoL) of clients with schizophrenia who resided in the community in Hong Kong.
Specific aim 1: To provide a profile of QoL in clients with schizophrenia.
Specific aim 2: To examine relationships between QoL and sociodemographic factors, such as gender, age, marital status, employment status and level of education.
Specific aim 3: To examine relationships between QoL and clinical factors such as mental status, number of hospitalisations and duration of illness.

A convenience sample of adults attending a psychiatric outpatient department was recruited over a seven-month period. Face-to-face interviews were conducted using a semi-structured interview schedule that included two rating scales to assess clients' mental condition, and to assess quality of life.

The results indicated that women reported less satisfaction with their quality of life than men, and unemployed people were the least satisfied. Most participants were least satisfied with their psychological health, financial situation, life enjoyment and sexual satisfaction. Although not generalisable, the authors concluded that the findings suggest a need to strengthen social and vocational rehabilitation for people with schizophrenia in Hong Kong.

Source: Chan and Wai Yu, 2004

Box 6.3 Example of a study with a hypothesis

This British quasi-experimental controlled trial took place in an inner-city health centre, where 400 homeless people registered at the health centre were entered into a 'three-arm' trial in a systematic (non-randomised) manner. The control group received usual care from the health centre and the two intervention groups were offered either health advocacy with a family health worker at the health centre when they registered, or outreach advocacy through visits to hostels and bed and breakfast hotels before they registered. The three groups had similar demographic profiles and no significant differences in morbidity at baseline.

The hypothesis tested was that a dedicated health advocacy service for homeless people can reduce the workload of GPs and other health workers. The hypothesis was supported, as the results indicated that outreach health advocacy successfully reduced the workload for primary care staff. Furthermore, health advocacy can alter patterns of help seeking by homeless people, and can address psychosocial issues at no extra cost.

Source: Reilley et al., 2004

Hypotheses

In some types of research a hypothesis, or hypotheses, are used to drive the research. The main types of research using hypotheses will be deductive studies that are trying to test a theory. These are normally studies that take a quantitative approach and most commonly, but not exclusively, will be experimental studies.

A hypothesis attempts to answer a question which has emerged from a research problem. A hypothesis goes further than a research question and predicts an outcome. This can make it a very powerful tool, as will be seen in Chapter 13. As well as predicting an outcome, the hypothesis is a statement about the relationship between two or more variables. The hypothesis statement will go as far as predicting the relationship between variables and, through testing the hypothesis, may or may not support the theory. There are two types of variables used in hypotheses: independent and dependent variables. Independent variables are those seen as a 'cause', which might be an intervention or treatment, and dependent variables are seen as the 'effect' or outcome. This is commonly phrased as a 'cause and effect relationship.

Using the earlier examples, the independent variable would be 'supported walking for 30 minutes' and the dependent variable would be 'the rate of infection'. Because hypotheses are expressed clearly with all the variables identified explicitly, we might end up with a hypothesis such as:

Young people, aged 12–16 years, with more than 20 per cent lower limb burns who have a supported walking programme of 30 minutes per day will have a reduced wound size within 10 days of injury than those who are placed on bed rest for 10 days following injury.

In this example, the supported walking programme and bed rest are the independent variables (cause) and wound size (effect) is the dependent variable.

A hypothesis can also be stated as a 'null' hypothesis, which begins 'There is no difference …'. The null hypothesis states that there is no relationship between variables. It is used predominantly in research where there are to be tests of statistical significance (see Chapter 22). Hypotheses are never 'proved,' or 'disproved'; rather they are supported or unsupported, accepted or rejected by the data.

Chapter 13 explains in more detail how hypotheses are used in experimental design studies but, for the purposes of thinking about the research question, it is important to note how hypotheses are much more detailed and specific and how they will predict an outcome. The hypothesis is the bridge between the research problem, as identified from a review of the literature, the research question, and an appropriate research design.

Defining the variables

A variable is a characteristic that varies between individuals and can be measured, for example, weight, age and gender. Some of the examples given earlier are variables: young people aged 12–16; wound healing and bed rest. Variables can change or be changed depending on the design of the study. They can be studied in isolation or in combination, depending on the design of the study. During the course of a study a new variable may arise which could affect the data collected. Variables are used in different types of research including experimental designs, surveys, correlational studies and epidemiological research. As noted earlier, it is important to define the specific terms, including variables, that are to be included in a study and express them precisely in the research question, aims or objectives.

Feasibility

As stated earlier, and as can be seen from Figure 6.2, it is essential at this early stage of the research process to consider the feasibility of the proposed study at the same time as identifying the research question. Any proposed study needs to be timely, and whether it is a good time to undertake such a study will become evident through reading around the proposed research topic. It must be self-evident that the research question being considered has not already been answered and that it is still relevant. At the same time it must be clear that there is value in trying to answer the question through the proposed study, that it will be cost-effective, that it is significant and that resources are available to conduct the study. One key resource is the availability of participants for a proposed study. There is no point posing valuable and significant research questions if access to participants is near impossible. In preparing the research question it is also important to involve others, particularly service users, patients and carers. Nurses may think it is an important question to try to answer through research but patients may have different priorities that need to be considered. Similarly, when a research topic does not readily fit in with an institution's research priorities there may be problems in getting permission to conduct the research. Furthermore, where funding is to be sought for a research project it is also worth considering whether the research topic will match any potential funders' research priorities.

Whether a proposed research study is feasible is also determined by ethical considerations. Chapter 5 provides an overview of the ethical principles that need to be considered when conducting research. However, it is essential that any proposed research starts from the premise of being ethical and be based on sound ethical principles. Furthermore, any ethics committee (NHS, social services or university) will expect a clearly set out main research question and any other **secondary research** questions. All proposals and protocols prepared for potential funders will also require explicit research questions. The research question is thus crucial.

Research questions and methodology adopted

Research questions should drive the chosen methodology for a research study. In the earlier example, there is an indication of what type of methodology might be used to answer the question. A hypothesis would lead to thinking of an experiment such as a randomised controlled trial comparing different types of mobilisation (bed-rest or walking for 30 minutes). A question such as 'How do patients move following lower limb burns and how does this influence wound healing?' might lead to an observation type of study that also has some wound measurement component. A research question such as 'Why are some patients better able to mobilise than others?' might lead to a study involving interviews with different groups of patients. Whereas a research question such as 'What is the lived experience of mobilising after lower limbs burns?' might suggest a phenomenological study.

In other chapters in this book there are debates about how the research may be driven by the particular beliefs of the researcher and may lead to the asking of particular research questions that will be answered by a particular approach to the research. For example, a researcher with a scientific background might pose a research question that leads to the prediction of a specific outcome (a hypothesis) and an experimental study. Conversely, a researcher influenced by interpretism/naturalism might pose a research question and suggest a methodology where the researcher and the researched are not objectively separated, such as in action research.

This chapter has focused on developing the research question at the beginning of the research process and then designing an appropriate study to answer the question or meet the aims of the study. Although the background, experience and expertise of the researcher are clearly important, it is the research question that should drive the research. In a profession such as nursing, that has such broad interests and is influenced by such a wide range of paradigms, it is inevitable that it will embrace an eclectic approach to research. However, it is crucial that the research design should be chosen to answer the research question.

Chapter summary

- A clearly defined problem or gap in current knowledge is an important prerequisite for any research and this is framed in the form of a research question.
- Developing a research question is the first stage in the research process.
- The research question:

  - identifies a gap in knowledge or a problem
  - focuses attention on directly relevant and significant issues that need to be researched
  - guides and focuses the research study
  - leads to an appropriate research design.

- The research question can be used for literature searching and undertaking systematic reviews and provides guidance for clinical audit.
- The research question is necessary for ethics review bodies and funding organisations to identify whether a study is justifiable and worth doing.
- Sources for research questions include clinical experience, professional issues, theoretical frameworks and policy imperatives.
- A research aim is a description of the intention or broad purpose of the research.
- Research objectives explain how the research question will be answered.
- A hypothesis is a statement of the expected relationship between or among the things being studied; it goes further than a research question and predicts an outcome.
- A variable is an 'object' that is being investigated in a research study and is considered to be capable of varying.

- A good research question is one that is clearly expressed and focused on a researchable problem.
- The research question is the driver in the choice of research methodology and design.

References

Beattie, A., Hek, G., Galvin, K. and Ross, K. (2004) 'What are the future career pathways in nursing and midwifery? A Delphi survey of nurses and midwives in the South West of England', *Nursing Times Research,* 9 (5): 348–64.

Björkström, E.A., Johansson, I.S., Hamrin, E.K. and Athlin, E.E. (2003) 'Swedish nursing students' attitudes to and awareness of research and development within nursing', *Journal of Advanced Nursing,* 41 (4): 393–402.

Blaxter, L., Hughes, C. and Tight, M. (2006) *How to Research,* 3rd edition. Maidenhead: Open University Press.

Carnwell, R. and Baker, S.A. (2003) 'A patient-focused evaluation of breast care specialist services in North Wales', *Clinical Effectiveness in Nursing,* 7 (1): 18–29.

Chan, S. and Wai Yu, I. (2004) 'Quality of life of clients with schizophrenia', *Journal of Advanced Nursing,* 45 (1): 72–83.

Edwards, A. and Talbot, R. (1999) *The Hard-pressed Researcher: A Research Handbook for the Caring Professions,* 2nd edition. Harlow: Longman.

Ekers, D. and Kingdon, D. (2003) 'Can cognitive behaviour therapy assist adherence to fluid restriction with dialysis patients: a case series', *Clinical Effectiveness in Nursing,* 7 (1): 15–17.

Funk, S.G., Champagne, M.T., Weise, R.A. and Tornquist, E.M. (1991) 'BARRIERS: the barriers to utilization scale', *Applied Nursing Research,* 4 (1): 39–45.

Henderson, E., May, C. and Chew-Graham, C.A. (2003) 'Binge eating disorder: general practitioners' constructs of an ambiguous pathology', *Primary Health Care Research and Development,* 4 (4): 301–6.

Hoffman. K., Donoghue, J. and Duffield, C. (2004) 'Decision-making in clinical nursing: investigating contributing factors', *Journal of Advanced Nursing,* 45 (1): 53–62.

Jelley, D., Scott, D. and van Zwanenberg, T. (2003) 'Copying GP referral letters to patients: the benefits and practical implications', *Primary Health Care Research and Development,* 4 (4): 319–28.

Jinks, A.M. and Bradley, E. (2004) 'Angel, handmaiden, battleaxe or whore? A study which examines changes in newly recruited student nurses' attitudes to gender and nursing stereotypes', *Nurse Education Today,* 24 (2): 73–156.

Lloyd-Williams, M., Kennedy, V., Sixsmith, A. and Sixsmith, J. (2007) 'The end of life: a qualitative study of the perceptions of people over the age of 80 on issues surrounding death and dying', *Journal of Pain and Symptom Management,* 34 (1): 60–66.

National Institute for Clinical Excellence (2003) *Pressure Ulcer Prevention*. London: National Institute of Clinical Excellence.

Reilley, S., Graham-Jones, S., Gaulton, E. and Davidson, E. (2004) 'Can a health advocate for homeless families reduce workload for the primary healthcare team? A controlled trial', *Health and Social Care in the Community*, 12 (1): 63–74.

Runciman, P. and McIntosh, J. (2003) 'Evaluation of the PATCH nursing service: partnership and training supporting children with complex needs at home', *Primary Health Care Research and Development*, 4 (4): 307–18.

Sackett, D.L., Richardson, W.S., Rosenberg, W. and Haynes, R.B. (1997) *Evidence-based Medicine: How to Practice and Teach EBM*. New York: Churchill Livingstone.

Sim, J. and Wright, C. (2000) *Research in Health Care: Concepts, Designs and Methods*. Cheltenham: Nelson Thornes.

Smith, E., Ross, F., Donovan, S., Manthorpe, J., Brearley, S., Sitzia, J. and Beresford, P. (2008) 'Service user involvement in nursing, midwifery and health visiting research: a review of the evidence and practice', *International Journal of Nursing Studies*, 45: 298–315.

Websites

Department of Health: www.dh.gov.uk has details about research funded by the Department of Health and any invitations to tender for new projects under their Research and Development pages.

Medical Research Council: www.mrc.ac.uk includes opportunities for projects funded by the Medical Research Council.

National Institute for Clinical Excellence: www.NICE.org.uk for details of published clinical guidelines and those in progress, and how to develop guidelines.

National Institute for Health Research Central Commissioning Facility: www.nihr-ccf.org.uk/site/docdatabase/rfpb gives guidance on the aims and scope for applications to the Research for Patient Benefit programme.

RDInfo: www.rdinfo.org.uk for guidance on how to start a research project, including a flow chart that guides the reader through turning an idea into a research question.

Service Delivery and Organisation Programme: www.sdo.nihr.ac.uk has details of research about the NHS Service Delivery and Organisation research programme. Also available is a checklist for researchers who are preparing proposals, with a section on research questions and research objectives.

Journals with good examples of research questions, aims, objectives and hypotheses

British Journal of General Practice
British Medical Journal
Clinical Effectiveness in Nursing
Health and Social Care in the Community
International Journal of Nursing Studies
Journal of Advanced Nursing
Nurse Education in Practice
Nurse Education Today
Nurse Researcher
Nursing Research

7

LITERATURE SEARCHING

Any research project starts from an idea, identification of a problem or something that a researcher wants to find out more about. Usually a researcher needs to gain more information before the idea, query or topic of interest can be refined into a project that is manageable and researchable. This process is helped by a review of the research literature that already exists. Searching for the literature that is relevant to a topic helps to refine a research question and should also confirm that it has not already been answered. The use of electronic databases has made the actual searching more convenient and faster. However, searching for relevant literature is a skill that has to be developed but will assist in keeping up to date with any relevant newly published literature as the research progresses.

The purpose of a literature review is to help to provide background information that gives a solid understanding of the research topic and a platform from which to develop an actual research project (Sim and Wright, 2000). A research literature review is essentially the same as any other literature review, but there will be more emphasis on locating the literature that can justify the conduct of further research on a given topic.

A literature review can be divided into two sections:

- Looking for literature that is appropriate to a specific topic.
- A balanced review of differing viewpoints or findings.

This chapter introduces the practicalities of searching the literature and outlines some strategies for successful searching.

Learning outcomes

This chapter is designed to enable the reader to:

- **Understand the steps involved in conducting a literature search**
- **Identify appropriate information to be retrieved when searching the literature**
- **Carry out a literature search of a topic in the reader's area of research/ practice interest**
- **Understand how to locate the relevant literature for a research question/topic**

KEY TERMS

Literature review, Literature search

Purpose of literature searching

Deciding where to begin searching the literature on a specific topic can be daunting. What must be remembered is that a **literature review**, whether as background for a research project or, for example, to identify best practice in a specific area, is *not* an attempt to identify every existing resource related to the topic of the research. Rather, the aim is to identify the *most relevant* resources (Gash, 2000). This requires the use of judgement to use or discard a particular resource and some familiarity with the general area of the research and research methods typically used in that area.

This means that the researcher needs to have a basic understanding of the specific research topic *before* embarking on the actual searching. This may sound contradictory, but without some insight into the research topic it will be very difficult to develop a research question, identify the terms for a search or make reasonable judgements about what to use or discard from the results of a search. Hopefully, a nurse researcher or group of nurses planning to undertake a research project will have a grasp of the key issues relating to the topic. However, for many research projects, the initial process of transferring an idea for research into an actual project begins with a general discussion about the topic that helps to increase the level of understanding about the area and how other researchers have approached the topic (Hek et al., 2000). This may include discussions with relevant and interested colleagues who can help to find the focus of the topic and so develop a clear research question. These informal discussions can assist particularly in refining search terms, and may even generate specific articles, references or contacts. Colleagues may have been involved in research on a related topic and be able to put you in touch with other researchers in the same area of interest or be willing to share papers and/or results. Others may have attended courses or conferences where the topic has been discussed and, again, be willing to share notes and conference proceedings. In addition, teachers and supervisors frequently have access to a wide variety of resources and/or individuals that can provide assistance in gaining more understanding of the topic. This type of discussion should really be undertaken before starting a **literature search** but it can also be useful in later stages of a search, particularly if the searching produces too few or far too many citations.

These initial discussions may also be able to stop you progressing too far with a topic that has already been very well researched or one that will be very difficult to research within the resources available, or where ethical considerations may make researching the topic impracticable.

Stages in the literature searching process

The main stages of the search, which are discussed below, include (Hart, 1998):

1 Confirming the research question.
2 Creating a set of search terms.
3 Deciding what are the most appropriate sources of information.
4 Performing a search.
5 Revising the search, as necessary, and replicating it in other sources.

Confirming the research question

As already suggested, before starting a search of the literature you need to determine what you are trying to find information about and what level of information is needed. It is important to remember that the aim of searching the literature for a research project is not to retrieve as many references as possible. The reason for searching the literature is to expose the *main gaps* in knowledge on the topic and identify the principal areas of dispute and uncertainty (Hart, 1998). The search should also give some guidance on the general patterns of findings from multiple examples of research in the same area and the types of research method that have been used by other researchers in the area. To do this, a clearly defined research question is essential, otherwise there is a risk of not finding relevant information (that is, citations) or of wasting a considerable amount of time.

How is a set of search terms created?

Having a clear idea of what you are looking for will help you to find relevant information and can save time by your not retrieving citations that are only loosely relevant to your topic. How a researcher generates a set of terms for a literature search depends on individual preferences. But it is usually a good idea to progress from general to specific concepts to avoid missing relevant information by making a search too precise initially.

A common way of starting to create a set of terms is to focus exactly on what you are looking for and break this down into keywords or concepts. For example: you are planning a study on the treatment of constipation in older people. The keywords in this example are *older people* and *constipation*. There are likely to be several ways of expressing these keywords – try making a list for yourself of alternative words, spelling variations and abbreviations. Below are some suggested search terms; these are the words or search terms that you will use to search the databases (though this is not a definitive list):

Constip*
Defaecation/defecation
Bowel function$
Bowel habit$
Bowel movement$

Older people/patient$
Elderly people/patient$
Geriatric$
Older adult$/patient$

Another way that is often used to generate search terms, which we have already encountered in the previous chapter, can be remembered as PICO (Sackett et al., 1997):

Problem
Intervention
Comparison (optional)
Outcome(s)

You may not always have a comparison, but you will usually be able to define patients or population, the intervention or treatment in which you are interested and the outcome measures (that is, the measured effect of the intervention or treatment).

P + I + C + O = the search question

For example: you are interested in 'the effectiveness of nicotine patches in helping adults to stop smoking'.

Using PICO:

What is the **P**roblem?
> = adults; cigarette smokers[1] for at least 3 years' duration.

What is the **I**ntervention (or treatment)?
> = application of nicotine patch or educational leaflet.

What is the **C**omparison (if any)?
> = nicotine patch versus educational leaflet.

What is the **O**utcome measure?
> = participants not smoking for at least one year.

Refining your search and setting boundaries

However you generate the terms for your search, you will need to refine these and set some boundaries; doing this will ensure that your search is comprehensive but not overwhelming.

There are a number of features used in databases that are worth understanding to make searching easier and effective. These allow you to use your own words and yet eliminate some of the problems you may encounter, such as:

- plurals, for example, child or children
- different spellings, for example, leukaemia or leukemia
- different terminology, for example, pavement or sidewalk
- prefixes, for example, prenatal, pre natal or pre-natal.

You can also use what are know as wild cards (*, ?) to search for spelling variations and plurals. For example:

leuk?emia to find leukaemia or leukemia
p*ediatrics will retrieve paediatrics or pediatrics
child* will retrieve children, child, as well as childhood and childish.

You can also truncate (for example, *, $) words to search for different word stems and word endings. The truncation symbol is usually an asterisk (*), but this may vary from one database to another. For example:

use comput* to find computer, computers, computing, computed and so on. (but comp* would also find compost!).

[1]You will have to decide if you are including pipe and/or cigar smokers.

In addition, you also need to specify how your keywords or search terms relate to each other. This is usually done by using what are know as Boolean Operators, that is, using the linking words AND, OR, NOT:

- **AND:** linking keywords with AND means that *all* keywords must appear in the search results.
- **OR:** combining terms with OR means that *any* of the keywords must appear in the search results. This will generate a larger set of results. You would use OR for linking alternative ways of describing the same subject, for example, older people OR elderly OR geriatric.
- **NOT:** used to *exclude* search terms; use with caution as you may remove too many results including those that are relevant!

Additionally, setting date limits for your search will make it more practical and ensure that you retrieve only citations that are up-to-date. It is important that the date range you set is realistic; a common convention is to set a 10-year limit to a search. However, you may wish to modify this if there are either an overwhelming number of citations or very few. Take care to check that it is your date range that is at fault rather than your search terms; your librarian will help you if this problem occurs.

It is also usual to limit your search to English-language publications for the purely practical reason of needing to be able to read the citations retrieved. Ordinarily this will not be a problem (unless you are doing a systematic literature review – see Chapter 18). However, if your research is in an area where most of the research literature has not been published in English, then it could be a disadvantage; for example, if the topic is about acupuncture, then using only English for a search will exclude the large body of Chinese literature.

Sources of information

Deciding what the most appropriate sources of information are is important for the credibility of your review. Essentially there are two sources of information: *primary* and *secondary* sources.

The researchers who carried out the original work on the topic produce *primary sources*. Primary sources are preferred over secondary sources because of the decreased potential for bias and distortion beyond the control of the researcher (Powers and Knapp, 1995). Primary sources are usually published as journal articles or abstracts from conferences.

Secondary sources make reference to the original research by someone other than the researcher. The source of data consists of summarisation of, or commentary about, primary data, such as in a literature review. Secondary sources are usually found within journal articles or textbooks.

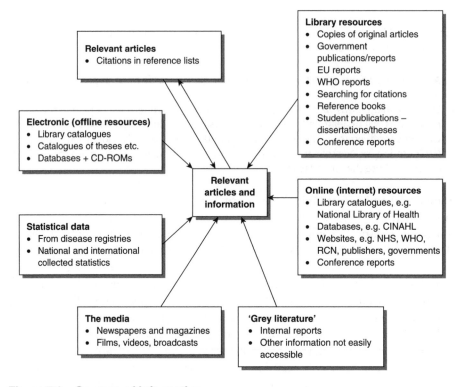

Figure 7.1   Sources of information

Relevant articles and information can be obtained from many sources; some of these are shown in Figure 7.1

Books generally represent the acceptance of an idea or method into the mainstream thought of that discipline. However, the time it takes to publish a book means that the information contained in it will be older than that found in journals, reports and so on.

To be relevant, journal articles need to be up-to-date, although it is possible to trace how trends have changed by reviewing older articles. It is also important to remember that not all articles meet academic standards. Most journal articles are now peer reviewed, which gives a sense of quality assurance, but this does not take away from the reader the need to make his or her own judgement about the quality of the research being described (Gash, 2000).

Papers in the form of conference proceedings have the advantage of being timely and present the very latest thinking/research on a particular topic. There may, however, be a disadvantage in that there may not have been time for the ideas presented to become fully accepted by the peer review process (Hart, 1998). Quality control may not be as rigorous as that of peer reviewed journals, though it is usual for there to have been some peer review prior to a paper being accepted for presentation at the conference.

Reports – research reports, technical reports, development reports, government reports – present details of research from a specific project. This is a growing body of literature that provides a good source of current tabular, graphic and statistical material. However, not all reports will be in the public domain and it may be difficult to obtain the full report, and they tend to be confined to science and technology although this may be changing.

Dissertations and theses – undergraduate, Master's, MPhil, PhD – are an important source of primary material because they should contain original work and meet a minimum academic standard. It can be difficult to obtain copies and you may have to consult them in the library where the dissertation/thesis is held.

Exactly which sources to use will depend on your research question, the time you have available to perform a search and review the literature retrieved, and what search resources you can access. You should, however, always remember that the quality of the information you obtain will vary. The next chapter discusses how to assess the quality of the articles you retrieve.

Performing a search

Actually performing a search has become much easier with the advent of electronic databases. These are huge bibliographic files that can be accessed electronically either via an online search (using the Internet) or from a CD-ROM (using computer discs that store the bibliographic information).

There are many bibliographic (electronic) databases that can be accessed by nurses, the majority of which have user-friendly programmes that are menu driven with on-screen support that makes retrieving a reference relatively easy. Furthermore, most university and NHS libraries also offer training sessions on using the most popular electronic databases; it is very useful to learn your way around these search resources.

The main electronic search resources that hold references on nursing studies include:

- CINAHL (Cumulative Index to Nursing and Allied Health Literature)
- British Nursing Index
- Allied and Complementary Medicine
- MEDLINE (Medical Literature Online)
- Cochrane Database of Systematic Reviews
- EMBASE (the Excerpta Medical database)
- PsychoINFO (Psychology Information)
- National Research Register

- ReFeR (Department of Health Research Findings Register)
- CancerLit (Cancer Literature)
- Dissertation Abstracts online

All of the above databases can be accessed via the National Library for Health at www.library.nhs.uk. The most useful databases for nurses are probably CINAHL, British Nursing Index and MEDLINE.

Steps for searching and retrieving citations using CINAHL

The Cumulative Index to Nursing and Allied Health Literature or CINAHL covers references to over 1,200 English (and other languages) nursing journals, as well as book chapters, nursing dissertations and some conference proceedings for nursing and allied health fields. Abstracts are available for many of the journals and, depending on your access rights, you may also be able download the full text of some articles.

You can access the CINAHL database via the National Library for Health website www.library.nhs.uk. This gives you a list of databases, for example:

Click the **advanced search** beside CINAHL to select this database to enable you to start searching.

- **Step 1: Starting the search** For this example we are going search for information about 'the use of laxatives in the management of constipation in elderly patients'. The logical way of searching is to search for one subject at a time: type **constipation** into the search box. You also need to make sure that 'Thesaurus mapping' is ticked, and then click **search**.

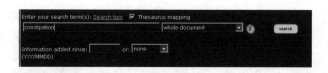

- **Step 2: Thesaurus mapping** This will take you to the thesaurus mapping where you will see a list of subject headings. Locate the subject heading closest to what you typed – here there is a 'constipation' subject heading, so just click on the word CONSTIPATION.

- **Step 3: Thesaurus Tree** Now you will see a Thesaurus Tree which shows subject headings or descriptors related to the word (**constipation**) you selected. This gives you an opportunity to broaden or narrow your search down to more specific subjects if you need to.

  – *Explode* offers you the chance to get all citations on constipation and any narrower subjects associated with this subject.
  – *Major descriptors* means that you will get citations where constipation is **one** of the major subjects, and if you do not tick this box you will also get citations where constipation is a minor subject in the article.
  – *Subheadings* relate to specific aspects of a subject that will help you to focus on your subject, for example, diagnosis, aetiology. When you want to do a focused search, simply tick the box in the subheadings column next to constipation to view what subheadings are available, make your choice and click [search] to continue. This will return you to the opening screen and the result of your search.

  For our example, because we are interested in the management of constipation, we want citations where constipation is the major subject, so tick the major descriptor box for CONSTIPATION and click on [search] and this will take you back to the opening screen and you will see the result of your search.

- **Step 4: Repeat the steps** The next step is to repeat the process, this time using the term **laxative**. Because we are interested in the use of laxatives for the management of constipation, this time we need to use a subheading, so tick the *drug therapy* subheading.

  When you have completed these steps you will have a set of results something like the one shown below.

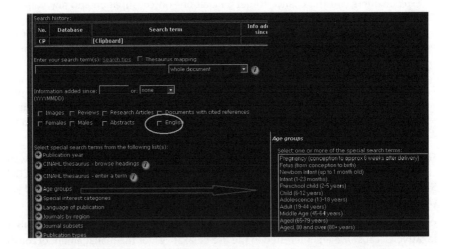

- **Step 5: Combining**   The results are for each subject separately, which is not very useful for our review. So the next step is to combine the searches to give the citations applicable to our search question.

  The citations for constipation as the major subject are in line 2 and those for laxative and drug therapy are in line 4. To combine the results of these searches we simply type 2 and 4 as our search terms. At this time we can also untick the box for thesaurus mapping and then click **search**.

- **Step 6: Refining your search**   If you recall, our search question was about 'the use of laxatives in the management of constipation in elderly patients'. So far we have retrieved citations about constipation and laxatives but have not related this to elderly patients. We can do this by using *special search terms*, which you can find in the section below your search results. To select *elderly patients* click on **age groups** and a pop-up box appears. Select the age groups that apply – here you have to decide the age ranges for the search, that is, whether to include the 'middle age' group in order to capture those between 60 and 64 years. Once you have selected the age groups, click on **search** to add these to your search list.

At this stage you may also wish to set limits to the years of publication and limit your search to English language publications. To limit your search to English, just click the box and to set the limits for year of publication. Follow the same procedure that you used to select the age groups once you have decided how far back you wish to go for your review, for example 2000–2007.

These will all appear as additional lines on your search results. To complete the search, combine the lines as before to give you a final search result for English-language publications between the years 2000 and 2007 about 'the use of laxatives in the management of constipation in elderly patients'. The number of citations is shown in the results list; in this example 63 were obtained, and you have finished your initial search!

What to do with your results

Clicking on ███████ in the final line of your search will show you a list of citations and you can start to determine which articles are really relevant to your research topic.

You can at this stage save the whole list of citations by clicking on ██████. When you are at this initial stage of your search, it is always a good idea to save the complete list as a reference – you may never need to refer back to this list, but it will avoid having to repeat the same search at a later stage.

Or you may wish to review the full list and highlight those citations that appear to be relevant by ticking the box next to it on the left-hand side. To display the citations you highlighted once you have finished reviewing the complete list, scroll to the bottom of the page and choose your display format ('medium' is the default setting) and click on the ██████ button. This will allow you to review your choices and to save in a variety of formats. Using the FULL display format will give you the abstract and references (and, if available, access to a full text copy of the article).

Saving and e-mailing your search

Using the box at the bottom of your screen gives you a variety of options for saving your search with or without your search strategy.

Revising the search and replication in other sources

Having your search as a PDF document can be very useful, but if you want to save your results as a word document choose RTF, click on [save] and follow the instructions on the screen. Alternatively, you can e-mail your results by clicking on the e-mail button and following the instructions given, making sure that you select the delivery format (same as the display format) and output format *before* you click on [deliver]!

Note:

- When you access CINAHL (or any of the other databases) via the National Library for Health website, details of where you can retrieve the abstract (usually online) or article are included.
- There are more detailed guides available for each of the databases when you go online.

By now you should have a list of citations that appear relevant to your topic, that is, a list of titles. The next stage of the process is to review the abstracts of these articles to check that they really do relate to the topic you are researching, and then obtain copies of these articles. This is the main way of ensuring that you retrieve only those articles pertinent to your topic and hence literature review. This process should narrow down the number of articles that you need to appraise in order for your literature review to be comprehensive.

However, for your search to be as comprehensive as possible you need to search more than one database, using the same search strategy for each database. This may yield some of the same information but it also ensures that you are less likely to miss an article that is relevant to your research topic.

Too many or too few results from a search

What you actually get from your search in numbers of citations and relevant articles is dependent on you having chosen appropriate search terms and on whether there is published literature that is relevant to your question.

Too many results are not uncommon when you first start searching, and this is often because you are afraid of missing something. However, getting too many results can be overwhelming, so you need to set some limits in order to make the information you retrieve more manageable. As indicated earlier, you can do this by setting publication date limits, using the thesaurus and combing searches using Boolean operators. If there are still too many results, you may want to consider selecting publications that review only higher-quality research studies.

Too few results is very frustrating, and there can be a number of reasons for this. The first step is to ask a specialist librarian or a tutor for advice. However, it may be that there is very little published literature relating to your topic. If this is what you suspect, then it is worth checking to see if you can find out about 'research in progress' that may be relevant. This may influence whether you start your own research and may guide you to potential collaborators and/or advisers.

Two useful databases that you can search for details of ongoing research are:

- *The National Research Register (NRR)*: This holds details of all research projects approved by the NHS and includes records of ongoing and recently completed projects. It can be accessed via the National Library for Health website or www.nrr.nhs.uk.
- *The Health Technology Assessment (HTA) programme*: The HTA is a national programme of research funded by the Department of Health R&D programme. It makes available to all NHS staff high-quality research evidence about the effectiveness and cost-effectiveness of all types of healthcare interventions. Details of reports in progress are included at www.ncchta.org.

Also, some older published research may not yet have been entered onto electronic databases, and you will only find this by trawling through the journal stacks in a bio-medical library.

Alternatively, it may be that your search terms are inappropriate or you have set too strict limits for your search. You should consider revising these and then redoing your search.

Getting unexpectedly few results can be worse than getting no results at all. It may appear satisfactory but have you really done a *good* search? Once you are happy that you have done a good search you need to review the abstracts and decide which articles you wish to retrieve in full so that you can start the next stage in the literature reviewing process. This is considered in the next chapter.

Chapter summary

- A literature review helps to provide background information for a research topic and assists the development of an actual research project.
- A literature review can be divided into two sections:
  - looking for literature that is appropriate to a specific topic
  - a balanced review of differing viewpoints or findings.
- The purpose of a literature review is to find the resources most relevant to the topic.
- Having a clear idea of what you are looking for *before* you start searching is cost-effective in terms of time and effort.
- You need to devise a search strategy that accurately reflects your research question before you start searching the databases.

- Searching electronically can increase the speed and convenience of literature searching.
- Primary sources of evidence come from researchers who carried out the original work on the topic.
- Secondary sources consist of summarisation of or commentary about primary data and refer to the original research.
- There is a range of different sources that can provide access to relevant articles.
- Always search the literature in a systematic way and keep a record of the searches you have conducted.
- The abstracts of articles identified by a search need to be reviewed to ensure that only articles pertinent to the topic are retrieved.
- Searching for articles is only one stage of the literature reviewing process.

References

Gash, S. (2000) *Effective Literature Searching for Research.* Aldershot: Gower.

Hart, C. (1998) *Doing a Literature Review.* London: Sage.

Hek, G., Langton, H. and Blunden, G. (2000) 'Systematically searching and reviewing literature', *Nurse Researcher*, 7: 40–57.

Powers, B. and Knapp, T. (1995) *A Dictionary of Nursing Theory and Research.* London: Sage.

Sackett, D.L., Richardson, W.S., Rosenberg, W. and Haynes, R.B. (1997) *Evidence Based Medicine: How to Practice and Teach EBM.* New York: Churchill Livingstone.

Sim, J. and Wright, C. (2000) *Research in Health Care: Concepts, Designs and Methods.* Cheltenham: Nelson Thornes.

Websites

Health Technology Assessment (HTA) Programme: www.ncchta.org

National Library for Health: www.library.nhs.uk

National Research Register: www.nrr.nhs.uk

8

CRITICAL APPRAISAL

Reviewing the research that has already been conducted is an important part of the research process, known as a literature review, and can be undertaken for a number of different purposes, such as supporting a research proposal or as part of a study report. The first step of this process, searching for the literature or assembling the evidence, is discussed in Chapter 7. The next stages in the preparation of a literature review are to start to draw some conclusions about the body of research that has been reported and make judgements about the quality of that original research. This involves assessing the research through a process of critical analysis and evaluation and is known as critical appraisal.

Critical appraisal of the evidence, or analytical evaluation of the research relating to a topic, is the unravelling of the reasoning that informs the research and arguments (Hart, 1998). This is, effectively, a two-stage process of reading analytically and then appraisal or synthesis of the information that you have gained from your reading. This chapter describes what reading analytically entails and offers guidance on how to critically appraise or evaluate different types of research study.

Learning outcomes

This chapter is designed to enable the reader to:

- **Recognise what is involved in reading analytically**
- **Be able to identify the findings of a research study that will be relevant to a specific topic of enquiry**
- **Recognise the different questions that need to be asked when critically appraising qualitative and quantitative research and literature reviews**

- Appreciate researchers' interpretations of the data presented in published reports
- Understand the role of critical analysis in research and evidence-based practice
- Be able to carry out a critical appraisal of a peer-reviewed paper

---

KEY TERMS

Critical analysis, Critical appraisal, Critique, Diaries, Purposive or purposeful sampling, Qualitative research, Quantitative research, Reading analytically, Synthesis

---

Why is a critical appraisal needed?

Critical appraisal is a structured process of identifying and evaluating the merits and/or value of research. No research study will be perfect; therefore, all research may be critically evaluated. However, the critical approach must be thoughtful and thorough. It is important to be realistic about our ability to evaluate research, and recognise that research is ongoing and cumulative in the sense that it can always be improved, refined and expanded. By being critical of the research of others we can learn to discriminate between 'good' and 'bad' research. This will also help the development of our own ideas about what and how we can do research. Being critical involves making decisions about the merit or value of a piece of research, and by applying 'careful judgement' both the good and bad points of the research can be considered or appraised.

There are a number of reasons why a critical appraisal of published research is necessary:

- Researchers may make unjustified claims about what can be done or changed on the basis of their findings. There may be alternative ways of interpreting the results of a study that may not have been considered by the researcher(s).
- The process of peer review of published papers acts as a procedure of quality control in many academic journals. This may be a very rigorous process, with papers being scrutinised by independent reviewers as well as the editorial team.
- Independent reviewers will usually be specialists on the subject area and, when appropriate, include statisticians. However, the peer review process is not infallible and readers/researchers should be able to make their own judgements about the quality of research. Just because a paper has been published does not guarantee that the findings are 'correct'; mistakes can be made and there will always be a risk of researcher bias. Bias in this context refers

to a tendency to misrepresent (intentionally or unintentionally) or any influence or action in a study that might distort the results of a research study.

- Most experienced researchers will be aware of the limitations of their published reports and will often demonstrate their own critical appraisal skills by using them to refine their understanding of the topic or methods or potential practical application of their research.

- Appraising how other researchers have approached a topic assists our own thinking about it and what may be appropriate methods of investigation.

- Research is of little value unless it somehow influences practice. This means that nurses need to be able to evaluate effectively to determine whether findings should be implemented. There should also be dialogue between practitioners and researchers so that practice changes happen in response to available evidence rather than simply because it seems like a good idea and/or is fashionable.

Critical appraisal is an evaluation of the strengths and limitations of the research report being reviewed. It should reflect an objective, balanced and thoughtful consideration of the validity and significance of the research under considera-tion. Critical appraisal is not a denigration of the study or the researcher(s') ability and the focus should be on the study itself, not on the individual(s) who carried out the research and published the findings. Any implications arising from the identification of strengths and limitations should be discussed with ref-erence to research literature. The first step of critical appraisal is to read the research analytically.

What is reading analytically?

Reading analytically is an active process concerned with learning to think, and hence read; that means using mental processes such as attention, categorisation, selection and judgement (Cottrell, 2005). This type of reading is often seen as moving from the general to the particular by skim-reading first and then re-reading to build up more understanding of what is being reported. It is a very different technique from reading a novel or a textbook where the aim, for the latter, is the acquisition of knowledge and learning. Reading analytically has the purpose of producing an evaluation of the (research) on a topic and is not something that can be done adequately in one reading or in a short time period (Hart, 1998). A researcher should expect to be regularly reading and reviewing the literature throughout any research project. This will not only increase understanding of the topic, but will also help in the development and maintenance of analytical reading skills.

The focus for analytical reading is the identification of arguments, and good ana-lytical reading is associated with an ability to recognise good or well-presented arguments (even if you disagree with them) and poor arguments (even if they support your own perspective). Effectively, to read analytically a sceptical approach has to be taken, that is, one that politely doubts the perspective being reported. This will include recognising that a research report does not give the full picture of the study and should prompt a highlighting of the elements of a study that are concerning or problematic as well as those aspects that have been well done. What the analytical reader, and critical appraiser, wants is evidence that the research is substantive and that methodological decisions are appropriate (Polit and Beck, 2006).

Deciding which of the published research to review was discussed in Chapter 7, but it is still likely to give what may be a daunting number of articles/texts to read and if each were read fully it would take a very long time. However, in order to produce an effective review it is necessary to evaluate each research paper separately. This will include reading the article and making notes. What a reviewer has to do is develop a way of being selective so that it is possible to get the essence or general idea of the arguments and be able to pull out the main points quickly. Maslin-Prothero (2005) suggests that there are three different levels of reading – scanning, in-depth reading and inferring:

- *Scanning/skimming* is used to help decide whether an article is relevant to the specific topic being investigated. This can also serve to identify which sections of a text or article require more careful reading. This can be done as part of searching the literature.
- *In-depth reading/re-reading and inferring* are necessary to achieve understanding and consideration of possible application of the literature to the 'real world', that is, clinical practice. Again, there is a need to be selective. The concentration should be on the sections that take an argument forward or summarise.

Being selective about what is read, that is, not reading a whole article or chapter in a book, is not taking a short-cut. As a researcher and reviewer you still need to gain enough understanding about your topic and related research to be able to criticise and summarise intelligently. This means being able to give a broad picture as well as focusing on those parts of the research literature that are of particular significance.

The reasoning or arguments presented in any research report, including the adoption of research design, interpretation of data and recommendations, should lead towards the end-point or conclusion, that is, the reasons support the conclusions. There is a need, however, to consider what the argument is predicated on, or what the underlying point of view is, and how this may impact on the conclusions reached. It is possible for the basis of an argument to be true or false and a reader needs be able to determine whether the arguments or reasonings actually support the conclusions. Flaws in reasoning can arise in a number of ways; for example, misinterpretation of results by using an inappropriate statistical test or assuming that one thing must be the cause of another when not all of the relevant variables have been considered (inappropriate linking of cause and effect). Researchers may not always recognise their own flaws or that their arguments are predicated on erroneous or out-of-date assumptions; for example, the research was predicated on the assumption that all registered midwives are also registered nurses.

The aim of analytical reading is to 'unpack' a research project in order to be able to understand how the conclusions were reached and whether these are logical (Hart, 1998).

Synthesis

Being able to recognise arguments is central to any **critical analysis**. Integral to this is the unpacking of the constituent parts of what the author(s) has presented in order to be able to infer or determine the relationship between them. **Synthesis** is rearranging the elements derived from your analytical reading to the actual identification of the relationships between the different elements. A research report attempts to convince others of the **reliability**, **validity**, **trustworthiness** or **rigour** (depending on the methodology used) of the study, and critical analysis draws on the reader's knowledge and experiences to integrate these with other types of evidence to determine whether the arguments are convincing. Synthesis means being able to assess the arguments set out in the text, give reasons for beliefs and actions, analyse and evaluate one's own and other people's reasoning and devise and construct better reasoning.

This process of synthesis can be achieved by using the following technique as you read in depth after scanning:

1 Circle ⬭ any inference indicators (keywords to look for are: thus, therefore, so, hence, should).
2 Look for and underline any conclusions that follow on from these inference indicators.
3 Place in brackets [ ] any stated reasons for these (keywords to look for are: because, for, since).
4 Attempt to summarize the author's arguments at this stage. If there is no clear argument, ask what point(s) the author(s) is trying to make and why.
5 Look at the conclusions again – remember there may be interim as well as final conclusions. Typical indications of a conclusion are the use of the following words: therefore, thus, hence, consequently, and so on. Take care not to confuse a summary or formulation provided by the author of their argument so far with a conclusion.
6 Taking the main conclusion, ask what reasons are presented in the text for believing this conclusion or why you are being asked to accept this conclusion. Typical indications of reasons are words and phrases such as: because, since, it follows, and so on.
7 The reasons provided for the argument can be ranked into a structure. Go through each reason (R) and ask whether it is essential or secondary backing for the argument. From this you will be left with the core reasons for the argument. You should then be able to construct an argument diagram with the following structures:

R1 + R2 = (therefore) conclusion [for joint reasons]
R1 or R2 = (therefore) conclusion [for independent reasons]

Variations on these structures are common. For example, a main conclusion may be supported by an interim conclusion and several basic reasons. This would give an equation something like this:

R1 + R2 = (therefore) interim conclusion
R1 or R2 = (therefore) main conclusion.

(adapted from Hart, 1998)

This stage is analysis rather than evaluation but should, with practice, enable you, as a reviewer, to extract the details of any argument. At this stage you do not need to consider whether the reasons are sound.

Reading retrieved articles

Alongside identification of the arguments being presented, there is also a need to ask questions about the research and its context. These questions should be systematically asked of each article being reviewed as you read.

Exactly how and what questions should be asked is down to personal choice. However, before starting to read and ask questions about the paper, any reviewer needs to consider whether they have sufficient grasp of the research process to be able to evaluate this study. Unfamiliarity with specific research methods is acceptable, but a basic understanding is necessary in order to be able to identify the good and bad points used in a particular study. It is also important to have an understanding of the terms used in the report. Background reading prior to starting a literature review on a topic will help to develop a broader understanding and enhance your ability to evaluate a paper. When reading a research report it is essential to ensure familiarity with the terms being used, otherwise there is a real risk of gaining only a superficial understanding of the study, which gives an inadequate basis for evaluation.

There are numerous guides available to help reviewers to **critique** research studies and these generally provide a set of critiquing questions that can be used to help evaluate published reports. These guides, understandably, differentiate the types of questions that are appropriate for the different types of research and review articles. There are, however, some questions that are generalisable to all research reports and some that are more important than others. Generally, questions relating to method and statistical analysis are very important in assessing the integrity of the research compared with questions about the literature review. The guide questions focus on the different elements of the research process and usually follow the structure of research reports:

- Title
- Abstract
- Literature review
- Method
- Results
- Discussion and interpretation
- Recommendations

These questions will often be worded in a way that prompts a simple 'yes' or 'no' answer. The expectation is that a 'yes' response demonstrates a strength and a 'no' is indicative of a limitation. Ideally, the answer in all cases will be 'yes', and a study that has a large number of 'yeses' is likely to be stronger than or superior to one that has only a few 'yeses' (Polit and Beck, 2006).

However, it is very important to acknowledge that the questions are posed to stimulate the reviewer to consider the implications of what the researcher has done. Any critique will need to identify more than the strengths or limitations of the study. Each relevant issue will have to be discussed; for example, if you answered 'no' to the question about whether participants were fully informed about the nature of the research, you should consider (and then discuss in the actual review) what impact this may have had on recruitment and results obtained. Although guidelines are useful, especially for novice reviewers, it is important to remember that they tend to be generic for the type of research and will not necessarily include all questions appropriate for a specific research design. This means that reviewers have to use their own judgement about whether the guidelines are sufficient for the type of study being critically appraised.

Quantitative research critique questions

Table 8.1 presents guidelines for use when appraising **quantitative research** reports. The questions suggested are basic and broadly applicable to quantitative research and so not all of them will be relevant to each study being reviewed. Some of the questions will not permit wholly objective responses; for example, there may be disagreement about the best research design for a study or which statistical test is most appropriate. This requires a reviewer to express an opinion and this should be based on sound principles gained from an understanding of research and reading about research. An effective appraisal involves asking questions about all aspects of a published report.

Global issues

Writing style

Research reports should be well written, that is, well organised, grammatically correct, concise and the use of jargon avoided where possible. Remember, though, that authors

Table 8.1 General guidelines for critiquing a quantitative research study

Element of the report	Questions
Global issues Writing style	• Was the report well written – grammatically correct, jargon use avoided and well organised? • Was the report written in a way that enables you or a practising nurse to understand the study and its findings? • Was there sufficient detail to enable critical appraisal?
Author(s)	• Do the researcher(s') qualifications/position indicate a degree of knowledge/experience in this particular field?
Title	• Was the title clear, accurate, unambiguous and did it indicate the research question?
Abstract	• Does the abstract give a clear overview of the study and summarise the main features of the findings and recommendations?
Introduction Purpose/research problem	• Was the purpose of the study/research problem clearly stated? • Was a quantitative approach an appropriate way of answering the problem?
Logical consistency	• Does the research report follow the steps of the research process in a logical manner?
Literature review	• Does the review give a balanced critical appraisal of the literature? • Was the literature up to date, original and mainly from primary sources and of an empirical nature? • Does the literature review identify a firm foundation for the new study?
Theoretical framework	• Has a conceptual or theoretical framework been identified? If not, is the absence justified? • Was the framework adequately described and appropriate?
Research question or hypothesis	• Was the research question or hypothesis clearly stated? If not, is the absence justified? • Does the question reflect the information presented in the literature review and conceptual framework?
Objectives	• Are the objectives clearly stated?
Method Research design	• Was the design clearly identified and sufficiently rigorous, given the study purpose? • Were appropriate comparisons made to enhance the interpretability of the findings?

(Continued)

Table 8.1   *(Continued)*

Element of the report	Questions
	• Were any threats to the internal and external validity minimised by the choice of design? • Does the design offer the most accurate, unbiased, interpretable and replicable evidence possible?
Population and sample	• Was the target population clearly identified? • Were there major differences between the target and accessible population? • How was the sample selected, and was it representative? • Were the inclusion/exclusion criteria clearly identified? Does the sample reflect these? • Was a sampling frame employed? • Are there any concerns about the integrity of the sampling frame? • How was the sample size determined, and was it appropriate for the study? • What sample size was achieved? Did it achieve the numbers recommended by a power calculation? • How was the sample selected? • Was the method of sampling appropriate to the design? • Were there any biases in the method of selection and were these acknowledged? • Were there any limits of generalisation of the findings from the sample to the population?
Ethical considerations	• Were the participants fully informed about the nature of the research? • Was the autonomy/confidentiality of the participants guaranteed? • Were the participants protected from harm? • Was ethical approval given for the study?
Data collection and measurement	• Were the data collection strategies described? • Were the methods of data collection appropriate? • Did the researcher ask appropriate questions or make relevant conservations for the topic? • Were sufficient data gathered? • Were data collection and recording procedures adequately described? • Did the researcher describe and discuss how rigour was assured? • Were data collected in a way that minimised bias by appropriately trained staff?

(Continued)

Table 8.1 *(Continued)*

Element of the report	Questions
Data analysis/results	• Did the researcher follow the steps of the data analysis method described? • Did the analysis yield an appropriate outcome, e.g. thematic pattern, theory and taxonomy? • Were the strategies of data analysis described and compatible with the research tradition? • Were the findings presented appropriately? • Do the themes appear to reflect the data meaning? • Did the analysis provide insight into the phenomenon being investigated?
Discussion	• Were all major findings interpreted and discussed? • Were the findings linked back to the literature review and the study's conceptual framework? • Was the original purpose of the study adequately addressed? • Were the interpretations made within the limitations of the study?
Recommendations and implications	• Was a recommendation for further research made? • Were any implications for clinical practice discussed?
References	• Were all the books, journals and other media alluded to in the study accurately referenced?

will often be restricted by word limits in any published report and expected to conform to the style of the journal publishing the report. This should not, however, result in a lack of information that makes comprehension of the report difficult. A report's style should encourage the reader to read the whole report (Polit and Beck, 2006).

Author(s)

You should judge each research report on its own merits and not assume validity and reliability on the basis of the author(s') qualifications and experiences. However, the author(s') qualifications and job title(s) can give an indication of the researcher(s') knowledge and expertise in the topic being investigated.

Title

The title should unambiguously suggest the research problem/purpose of the study and its population. Titles that are too long or too short can be confusing or misleading (Parahoo, 2006).

Abstract

The abstract should provide a concise overview of the research and a summary of the main findings, conclusions and recommendations. Ideally, the abstract will also include brief details of the study, method, sample size and selection, though this may not always be possible because of imposed word limits.

The aim of any abstract is to provide the reader with sufficient information to be able to determine if the study is pertinent to their topic of enquiry and whether or not to continue reading (Parahoo, 2006). Abstracts are very important because they are usually the main section of a report that is read to determine whether the research is in fact relevant for a specific review.

Introduction

Purpose/research problem

The research problem, or purpose of the study, is frequently presented as part of the introduction of a research report. It should give a broad indication of what has been studied/investigated (Polit and Beck, 2006). Remember that broad problems often have many aspects that will need to become more focused before they can be researched.

Logical consistency

The reporting of a research study should follow the steps in the research process itself, and if this is done then a logical progression will be presented. This means that a reader will see clear links between the purpose of the study that follow through all other sections of the report.

It is essential when reporting results to ensure that anyone reading the report understands the terms and concepts used for the research. To ensure this understanding, any concepts or terms referred to should be clearly defined (Parahoo, 2006).

Literature review

The aim of the literature review in a research report is to identify any gaps in the literature relating to the problem and to suggest how the study attempts to fill or partially fill those gaps. It should also assist in further defining the research question and can be very useful in explaining how a broad problem has evolved into the study that is being reported (Parahoo, 2006). The literature review should demonstrate an appropriate depth and breadth of reading around the topic being studied and assist in confirming the appropriateness of the study methodology.

Any studies included should be up to date, that is, certainly not more that ten years old and preferably not more than five years old. Exceptions can be acceptable for topics where there is a paucity of research, or where there is a seminal or very significant study that remains relevant to current practice. Reference to some historical as well as contemporary literature is expected, as this will give a context to the topic. The majority of the literature in the review should usually be empirical data from the original source rather than from a secondary source or anecdotal evidence.

A good review will identify the keywords and details of databases used to conduct the search, with the themes that emerged from the literature then being presented and discussed (Carnwell and Dalg, 2001). The data from previous research should be presented to demonstrate that it has been reviewed critically. The strengths and limitations of the studies should be highlighted, and the findings of the different studies also compared and contrasted (Hart, 1998).

Theoretical framework

Theoretical frameworks are a concept that both novice and experienced researchers find confusing. In many quantitative research studies the research problem is not linked to a specific theory or concept (Polit and Beck, 2006). This means that a reviewer has to first determine whether the study actually has a theoretical or conceptual framework. If there is no framework, consideration of the level of contribution to knowledge by the study has to be made. Nursing can be criticised for its lack of theoretical foundations. However, it has to be acknowledged that much of the research is so pragmatic that the adoption of a theory will not enhance its usefulness (Polit and Beck, 2006). If a theoretical framework is presented, then it should be clearly identified and explained to the reader.

Research question or hypothesis and objectives

The research question and/or the research hypothesis should link with the initially stated purpose of the study or research problem. The report should clearly present a statement of purpose, research question and/or hypothesis. They should be congruent with the information presented in the literature review. The objectives should explain in some detail what the study expected to achieve (Parahoo, 2006).

The use of research questions, hypotheses and objectives is dependent on the type of research being reported. Some descriptive studies may not identify any of these items but simply refer to the purpose of the study or the research problem; others will include either aims and objectives or research questions and studies of relationships that exist between two or more variables, and will use either a research question or hypothesis. A hypothesis and a null hypothesis, identifying the variables to be manipulated, should be clearly stated in reports of experimental and quasi-experimental studies.

Method

Research design

The most important consideration for evaluating a research design is whether the design enables the research question to be answered (Polit and Beck, 2006). Essentially, this means asking whether the design selected matches the aims of the research. You would not expect an experimental design to be used when the purpose of the study is to explore or describe a phenomenon. Similarly, when a study is aimed at identifying the extent or range of a problem, a non-structured or flexible design would raise the possibility of bias and lack of rigour. The main questions to ask relate to whether the design offers the most accurate, unbiased, interpretable and replicable evidence possible (see Chapter 11).

Population and sample

A decisive factor in determining the adequacy of a quantitative research study is the degree to which a sample represents the population it was drawn from (Polit and Beck, 2006). Critiquing questions are aimed at identifying how generalisable the findings are likely to be. This means that a reviewer needs to be able to clearly identify the target population and how the sample was selected. The size of the sample is also important, as small samples give rise to the possibility of over-representation of small subgroups within the target population. For example, if, in a sample of registered nurses, 40 per cent of the respondents were males, then males would appear to be over-represented in the sample, thereby creating a sampling error. In addition, the report should clearly identify what criteria were used to include or exclude participants, how the sample was selected and how many were invited to participate (see Chapter 19).

Ethical considerations

Any research involving human beings should be conducted ethically, and in health-care where research participants may be particularly vulnerable there is even more of an imperative for ethical conduct in research (Sim and Wright, 2000). The onus when critiquing a research report is to confirm that ethical principles have been applied. Essentially, the reviewer needs to ask whether participants were told what the research entailed, how their anonymity and confidentiality were protected and what arrangements were in place to avoid preventable harms.

Health and social care research has to be approved by an ethics committee and the institution where the research is conducted before research can be undertaken. Any research report requiring ethical approval should state that this was given, and ideally which committee gave the approval (see Chapters 4 and 5).

Data collection and measurement

There are a number of strategies that can be adopted when collecting data in a quantitative study. In order to be able to assess whether data collection was appropriate, sufficient detail has to be included in a report to enable judgements. Alongside there should be an indication of how any data collection instrument was designed. Researchers usually have the choice of using an existing instrument or developing one specific to their study. It should be clearly stated whether a study-specific or an 'off-the-shelf' data collection instrument has been used. In either case, it is essential that the data collected actually will elicit accurate information, help achieve the goals of the research and that this demonstrated in the report. It should, however, be remembered that existing instruments are often in the form of standardised tests or scales that have been developed for a purpose other than that of the study being reported. This requires the researcher to provide appropriate evidence in relation to the validity and reliability of the instrument (Polit and Beck, 2006) and its appropriateness for the current study. Validity is described as the ability of the instrument to measure what it is supposed to measure, and reliability refers to the level of consistency of values measured under specified conditions (Sim and Wright, 2000). It is important to recognise that if an instrument has been modified or used with a different population, then previous validity and reliability will not be applicable, and details of how the reliability and validity of the adapted instrument was established should be explained (Polit and Beck, 2006). This may mean that details of a pilot study are included to clarify validity and reliability of the chosen instrument. Any adjustment made following a pilot study should be explained and justified.

The report should also include an outline, in clear logical steps, of the process by which and by whom the data was collected and details of any intervention used.

Data analysis and results

Reviewing the data analysis section of quantitative research studies is often seen as a daunting process because it is associated with an apparently complex language and the notion of statistical tests. A report should state clearly what statistical tests were undertaken, why these tests were used and the results. A useful guide is to remember that descriptive studies only use descriptive statistics and correlational studies, quasi-experimental and experimental studies use inferential statistics (Clegg, 1990). Statistical significance helps to identify whether a result could be due to chance rather than to real differences in the population. The convention in quantitative studies is to identify the lowest level of significance as $P<0.05$ (see Chapter 22). The percentage of the sample of study participants is important to any consideration of the generalisability of the results, and participation of at least 50 per cent of the sample is required to avoid a response bias (Polit and Beck, 2006).

The results should be presented in a way that makes it easy for readers to interpret them for themselves. The use of tables, charts and graphs is an acceptable way of summarising results. These should be accurate, clear and link into the text appropriately.

Discussion

The discussion of the findings should have a logical link with the presentation of the results and should relate to the literature review and, where appropriate, the conceptual framework in order to put the study in context. If the hypothesis appeared to have been supported by the findings, this should be developed in the discussion. All major interpretations or inferences drawn should be clearly identified and discussed. The significance of any findings, particularly generalisability, should be stated and considered within the overall strengths and limitations of the study (Polit and Beck, 2006).

Recommendations and Implications

Finally, the report should indicate opportunities for relevant and meaningful further research on the topic. It is expected that the discussion section will have explored some of the clinical significance and relevance of the study. However, implications of findings and recommendations for practice should be made with caution and will obviously depend on the nature and purpose of the study.

References

The research study should conclude with an accurate list of all the books, journal articles, reports and other media that were referred to in the report (Polit and Beck, 2006).

Qualitative research critique questions

As with a quantitative study, critical analysis of a qualitative study involves an in-depth review of how each step of the research was undertaken. **Qualitative research** is essentially an assortment of various approaches that have commonalities as well as differences (Parahoo, 2006). However, although the different philosophical stances of the various qualitative research methods generate discrete ways of reasoning and distinct terminology, there are many similarities within these methods. This, alongside the subjective nature of qualitative research, gives rise to an assumption that it is more difficult to critique. Table 8.2 presents guidelines for use when appraising qualitative research reports.

Global issues

The questions to ask about writing style, author, title and abstract of a qualitative research study are the same as those asked about quantitative studies as described in the previous section.

Introduction

Statement of the problem

Many qualitative research studies are characterised by the abstract nature of the topics examined and hence the particular experience may be interpreted differently by another individual, or by the same individual under different circumstances, for example, when in pain. These abstract encounters or experiences are known as 'phenomena' (Polit and Beck, 2006), and the phenomenon being investigated needs to be clearly explained in a research report.

There should be an explanation of why the study needs to be undertaken and what information could be expected to arise from conducting it. This should also include a statement of how it will contribute to the general body of understanding of the phenomenon.

The use of a qualitative approach and the qualitative methodology to be used also need to be justified.

Literature review

The role of a literature review is to give an objective account of what has been written on a given topic. Qualitative methodologies vary with regard to the conduct of

Table 8.2 General guidelines for critiquing a qualitative research study

Element of the report	Questions
Global issues Writing style	• Was the report well written – grammatically correct, jargon use avoided and well organised? • Was the report written in a way that enables you or a practising nurse to understand the study and its findings? • Was there sufficient detail to enable critical appraisal?
Author	• Do the researcher(s') qualifications/position indicate a degree of knowledge/experience in this particular field?
Title	• Was the title clear, accurate, unambiguous and did it indicate the research question?
Abstract	• Does the abstract give a clear overview of the study and summarise the main features of the findings and recommendations?
Introduction Statement of the problem	• Was the phenomenon to be studied clearly identified? • Was the phenomenon of interest? • Was a qualitative approach an appropriate way of answering the problem?
Literature review	• Has a literature review been undertaken? • Does the review give a balanced critical appraisal of the existing body of knowledge relating to the phenomenon? • Does the literature review identify a firm foundation for the new study?
Theoretical framework	• Has a conceptual or theoretical framework been identified? • Was the framework adequately described and appropriate?
Methodological and philosophical underpinnings	• Has the philosophical approach been identified? • Has the philosophical basis and underlying tradition been explained?

(Continued)

Table 8.2 *(Continued)*

Element of the report	Questions
Research question	• Was there an explicitly stated question? If not, has its absence been justified? • Was the question consistent with the study's philosophical basis, underlying tradition and conceptual or theoretical framework?
Method Research design and research tradition	• Does the research tradition (if there is one) harmonise with the method of data collection and analysis? • Was the time in the field adequate? • Was there an appropriate level of contact with participants? • Was there evidence of reflexivity in the design?
Sample	• Were the sampling method and sample size identified? • Was saturation of data achieved? • Was the sampling method appropriate? • Were the population and setting adequately described and appropriate for informing the research?
Ethical considerations	• Were the participants fully informed about the nature of the research? • Was the autonomy/confidentiality of the participants guaranteed? • Were the participants protected from harm? • Was ethical approval given for the study?
Data collection	• Were the methods of data gathering adequately described and appropriate? • Were the question asked, and observations made and recorded in an appropriate way? • Were the data gathered of sufficient depth and richness? • Were data collected in a way that minimised bias by appropriately trained staff?
Data analysis/results	• Was there a description of the methods used to enhance trustworthiness of data? • Were the data management and analysis methods adequately described? • Was the strategy used for analysis consistent with the research tradition and appropriate for the type of data collected? • Was the original purpose of the research adequately addressed?

(Continued)

Table 8.2   *(Continued)*

Element of the report	Questions
	• Were the themes or patterns logically connected to form an integrated picture of the phenomenon?
Conclusions/implications and recommendations	• Were the importance and implications of the findings identified? • Are recommendations made to suggest how the research findings can be developed?
References	• Were all the books, journals and other media alluded to in the study accurately referenced?

a literature review before the data collection period. Equally, there is debate about whether the conceptual framework should come before data collection and data analysis.

When critiquing qualitative studies, the reviewer has to decide whether the researcher has justified the chosen approach. For example, a major premise of grounded theory is that data are collected in isolation from any predetermined theory or conceptual framework. Therefore the literature review is undertaken once the data have been collected. The basis for this type of approach is to explore concepts embedded in the data, thereby allowing theory to be generated from the data rather than vice versa (Sim and Wright, 2000). A similar approach is often employed in phenomenological investigations where the literature review may not be carried out until the data analysis is complete. The aim is to ensure that the findings actually reflect participants' experiences and are truly grounded in the data (Burns and Grove, 2001).

When critiquing qualitative research studies, the literature review should be appraised in the context of the particular methodology used because the existing literature provides both the basis for research and the context for interpretation (Meadows, 2003). So that where it was appropriate for the literature review to be done only after data collection, the report should identify how the process was achieved and the way the literature was used to determine similarities with, or differences from, the research findings. A literature review carried out before data collection and analysis should follow the usual remit of giving a comprehensive and balanced account of previous work. This will include identification, where appropriate, of relevant themes, conceptual models and theoretical frameworks that give a sound background to the research.

Theoretical framework

Many qualitative studies are described as inductive or theory-generating research, meaning that the purpose is to develop theory rather that to test a theory, and is linked with grounded theory, ethnography and phenomenology. The adoption of such a stance should be justified, for example where little is known about the phenomenon under study or where existing theories do not seem to provide the answer (Polit and Beck, 2006). Other qualitative studies may use known theories to 'frame' their studies in order to establish boundaries or parameters and to guide the different stages of the study (Parahoo, 2006) (see Chapter 14).

Methodological and philosophical underpinnings

It is important to recognise that the major qualitative approaches differ in their disciplinary or philosophical origins that incorporate a set of beliefs about knowledge and how this knowledge is developed. Thus the focus and manner in which sampling, data collection and analysis are undertaken will vary in relation to the approached used. For a reviewer to be able to establish coherence and congruence, the chosen approach should be outlined and justified.

Research question

In qualitative research, the research question reflects the identified phenomenon of interest that is directing the progress of the research. It is important to recognise that a qualitative research study does have some limits; for example, if post-operative pain is being investigated, then it is essential to identify how and which aspect the research is focusing on, and details of how the particular focus was determined should be given.

Depending on the type of qualitative approach adopted, for example grounded theory, the research question may be modified as new data bring new direction to the phenomenon of interest. Any modifications should be explained and justified in the report.

Method

Research design and research traditions

Actually evaluating qualitative research design can be difficult (Polit and Beck, 2006). Some of this is because decisions about design will not always be documented. There should, however, be an indication of whether a study has been conducted within a particular research tradition, possibly allowing a reviewer to reach some conclusions about the study design. For example, in a grounded theory study, was the data analysed as the study progressed to permit constant comparisons? The report should also give details of reflexivity.

Reviewers also need to be able to identify whether the researcher(s) spent an adequate time in the field or with study participants to gain a true picture of the phenomenon under investigation.

Sample

Participants are usually recruited to a study because of their exposure to, or their experience of, the phenomenon in question. The aim is to ensure richness in the data collected and is referred to as **purposive** or **purposeful sampling** (Sim and Wright, 2000). **Theoretical sampling** is frequently used in grounded theory. This type of sampling involves determining the sample as a result of themes that emerge from the data analysis, and the researcher then explores these themes in more depth and/or develops a theory from these data (see Chapter 19).

Qualitative research is often criticised because the findings are not generalisable as a consequence of the use of small samples. Instead, data collected from participants builds on the information from earlier participants and the accumulated data can then offer a significant depth of information about the phenomenon. Data are usually collected until no new material is emerging, that is, data saturation has been reached, and at this stage data gathering is usually stopped (Parahoo, 2006).

Ethical considerations

The onus when critiquing a research report is to identify that ethical principles have been applied. Essentially, the reviewer needs to ask whether participants were told what the research entailed, how their autonomy and confidentiality were protected and what arrangements were in place to avoid preventable harms. Health and social care research has to gain an ethical committee and institutional approval before the research can be undertaken. Any research report requiring ethical approval should state that this was given, and ideally which committee gave the approval.

In qualitative research the commonly used data collection tools include interviews and participant observation, and as a result anonymity is not possible. There is, therefore, even more of an imperative to assure participants that their identities will not be revealed in any research report (Parahoo, 2006). The role of the interviewer is to encourage participants to 'open up' and discuss their experiences of the phenomenon. Because of this there will always be the possibility of unintended disclosure of personal information by participants, or uncomfortable experiences relating to the topic being studied may be reawakened. As a result, consent needs to be a process of continuous negotiation with participants to ascertain their agreement to continued participation (Polit and Beck, 2006). It should also be recognised that in qualitative research, ethical issues often arise at different stages and may be discussed in a report when they arise, rather than under a specific heading.

Data collection and measurement

There are a number of strategies that can be adopted when collecting qualitative data, including interviews (semi-structured and unstructured), participant observation, written texts such as **diaries** or emails, and historical or contemporary documents. The rationale for the chosen method of data collection should be described in sufficient detail to give a reviewer an overview of the process. It should be evident from the discussion that the researcher has adhered to the processes inherent in the particular approach being used. If a semi-structured interview format is selected, there should be an explanation of how the themes or questions were derived. For unstructured interviews, the initial question should be clearly linked to the purpose of the study. The rationale for the decisions about the type of interview, such as face-to-face or focus group, should be clearly presented and justified (see Chapter 21).

Data analysis/results

The process of data analysis is fundamental to determining the credibility of qualitative research findings. Essentially, it involves the transforming of raw data into a final description, narrative or identification of themes and categories. The means by which this is done is variable, with some researchers using generic data analysis tools whereas others use less structured and more creative approaches. What is important is that the process is described in sufficient detail to enable the reader to judge whether the final outcome is rooted in the data generated (Holloway and Wheeler, 2002). The description should enable a reviewer to confirm the processes of concurrent data collection and analysis, organisation and retrieval of data, as well as the steps in coding and thematic analysis. Any verification strategies used should be presented, for example member checking, that is, verifying with participants (see Chapter 23).

Rigour or trustworthiness is the means of demonstrating the plausibility, credibility and integrity of the qualitative research process. A study's rigour may be established if the reviewer is able to audit the actions and developments of the researcher (Polit and Beck, 2006). Burns and Grove (2001) suggest that the critique of qualitative research requires an appraisal of the rigour in documentation, procedural rigour and ethical rigour. Rigour in documentation ensures that there is a correlation between the research process steps and the study being reviewed. Procedural rigour refers to appropriate and precise data collection techniques and incorporates a reflective/critical component in order to reduce bias and misinterpretations. Ethical rigour refers to the confirmation that the study has applied ethical principles throughout.

The issue of transferability of a study should also be considered part of the appraisal process. This is determining whether the findings can be deemed relevant outside of the context of the study situation. Transferability is enhanced when the results are meaningful to individuals not involved in the research study.

Findings/results from qualitative studies can be represented as a narrative (story), themes, description of the phenomenon under study or an interpretive account of the understanding or meaning of an experience. However, the outcomes that are presented should be discussed in the context of what is already known. Care should be taken to ensure that exaggerated claims about the significance of the study and implications for practice are not made inappropriately.

Conclusions, implications and recommendations

The report should have a clear conclusion that places findings in a context that indicates how this new information is of interest, and its implications for nursing. These should assist in being able to contrast a reader's own interpretation of the findings with those of the researcher (Polit and Beck, 2006).

There should also be reference to any limitations of the study that will help put the research into context and enable judgements to be made about the need for, and viability of conducting, further research into the same phenomenon. Recommendations should include detail of how they may be developed in practice.

References

An accurate list of all the books, journal articles, reports and other media referred to in the study should be included in a reference list at the end of the study (Polit and Beck, 2006). This list can also be a good source of further reading and is very useful when undertaking a literature search on a related topic.

Systematic review critique questions

Although a systematic review is an objective critique of the literature available on a topic it cannot be taken for granted that a review is the most reliable source of information. Systematic reviews are only as good as the data available to them, and if the body of original research is of poor quality or very limited, then a systematic review will struggle to produce reliable results (Lindsay, 2007). It should also be noted that systematic reviews can be restrictive about the types of research that are included. Notably, Cochrane reviews tend to exclude qualitative studies, although there is an increasing demand for the inclusion of studies that investigate socially complex interventions, such as nursing care, that will often yield qualitative data or a mixture of quantitative and qualitative data. There is, therefore, just as much of a need to critically appraise a systematic review as any other research report.

Essentially, the appraisal of a systematic review is the same as for any other type of research; that is, you need to ask a series of questions. The following checklist is offered as a framework for appraising a systematic review.

1   *Did the systematic review address a clearly focused clinical question?*
    The question should be clearly defined since the reviewer(s) will have had to make dichotomous (yes/no) decisions about whether to include a potentially relevant paper, or reject it as irrelevant (Greenhalgh, 1997). However, it may not be stated as a question, for example: 'The aim of this review was to systematically review studies focusing on communication of end-of-life and prognosis with adults, and/or their caregivers in advanced stages of a progressive, life-limiting illness' (Parker et al., 2007).

2   *Were the terms or concepts used in the review defined?*
    This helps to confirm that you understand the terms used in the review and the interpretations placed on them by the reviewers. For example, Parker et al. (2007) define prognosis as including life expectancy, how illness may progress, potential future symptoms and functional ability. A systematic review report should also include details of the terms and combinations of terms used (Parahoo, 2006). This allows others the opportunity to replicate the search and a reader to identify whether there were gaps that might reduce the quality of the review.

3   *Were all the relevant databases identified and searched?*
    In a systematic review, the reviewer(s) are expected to be as comprehensive as possible in searching for studies (see Chapter 18, Box 18.2 for a checklist of data sources for a systematic review). The need to explore the 'grey' literature may be more pertinent for topics outside of mainstream healthcare, such as complementary or alternative therapies (Greenhalgh, 1997).

4   *Were inclusion and exclusion criteria stated?*
    This gives an indication as to whether the review considered all types of research study or concentrated on particular designs, such as randomised controlled trials (RCTs) and other types of clinical trial or experimental research.

5   *Was the quality of the included studies assessed?*
    Part of the function of a systematic review is to objectively assess the quality of each study. There should be a clear description of a scoring system or strategy against which each study was assessed. There is no set standard for assessing the 'true' quality of a research study and it is not uncommon for reviewers to devise their own scoring system. Such a system will be based on a mixture of generic (common to all research studies) and specific (to the field/area) aspects of quality. Greenhalgh (1997) suggests that each study should be assessed in terms of:

- Methodological quality: the extent to which the design and conduct are likely to have prevented systematic errors (bias)
- Precision: a measure of the likelihood of random errors (usually depicted as the width of the confidence interval around the result)
- External validity: the extent to which the results are generalisable or applicable to a particular target population.

6 *How was the evidence combined or summarised?*
Did the approach to the interpretation of the results appear sound and reflect the question of the review as well as the broader context of the question? If a meta-analysis was undertaken, was this a reasonable thing to have done?

7 *What were the conclusions of the review?*
When reviewing the conclusions, consideration should be made of whether they have been reached by means of what Greenhalgh (1997) refers to as a 'sensitivity analysis'. Sensitivity analysis consists of asking a series of 'what ifs'. These include what if: different inclusion and exclusion criteria were used; unpublished studies were included/excluded; study quality was assigned differently; studies using other research designs were included/excluded; and all patients unaccounted for were assumed to have died/been cured? If the responses to these questions make little difference to the results presented, then, according to Greenhalgh (1997), it can be assumed that the conclusions are relatively robust.

8 *Overall, do the findings help or confuse, and is the evidence presented sufficient to change practice?*
Understanding of the outcomes of a review is necessary for an assessment of its relevance for practice, or a research topic. As with any piece of research, a systematic review should include recommendations for further investigation and/or implications for practice.

Chapter summary

- Critical appraisal of the evidence or analytical evaluation of the research relating to your topic is the means by which the reasoning that informs the research and arguments can be unravelled.
- Critical appraisal involves reading analytically and synthesising the information gained from reading.
- Reading analytically requires the reader to attend, categorise, select and judge.
- Analytical reading is associated with an ability to recognise well-presented and poor arguments regardless of one's own perspective on the topic.
- Synthesis is rearranging the elements derived from analytical reading to the actual identification of the relationships between the different elements.
- Each study should be appraised in accordance with the type of research design used.

References

Burns, N. and Grove, S. (2001) *The Practice of Nursing Research: Conduct, Critique and Utilization*, 4th edition. Philadelphia, PA: Saunders.

Carnwell, R. and Dalg, W. (2001) 'Strategies for the construction of a critical review of the literature', *Nurse Education in Practice*, 1: 57–63.

Clegg, F. (1990) *Simple Statistics: A Course Book for the Social Sciences*. Cambridge: Cambridge University Press.

Cottrell, S. (2005) *Critical Thinking Skills*. Basingstoke: Palgrave Macmillan.

Greenhalgh, T. (1997) 'How to read a paper: papers that summarise other papers (systematic reviews and meta-analysis)', *British Medical Journal*, 315: 672–5.

Hart, C. (1998) *Doing a Literature Review*. London: Sage.

Holloway, I. and Wheeler, S. (2002) *Qualitative Research in Nursing*. Oxford: Blackwell.

Lindsay, B. (2007) *Understanding Research and Evidence-based Practice*. Tavistock: Reflect Press.

Maslin-Prothero, S. (2005) *Study Skills for Nurses and Midwives*. London: Baillière Tindall.

Meadows, K. (2003) 'So you want to do research: an overview of the research process', *British Journal of Community Nursing*, 8 (8): 369–75.

Parahoo, K. (2006) *Nursing Research: Principles, Process and Issues*. Basingstoke: Palgrave Macmillan.

Parker, S., Clayton, J., Hancock, K., Walder, S., Butow, P., Carrick, S., Currow, D., Ghersi, D., Glare, P., Hagerty, R. and Tattersall, M. (2007) 'A systematic review of prognostic/end-of-life communication with adults in the advanced stages of life-limiting illness: patient/caregiver preferences for the content, style, and timing of information', *Journal of Pain and Symptom Management*, 34 (7): 81–93.

Polit, D. and Beck, C. (2006) *Essentials of Nursing Research: Methods, Appraisal and Utilization*, 6th edition. Philadelphia, PA: Lippincott Williams & Wilkins.

Sim, J. and Wright, C. (2000) *Research in Health Care: Concepts, Designs and Methods*. Cheltenham: Nelson Thornes.

Suggested further reading

Burns, N. and Grove, S. (2001) *The Practice of Nursing Research: Conduct, Critique and Utilization*, 4th edition. Philadelphia, PA: Saunders.

Cottrell, S. (2005) *Critical Thinking Skills*. Basingstoke: Palgrave Macmillan.

Hart, C. (1998) *Doing a Literature Review*. London: Sage.

Lindsay, B. (2007) *Understanding Research and Evidence-based Practice*. Tavistock: Reflect Press.

Maslin-Prothero, S. (2005) *Study Skills for Nurses and Midwives*. London: Baillière Tindall.

Parahoo, K. (2006) *Nursing Research: Principles, Process and Issues*. Basingstoke: Palgrave Macmillan.

Websites

National Library for Helath: www.library.nhs.uk

Critical Appraisal Skills Programme (CASP): www.phru.nhs.uk/casp

9

LITERATURE REVIEWING

The starting point for any research is the identification of a gap in knowledge that a study is aiming to fill. In order to be able to do this, researchers have to review and evaluate the research that has already been done on the topic. Nurses and other health-care professionals also often ask questions about the effectiveness of different ways of delivering care, interventions and new products/procedures. The imperative driving these questions is the need to ensure that practice is evidence-based, and hence there is a need to examine research already conducted to be able to determine what is best practice. This reviewing of the existing body of evidence is an important part of the research process and can be undertaken for a variety of different purposes. The main purposes for research literature reviews are: to support a research proposal; to introduce a research report; as part of a dissertation or thesis; and as a freestanding review.

Chapters 7 and 8 described how to search for relevant literature and critically appraise the evidence presented by the literature. This chapter describes the different stages involved in preparing a research literature review that could be used for writing a proposal or a research report. The more complex processes of conducting and writing of systematic literature reviews is discussed in Chapter 18.

Learning outcomes

This chapter is designed to enable the reader to:

- **Recognise the purpose of a literature review in a research project**
- **Understand how to manage the information gained from reading effectively**
- **Be able to prepare a research literature review**

> **KEY TERMS**
>
> Critical appraisal, Literature review, Narrative review, Systematic review

What is a literature review?

A literature review is part of a research proposal, a section in a completed research study report, and can also be part of a journal article where it is sometimes called the introduction. Hart defines a literature review as:

> The selection of available documents (both published and unpublished) on the topic, which contains information, ideas, data and evidence written from a particular stand-point to fulfil certain aims or express certain views on the nature of the topic and how it is to be investigated, and the effective evaluation of these documents in relation to the research being proposed. (Hart, 2003: 3)

This type of **literature review** is sometimes called a 'narrative literature review' (Crowley, 1996). A literature review is a systematic framework that includes **critical appraisal**, is structured and goes into sufficient detail to make it possible for the reader to be able to replicate the review. A narrative literature review is different from a systematic review, which is essentially a review of a clearly formulated question that uses systematic and explicit methods to identify, select and critically appraise relevant research, and to collect and analyse data from studies that are included in the review.

Table 9.1 gives an indication of some of the differences between **narrative** and **systematic reviews.**

A literature review helps to focus on a research topic and, by so doing, enables the progressive narrowing that turns a topic into a practical and doable research project. Doing a literature review may be seen as a laborious and difficult aspect of the research process, but careful application when undertaking a literature review for a research project can avoid wasting effort on vague searching at a later stage.

What is the purpose of a literature review?

A literature review sets out to provide answers to the following questions:

- What is currently known about the topic?
- What are the main questions and problems that have been addressed to date?

Table 9.1 Distinctions between narrative and systematic reviews

	Narrative review	**Systematic review**
Focus	Often addresses a broad range of issues, and brings these together in an overview.	Usually focuses on a single specific question, without attempting to provide an overview of the topic.
Research question	When present, is usually descriptive in nature.	Usually explanatory.
Search strategy	Often unstated or implicit.	Explicit inclusion and exclusion criteria are used.
Selection of sources	Selective and subject to conscious or unconscious selection bias.	Comprehensive, with a deliberate avoidance of selection bias.
Nature of sources	Mainly published sources, including both theoretical and empirical papers.	Published and unpublished ('grey') sources; usually only empirical papers.
Assessment of sources	Sometimes, and not usually according to specified criteria.	Always, using specific criteria with the focus mainly on methodological issues.
Conclusions	Summative.	Summative or analytical (meta-analysis).

Source: Sim and Wright, 2000: 283

- What aspects of the topic have not been considered? What are the gaps?
- What are the major issues and debates about this topic?
- What research has previously been done?
- What are the origins and definitions for the topic?
- What recommendations for further research have previously been made but not acted upon?
- What methods have other researchers used to investigate this topic? Were some of these methods better suited to investigating this topic than others?

Overall, a literature review will question how the approaches to the above questions have increased our understanding and knowledge of the topic being researched. It should put the research question/problem into context and critically appraise the merits of the research. The results can then be written up to present a logical coherent case for pursuing the study or to provide an informed introduction of a research study report. The task of asking all of the above questions may seem rather daunting, but if approached in a systematic way it will be possible to construct a review that actually provides the answers.

How do you do a literature review for a research project?

Essentially, a literature review consists of first determining the exact topic of the review. This is more or less the same as deciding on a research question, though, as was discussed in Chapter 6, a literature review often helps to inform the development of a research question. Once the topic for the review has been decided upon, then the literature can be searched to find what research has already been undertaken on the topic. A search of the literature, as described in Chapter 7, enables articles relating to the topic to be retrieved. Each of the retrieved articles then needs to be read and critically appraised, as described in Chapter 8. The aim of these processes is to provide an account of the available research literature on the specified topic that will enable an evaluation and identification of the gaps in the existing research. Chapter 8 gives suggestions for the type of question that should be asked for the different types of research. Some researchers prefer to use a generic set of questions for the articles they appraise. This can be more appropriate when there is a diverse range of research methodologies in the literature being reviewed. A set of generic questions that can assist in critical appraisal is given in Table 9.2.

Table 9.2   Generic questions to ask about each section of a research paper

Section	Questions
1 Title	• Does the title provide a clear and unambiguous statement of the topic under investigation? • Is it concise and informative? • Is the type of approach used in the title e.g. a comparative study of; an ethnographic approach to; a double-blind cross-over; a pilot study?
2 Author/researcher	• Does the author have the appropriate background to enable him or her to conduct the study successfully? • Look for qualifications, role/speciality and place of employment associated with good research. • Multiple authors may indicate need for specialist expertise or team led by an experienced researcher who may have attracted funding. • An awareness of the researcher's background should improve understanding of the approach used and any assumptions that have been made but not necessarily stated in the report. For example, researchers with a clinical background are likely to have a different approach from that of researchers from an academic background investigating a ward-based problem.

(Continued)

Table 9.2   *(Continued)*

Section	Questions
3 Abstract	• Does this provide a clear summary of the research, i.e. problem being researched, methodology, significant results and conclusions? • This section is very helpful in identifying relevant articles when searching the literature.
4 Introduction	• Clearly identified problem? If the research problem is not clearly set out it will be difficult to interpret any findings. It is helpful if the actual research question is stated, but it does not always appear. Often the aims and objectives of the study are given and sometimes these do not really explain what question the researchers were trying to answer. • Is the problem researchable or have the researchers been unrealistic in their expectations of the outcomes from the study? For example, 'Does preparation of the ward prior to meals being served improve patient nutrition?' is a very interesting topic which could yield much useful data. However, it is very broad and inevitably there will be many factors other than ward environment that impact on patients' nutritional status. This would not be a realistic research question in a single study. • Rationale for choice of topic described? • Rationale for methodology described? • Depending on the approach, research aims and objectives or the hypothesis/null hypothesis stated, is this consistent with the topic under investigation?
5 Literature review	Not all research papers will have a literature review section/heading. Sometimes the review is included in the introduction or background. Whatever it is called, it should come before any detailed information about how the research was conducted and the results section. Specific questions to ask about the review include: • Does this indicate the author's familiarity with the topic under investigation? • Is it pertinent to the research topic? • Does it cover all the important aspects about the topic or have key references been omitted or ignored? • Does the review inform the theoretical origins as well as previous articles on the topic? • Are the references up to date? • Is it easy to follow or is there a lack of structure, making it difficult to understand the arguments? • Is there a summary of the key points that highlight the gaps the research aimed to fill?
6 Methodology/design/methods	• Methodology = approach taken, e.g. action research: is the approach clearly stated with an identifiable underpinning theory? • Research methods = the tools by which data is collected, e.g. pre- and post-intervention questionnaires, focus group interviews: are these described clearly?

(Continued)

Table 9.2   *(Continued)*

Section	Questions
	• Design = how the whole study hangs together: is it justifiable and is there a logical description of what the researcher planned to do and how it was actually done? • Is sufficient detail given to make it possible to repeat the study? • Are technical terms used, and if so are they defined or is it assumed that the reader will understand them? Some level of expertise has to be assumed, but authors should explain any very specialist terms or when there could be more than one interpretation of a term.
7 Sample selection	• Who or what makes up the study population, and are they appropriate? • Are the participants clearly defined? For example, if elderly people or children participated, are the age ranges explained and justified? • Are the inclusion and exclusion criteria stated and justified? • How was the sample selected, e.g. self-selection, convenience sample, randomly? • Does the author justify the selection? • Is the sample size explained and was the sample size appropriate? A comprehensive understanding of statistics is not required for this but rather an understanding of how sample sizes can be calculated and the sort of numbers of participants you would expect to see in different types of studies. (These issues are discussed in Chapter 19 of this book.) • Qualitative studies can use quite small samples, whereas quantitative studies usually require larger samples and statistical advice may be needed for the results to be statistically significant.
8 Data collection	• Is the way the data were collected described and discussed in enough detail? This should include justification for the choice of how data were collected which is robust enough to stand up to criticism. For example, if reminders were not sent to participants who failed to return questionnaires, were the reasons for this non-action explained? • Are the advantages and disadvantages of the method(s) discussed? • Are details given about the instruments or tools used, e.g. questionnaires, interview schedules and measurement scales? These details do not have to be comprehensive or necessarily include copies of the actual questionnaires. There should be just sufficient detail for the reader to understand the type of data being sought. For example: The questionnaire comprised two parts. To evaluate the patients' constipation status, a constipation visual analogue scale (CVAS) was constructed. This was an 8-point scale, where a score of 0–1 indicates no constipation, 2–4 indicates constipation and 5–7 indicates severe constipation. … For the management of patients' constipation, four further questions were asked to determine the advice provided, satisfaction with treatment, explanation of need for laxatives and patient preferences for laxatives.

(Continued)

Table 9.2   *(Continued)*

Section	Questions
	Patients' use of medication, specifically laxatives, opioids and other constipating medication, was collected from the patient records. (Goodman et al., 2005: 239)
	• This section should also include some reference to the reliability and validity of results for quantitative studies and plausibility and trustworthiness of findings for qualitative studies. • If justification of the research methods was not given in the methodology section, then it should be covered here, with reason(s) for choice of method(s) stated.
9 Ethics	• Is there evidence of approval from the appropriate ethics committee? • Are any ethical issues around the conduct of the research discussed? For example, if the research involved vulnerable groups, how were they protected? • Are the methods of participants' consent and how confidentiality was protected explained?
10 Results/findings	• Were the methods of data analysis appropriate for the research methods? • Is some raw data presented as well as the findings? • Are the results presented in a clear, concise, precise and logical manner? • Are the results sufficiently complete and detailed to answer the questions posed?
11 Discussion	• Are all the results discussed in relation to the original question/hypothesis? • Is it balanced and objective? • Does it draw on previous research findings and/or the literature review to explain, compare and contrast other results obtained? • Are any weaknesses and limitations in the study identified and, if possible, suggestions made as to how they might be overcome in the future?
12 Conclusions	• Do the results and discussion support these? • Are they confined the original purpose of the study?
13 Recommendations	• Are these practical, accurate and appropriate?
14 References	• Are they complete and searchable?
15 Appendices	• Are they arranged in either a numerical or alphabetical order? • Are these clearly marked and appropriate?

It is preferable to make notes about what the research reports say as each paper is read. An example of a pro-forma that could be used for compiling a record of what you gleaned from this reading is given in Figure 9.1. The important thing is to keep a record so that you can refer to what you found in the paper without having to re-read the paper.

What you actually decide to record will vary with each research project, but it is best to get into the habit of making a detailed note of everything read from the outset. The basic details that should be recorded are described in Chapter 7, Literature Searching. As each article is read it is useful to add comments to the basic information so that the evaluation and details of what has been read are all kept together. This is where storage on a reference database can be useful, but a paper-based system can be just as efficient. But whatever system is used, it is essential to keep a back-up copy – otherwise there is a real risk of having to repeat the search or re-read all of the articles.

The next stage is to evaluate the arguments. This is the process that moves on from simply presenting an account, albeit critical, of each article that provides a comprehensive picture of what has been reported from the different research studies. This involves not taking things at face value and offering opinions about what has been written. It also requires comparison between different papers and texts that indicates where there are differences, similarities, contradictions and deficiencies (or gaps in the research). This is an essential skill for a researcher and is best developed by adopting a systematic approach towards analysis of the arguments and then evaluation.

Evaluating the arguments

Evaluation, like all the other stages of critical appraisal, is essentially asking a series of questions. These should include:

1 How do we know that this is true? Is the source reliable? Was this a 'good' research study?
2 Are the findings of the research representative of the whole population rather than just the sample who participated in the research?
3 Does this correspond with what I already know about the topic?
4 Does this contradict other evidence?
5 What is missing? What are we not being told?
6 Are any other explanations possible?
7 Are any comparisons made appropriate?
8 Does the evidence support the author's reasoning?
9 Is there any additional evidence that strengthens or weakens the conclusion?
10 Does the reasoning support the conclusion? If not, can you state the way in which the move from reasons to the conclusion is flawed?

Use your answers from 1–9 to help you make your evaluation.

Author(s)	
Year of publication	
Title of article/book	
Journal name	volume: issue: pages:
Book publisher and edition	
Website address	Date downloaded
Research problem/question	
Type of study	Quantitative ☐ Qualitative ☐ Mixed ☐
Design	e.g. experimental, survey, grounded theory, phenomenology
Description of intervention	e.g. self-report questionnaire, observation, comparison of wound dressings
Sample	Size: Sampling method: Sample characteristics:
Key results/findings	
Recommendations	
Strengths: How does this advance our understanding of the subject? Are the hypotheses, methods, sample sizes or types of control for variables, recommendations appropriate? Ethics considered?	
Limitations: In what ways is it limited? When and where would it not apply? Are there any flaws in the research design and methods, sample size or type, or conclusions not based on results?	

Figure 9.1   Example of a critical appraisal record for a research article

What goes into a literature review?

Having completed a critical appraisal of the important papers relevant to the topic and evaluated the different arguments presented by the research, you are actually ready to start writing a critical literature review. This is basically a summary for use at two different stages in the research process: in the proposal to support the need for a research project and in the research report to justify the conduct of the study. The difference between these literature reviews is usually in the length. A literature review used in the final report will be expected to contain a detailed appraisal and be more up-to-date simply because it is written as part of an actual study. Whereas a literature review used in a proposal may be regarded as a précis of what will be included in a literature review of the study report. The aim for this review is to provide supporting evidence to convince, say, grant-making bodies, ethics committees and supervisors of the need for the research study.

There is no recipe for writing a narrative critical literature review. The aim is simply to convince the reader that the research study is necessary and represents the next step in knowledge-building for the topic. This means that it will discuss relevant findings, together, where appropriate, with a comment on the methods used and any strengths and limitations of the work. In this way it will be possible to demonstrate that there has been a considered and justified examination of what others have discovered and written about on a specific topic. It is not expected that a chronological approach for reviewing the literature will be possible, say by starting with the earliest work on the topic and progressing through to the latest publication. Similarly, it will not usually be possible to present an individual review of each paper in turn.

A literature review has to have a structure that follows a logical argument if gaps in the literature are to be highlighted. This means that it is more likely that it will be arranged in themes emerging from the literature or framed around certain research questions or identified problems. It also means that, although each study will have been critically appraised, not all aspects of each study will necessarily need to be included when writing the literature review. Remember, it is a summary of the work that has been done and not a comprehensive description of each research study. Suggested headings for a literature review are given in Figure 9.2.

There are also some conventions of language associated with writing in a critical review of research literature. For example, authors suggest, assert, argue, state, conclude or contend. A good way of developing an understanding of these conventions is to read a few critical reviews before embarking on writing your own critical literature review.

```
1   Introduction – overview of what will be covered by the review
2   Review of the key themes relating to the topic
3   Description of how each theme has been studied
4   Overview of studies and types of research design used
5   Results
6   Critical evaluation
7   Critical summary of current knowledge and gaps in the literature
8   Identification of research needs
9   Rationale for the study design
10  Overview and niche for proposed study
```

Figure 9.2   Suggested headings for a critical literature review

Referencing the research literature

In order to be able to discuss the research literature relevant to your project you will need to refer to the actual papers: this is called 'referencing' or 'citing'. It demonstrates and attributes the source of the information used, lends authority to the claims made and allows readers to refer to full copies of articles of interest to them.

It is possible to use too many or too few references; the aim is to achieve a balance and arrive at what are felt to be the appropriate number of references necessary to support the arguments being presented. It may also be necessary, in a review for a proposal, to take account of guidelines from grant-making bodies (when applying for funding) or regulatory authorities that will be reviewing your proposal. Suggestions of how to use and not use references are given below.

Use and abuse of references

References should be used to:

- justify and support your arguments
- allow you to make comparisons with other research
- express matters better than you could yourself
- demonstrate your familiarity with your field of research.

You should not use references to:

- impress your readers with the scope of your reading
- litter your writing with name and quotations
- replace the need for you to express your own thoughts
- misrepresent their authors.
  (Blaxter et al., 2006: 128)

There are several conventions available for referencing published work, and authors usually use one that they are familiar with and prefer, or follow the referencing style requested by a journal. Some of the electronic reference databases may be able to format your references in one of a range of different styles.

The two most commonly used conventions for referencing are by numbering (Vancouver) or by author and year (Harvard) in the text, with the full details of the reference only appearing in a list at the end of an article. Nursing journals such as *Nursing Times*, *Nursing Standard* and *Nurse Researcher* use the author and year style, whilst the *British Medical Journal* uses the numbering system.

Chapter summary

- A critical literature review provides an overview of the research available to support a research proposal and inform a research report.
- Narrative and systematic reviews are different and serve different purposes.
- A literature review helps to focus on a research topic.
- Critical appraisal is a structured process of identifying and evaluating the merits and/or value of research.
- When reading a research study, questions should be asked about each section.
- Evaluation of the literature involves giving a critical account and comparison of the different studies to highlight similarities, contradictions and gaps in the literature.
- When writing a literature review, the aim is to convince the reader that the research study is necessary and represents the next step in knowledge-building for the topic.
- All the literature used should be referenced using a recognised system.

References

Blaxter, L., Hughes, C. and Tight, M. (2006) *How to Research*. Maidenhead: Open University Press.

Crowley, P. (1996) 'Using an overview', *Ballière's Clinical Obstetrics and Gynaecology*, 10: 585–97.

Goodman, M.L., Low, J. and Wilkinson, S. (2005) 'Constipation management in palliative care: a survey of practices in the United Kingdom', *Journal of Pain and Symptom Management*, 29 (3): 238–44.

Hart, C. (2003) *Doing a Literature Review*. London: Sage. p. 3.

Sim, J. and Wright, C. (2000) *Research in Health Care: Concepts Designs and Methods*. Chelterham: Nelson Thornes.

Websites

Critical Appraisal Skills Programme (CASP): www.phru.nhs.uk/casp
National Library for Health: www.library.nhs.uk

10

WRITING A RESEARCH PROPOSAL

Nurse researchers are often required to submit a **research proposal** for a variety of audiences. These can include proposals for local research monies or development opportunities, those sent in response to external funding calls, to meet ethical approval requirements or as part of academic assessment requirements. Frequently proposals are required when seeking staff development funding support for academic study. Applications for doctoral study usually include a research proposal that outlines an intended research project or publication plan (Locke et al., 1999). Though many of the elements discussed in this chapter may have some relevance for potential doctoral students, they are specifically directed at those responding to a competitive tendering process in order to secure research monies to complete a specific piece of research.

In developing a research proposal, the nurse needs to consider how best to prepare the application and make decisions about its content. University-based researchers responding to calls from external bodies will also need to consider using **full economic costing** packages to generate predicted project costs.

In this chapter we outline the steps involved in preparing to submit a research proposal for funding. We review the likely structure such a proposal would follow, identifying key information that might be provided to support an application. We also discuss the use of full economic costing to cost research undertaken by universities.

Learning outcomes

This chapter is designed to enable the reader to:

- Understand the steps involved in preparing a research proposal
- Appreciate the role of a research proposal as a mechanism for applying for research funding

- **Discuss the probable content of a research proposal**
- **Understand the function and details of full economic costing**

KEY TERMS

Full economic costing, Research proposal

Preparing the application

Identifying funding opportunities

Information about research bidding opportunities can be presented through a number of forums and mechanisms. Often advanced intelligence is received through specific networks operating within a specialist field. Funding calls can be advertised in the press or emailed to specific mailing lists. Most organisations funding research advertise new research opportunities on their websites. In the UK these include the Association of Medical Research Charities (www.amrc.org.uk), the Economic and Social Research Council (www.esrc.ac.uk) and the Wellcome Trust (www.wellcome.ac.uk), along with a number of other funders. Universities will often employ staff to collect a list of funding opportunities to circulate to key research staff, and a similar system operates within the NHS, the world's largest publicly funded health service, through the research and development units. Organisations such as the Higher Education Academy (HEA), who help institutions, discipline groups and all staff to provide the best possible learning experience for their students, have a Health Science and Practice (HS&P) subject centre that provides a newsletter to members highlighting research opportunities. The Royal College of Nursing, the body in the UK that represents nurses and nursing, promotes excellence in practice and shapes health policies, has a Research Society that also provides a regular update of research opportunities (www.man.ac.uk/rcn/).

Not all research funding opportunities are advertised as part of specific funding rounds. A number of charities and other healthcare organisations have identified monies available to support research related to their specialism. Researchers can submit more general proposals that relate to the aims of the funding body, one example being the Resuscitation Council (UK) (www.resus.org.uk) who fund a variety of research projects in the field of resuscitation through small grants.

At present, nursing research doesn't have a specific funding body, and though there are a number of funding opportunities the competition is often high. Those proposals most likely to succeed meet the aims and objectives of the call, are succinct and focused, have relevance and demonstrate an ability to complete the research. Writing proposals is a skill and one that requires development over time. A number of strategies can be employed to maximise success, though it should be remembered that funders for a variety of reasons reject a number of proposals (Goldblatt, 1998). Learning from rejection is important, so any opportunities for feedback should be sought.

Background work

When a call is received it is important to consider if the research relates to an existing research record and how a current profile can support the proposal. A proposal is more likely to be successful if the researcher can demonstrate a clear area of expertise in the field and present a profile of previous research and publications that relate to the call. At this stage it is worth considering who may form the research team. Depending on the scope of the bid, strategic decisions may need to be taken regarding the composition of any bidding team. Woods (2000) suggests that partners may be required for healthcare research. Most research projects will involve more than one person, attracting a team who bring different strengths to the proposal. For example, healthcare research may benefit from a team composed of a number of different healthcare professionals, reflecting an interprofessional approach. Collaboration between healthcare providers and university staff may be helpful. Research can often benefit from user involvement, national or international links, and European funding requires the inclusion of different European-based partners.

It is also important to clarify the aims and objectives of the call, visiting websites or accessing other background information. It may be possible to speak to the funders to ascertain further detail. Some funders, such as the Joint Information Systems Committee (JISC) who fund e-learning-based research, run Town Planning meetings and invite possible bidders to attend sessions that provide further bid information and opportunities to ask questions. Funders may also offer an opportunity to attend a community of professionals, whose members may work together to produce a bid.

The bid should also be discussed internally, with Research and Develop departments or within local research communities. It is also important to alert the institution of a possible bid opportunity so that appropriate departments and staff can offer help with reading though proposals, funding advice and can ensure that any internal processing systems are followed.

Planning the writing

Often the time to respond to a call is limited, though this will vary according to the funder and the details of the bid. A number of funders request expressions of interest that can be a couple of pages in length. Full bids can take some time to develop, though often the available response time is less than a month. It will be important to look at what material is readily available to support the bid. For example, can a previous academic paper or literature review be updated for use? The guidance for proposal submissions varies across funders, and any submission not meeting these is likely to be discarded. It will therefore be crucial to follow the guidance and either allot members of the team to undertake the development of parts of the bid or agree some sort of writing programme.

Content of the proposal

The content and presentation required is likely to be outlined by the funder. This may be very prescriptive and should be followed, as failure to meet the requirements set out in the call can to lead to it being discarded without consideration. Often funders provide headings that need to be used and identify a word limit. There is usually the requirement to submit supporting CVs and often a need to demonstrate support from employers and any partner organisations involved in the bid. The Economic and Social Research Council, the UK's leading research and training agency in economic and social research, provides one suggested template with accompanying guidance notes on how to write a good application (www.esrcsocietytoday.ac.uk). The proposal example in Figure 10.1 was written in response to an HEA HS&P subject centre call to scope e-learning use in health science and practice disciplines (www.health.heacademy.ac.uk). Looking at the structure of this, it includes the project title, details of the project team, introduction, aims and objectives, methodology, areas of learning and teaching to be addressed, outcomes, timetable for completion, evaluation and dissemination strategy, budget and signatures. The CV of the lead investigator was also required. The requirement to demonstrate areas of learning and teaching to be addressed is a specific requirement of an HEA HS&P bid and relates to their aims and objectives as an organisation that supports learning and teaching development in higher education.

In developing a proposal it should be remembered that its function is to provide clear justification of the need for the study and detail how the study will be completed in order to achieve the aims and objectives and address the research questions or problems. The proposal is therefore likely to include:

- Research problem and background
- Aims and objectives
- Research methods
- Data collection
- Data analysis
- Ethical approval issues
- Project team and management
- Outputs
- Dissemination
- Budget (see full economic costing)
- Curriculum vitae

Higher Education Academy

Subject Centre for Health Sciences and Practice

Application for Mini-Project Funding

1. Title of project

Scoping e-learning; use and development in Health Sciences and Practice

2. Project leader

Title		Forename		Surname	
Current post					
Full address	(Details omitted)				
Telephone				Fax	
E-mail					

3. Project partners (if any)

Name	Department and Institution
a) (Details omitted)	
b)	

Figure 10.1   Research proposal (printed with the permission of the Higher Education Academy Health Sciences and Practice Subject Centre)

4. Description of project

Introduction

For the purpose of this study an inclusive definition of e-learning will be employed that encompasses all learning delivered electronically (Glen and Moule, 2006). The uptake of e-learning has been variable within Health Sciences and Practice (HS&P) disciplines across the UK. This may be related to organisational strategy and access to hardware and software. Additionally, confidence in use, IT skill development or personality characteristics can impact on adoption.

The [name omitted] University is well placed to complete this research. The [name omitted] Faculty has developed expertise in the design, implementation and research of e-learning, including a number of funded research and development projects [web link omitted], follow link to [research centre omitted].

a. Aim

To scope the use of e-learning within Higher Education Institutions (HEIs) across the UK in the HS&P disciplines.

b. Objectives

Are to:

- Conduct a comprehensive survey of e-learning implementation.
- Explore factors influencing adoption and use, identifying drivers and barriers.
- Review the employment of e-learning within curricula that represent a range of learning and teaching models.
- Identify, explore and compare cases from exemplars and late adopters to make explicit barriers to implementation and good practice.
- Make recommendations for future practice.

Methodology

A mixed methodology is proposed, using an initial survey and case studies.

(Continued)

Sample

Using existing HS&P databases, all HEIs providing education to the HS&P disciplines within the UK will be surveyed to identify cases of exemplars and late adopters.

Design

There will be two phases to the project:

Phase 1: Quantitative survey data will be collected via a questionnaire adapted from existing open access tools developed in the Joint Information Systems Committee (JISC)-funded Managed Learning Environment study (www.mlestudy.ac.uk/). This will enable access to a representative population, using a previously validated measure. Data will be analysed using descriptive statistics.

Phase 2: Four case study sites will be identified from the relative level of integration of e-learning identified in the survey, to encompass exemplar and late adopters. Case study research will allow the local examination of e-learning practice (Yin, 1994). Through review of relevant data sources and interviews with key staff and students we will explore current policies and practices. Qualitative data will be analysed thematically (Miles and Huberman, 1994).

Ethical issues

Phase 1: Completion and return of questionnaires will be taken as implied consent.

Phase 2: The research team will secure appropriate ethical approval as required by each HEI.

All data collected will be stored in accordance with best practice. The confidentiality and anonymity of all participants will be observed.

c. Areas of learning and teaching to be addressed

The results of the scoping are expected to identify areas where e-learning is likely to impact on the student learning experience, such as:

- Access to bibliographic information.
- Course information provision.
- Issues relating to learning and teaching online.
- Use of e-technology to support communication.

d. Outcomes

Will include the identification of:

- current use of e-learning in HS&P disciplines
- factors that can influence the adoption of e-learning
- resource implications for supporting e-learning delivery
- suggestions from the HEIs as to how the development and implementation of e-learning could be improved
- good practice guidelines that can inform HEI policy and practice development
- evidence for use in the development of further Quality Assurance Agency (QAA) and benchmark standards for e-learning
- summaries of research findings for the case study sites
- recommendations for future development of e-learning strategies and products.

e. Timetable for 2007

January–February	Adapting questionnaire. Accessing sample for phase 1.
March–April	Data collection phase 1 (start analysis).
May–August	Conduct data analysis phase. 1. Identify sample phase. 2. Ethics approval as needed. Interim report for HS&P Subject Centre.
September–October	Phase 2 data collection.
November–December	Data analysis phase 2 data. Final report for HS&P Subject Centre. Summary report for case study sites. Abstracts for presentation at conferences, e.g. Association for Learning Technology Conference (ALTC), Festival of Learning 2008.

(Continued)

f. Evaluation and dissemination strategy

The evaluation and progress of the research will be conducted through the Centre for Learning and Workforce Research advisory group.

Dissemination will be through:

- Project website at the university and HS&P Subject Centre.
- Final report for HS&P Subject Centre.
- Summary of the case studies report available to the sites and on the website.
- Publications in peer-reviewed journals.
- Report for the HS&P Subject Centre Newsletter.
- Abstracts submitted to relevant conferences .

Year 2 funding opportunity

We would welcome the opportunity to disseminate the good practices seen, particularly to the late adopter case study sites, and evaluate the effect of this on student learning.

References

Glen, S. and Moule, P. (eds) (2006) *E-learning in Nursing*. Basingstoke: Palgrave.

Miles, M. and Huberman, A. (1994) *Qualitative Data Analysis*, 2nd edition. Thousand Oaks, CA: Sage.

Yin, R. (1994) *Case Study Research: Design and Methods*, 2nd edition. Thousand Oaks, CA: Sage.

5. Budget

The budget headings provided below are only a guideline. It is not necessary to enter a figure for every heading if not appropriate. Overheads (including hardware and software) will not be covered.

Time release	£ 3,980
− Number of hours/rate of pay − Project Lead, 5 days − Senior Lecturer, 4 days − Research Associate, 9 days − Statistician 2 days	
Administrative/secretarial support 80 hours (including tape transcription)	£ 1,002
Other assistance (please specify)	£
	£
	£
Training and professional development	£
Travel and subsistence* Travel − case study sites for interviewing and documentation review − overnight stay at two case study sites − train ticket, Festival of Learning conference attendance	£ 2,000 £ 90
Materials − Production of questionnaire survey for 900 departments and postage	£ 576
Other costs (specify) Conference attendance September 2008 **Please note that the university will be meeting additional costs (travel and conference fees for an additional delegate, production and dissemination of reports, costs associated with the advisory group meetings and additional time for each named researcher). Total contribution £ 3,732)**	£ 350
Total	£ 7,998

*Please include in your travel budget costs of attending an initial Project meeting and attendance at our Festival of Learning

(Continued)

6. Name and signature of project contact	

7. Signature(s) of Head(s) of Department(s) in which project is to be undertaken

Heads of participating departments should sign indicating their support for the application and confirming that the grant will not be top-sliced.

Name	Department/Institution
a)	
b)	
c)	
d)	

Figure 10.1   Research proposal (printed with the permission of the Higher Education Academy Health Sciences and Practice Subject Centre)

Increasingly the funder of health and social care research will also expect user involvement in the research, and including reference to this in the proposal is helpful. It may, for example, include having users involved in designing the research, in its implementation or as members of an advisory or steering group for the project. The decision to involve users needs to be taken early on, especially if they are to form part of the research team. There are also implications for the research budget, which may need to include user costs (DoH, 2002).

Research background, aims and objectives

Robson (2002) suggests that a vague presentation here will contribute to the rejection of the proposal. This part of the proposal needs to present the existing research in the field and give justification for the research. In nursing research it may be possible to argue the potential benefits to nursing care and patient experience. The background should be used to demonstrate the bidder's expertise, referencing publications and highlighting experience in the field. An opportunity to refer to work of potential scrutineers should be taken, and it is important to demonstrate a wider and current knowledge base. A word limit may be imposed on this section and therefore any inclusions must have relevance. It may also be possible to make a statement here about the credibility of the research team and their ability to complete the research, as in Figure 10.1. Clarity will also be aided if the research aims and objectives are set out in achievable terms. Funders will always be concerned that the expected outcomes are achievable within the timeframe and budget set out.

Often the call will include the aims and objectives the funders want to achieve which can aid the researcher. For example, the aim and objectives of the HEA HS&P call were clearly laid out to include a survey of e-learning practice in HS&P and identification of cases of late and early adopters of e-learning. These therefore appear within the proposal objectives. It may also be helpful to review the general philosophy, aims and objectives of the funding body and to reflect these within the proposal. It is important to reiterate the need to write achievable aims and objectives and to ensure that the remainder of the proposal demonstrates how these will be met.

Proposed investigation

The proposal needs to make clear what kind of research design is going to be used and outline the stages of the research. This detail needs to be presented in the opening lines with a rationale for the adoption of particular approaches if required. Details on a number of research designs and methods are presented in Chapters 11, 13–17, 20, 21 and can be used to support proposal writing. The amount of detailed description required on the methods, sample, data collection and analysis will depend on the funder. There should be sufficient information presented to make clear how the sample will be selected and composed, how data will be collected, from where and by whom, and clear statements about the processes of data analysis should be provided. The funders need to understand what sampling approach will be used (see Chapter 19) and sample size, and be confident that the sample can be accessed within the timeframe. It would add strength to the proposal if the bidders can demonstrate previous use of the suggested methodologies and convey an understanding of the strengths and weaknesses of the approaches suggested.

The bid may suggest the need for pilot work to test out data collection approaches or tools. It may also identify the involvement of a statistician to support the analysis of numerical data and refer to a power calculation to support sample size generation. It should be clear to the funders that the design, sample, methods of data collection and analysis are consistent with the aims and objectives of the study. For example, in the Figure 10.1 proposal, the objectives include a survey and the identification of early and late adopters of e-learning. They also suggest that good practice will be identified. To support this, the design includes the administration of a survey across universities delivering to HS&P and a second phase of case studies that will explore early and late adopters and extract examples of good practice.

Ethical issues

Much research conducted within healthcare will require ethical approval to meet research governance requirements (see Chapters 3 and 4). Some funders require evidence of ethical approval prior to proposal review, such as the Resuscitation Council (UK). The proposal will need to outline the ethical approval processes that will be put in place and identify these in the project timeline. Nursing research is likely to meet the requirements for researching ethically in the UK set out by the Research Governance Framework for Health and Social Care (DoH, 2005) and seek approval from the National Research Ethics Service (NRES) (www.nres.npsa.nhs.uk/) (see Chapter 4). This will address how issues such as the provision of participant information and informed consent will be managed. Additionally, the proposal can outline processes in place to manage and store research data in line with the Data Protection Act, which makes new provision for the regulation of the processing of information relating to individuals (HMSO, 1998).

Project management

Most funders want to be confident that the planned work is likely to be completed in the funding timeframe, often one or two years. To help funders make this judgement, a timeline of work or a Gantt chart should be included. Figure 10.1 suggests a work schedule for a 12-month project. This provides a plan of work and highlights the key activities. Depending on the funder, a more detailed plan of work may be required. The funder may also want to see evidence that the schedule will be monitored by a steering group or advisory body and can request feedback on progress in a formal interim report. It is advisable to write an initial plan of work that is realistic. A project lasting one year should expect to spend three to four months gaining ethical approval, accessing a sample and preparing for data collection, a further three or four months should be spent collecting and analysing the data, with the final months used for collating and presenting the results.

The funders will also need to be confident that the research team has the skills and expertise to complete the research. The curriculum vitae of the project manager will be reviewed and possibly those of the project team members. Where a more novice researcher is leading a proposal, it will be important to demonstrate that research support and mentorship is in place. This may come from the mentorship of a more experienced researcher or through a steering group.

Dissemination

The outputs from research are becoming increasingly important to funders in health and social care. Not only is the generation of a report, conference papers and publications expected, but other forums of dissemination can be supported. These might include hosting a website related to the project, holding events that will disseminate the results to relevant professional groups and providing reports in various formats that might be more applicable to users and other consumers of research. The report can also be produced as a DVD, and the executive summary can be made available as a podcast. The project may have other outputs such as toolkits, teaching materials or new developments. The dissemination of these will need some consideration and the distribution or marketing may be governed by a contractual agreement made with the funder at the outset of the project. Issues of intellectual property rights will need consideration as it is important to know who owns the copyright of any products. Often these are owned by the institution(s) employing the research team, though agreements can be in place that reward the individual employees. In research projects where such issues are likely to arise, legal advice should be sought.

Curriculum vitae

The proposal will need to include the curriculum vitae (CV) of the lead investigator at least, and possibly require a two-page submission from each member of the team. These can be gathered at the early stages of developing the proposal. A template may be offered that should be used by all involved. Alternatively, if no template is suggested, the format of the following headings may be used:

- Name and contact details
- Current employer and position
- Employment history
- Educational qualifications
- Research experience
- Relevant publications
- Conference presentations

The CV must include those aspects of research activity and experience that are relevant to the bid. It should support the application and demonstrate research capability.

Full economic costing

Full economic costing (fEC) relates to the costing and charging of research undertaken by universities in the UK. It is a research costing methodology introduced by the government in 2005 following the Transparency Review that was originally instigated in 1998. The review was undertaken to demonstrate the full costs of research and other publicly funded activities in higher education. It was completed to improve accountability for the use of public money. Policy documents (HM Treasury, 2002a, 2002b) state that government departments and other purchasers of contracted research undertaken by universities must expect to pay the larger percentage of the costs of their research.

The costs relate to three areas:

- Directly incurred costs: costs directly related to the project including research assistant pay, travel, subsistence, equipment, external consultants, consumables, printing and stationery, IT hardware and software.
- Directly allocated costs: the principal investigator and co-investigator costs, estates and other directly allocated costs such as major facilities, centrally sourced technicians.
- Indirect costs: contribution to centrally shared costs.

The use of fEC is mandatory and most universities have access to web-based sites that enable calculation of the total cost of research based on the input of directly incurred and directly allocated costs. Any nurses undertaking research within universities or as part of a university based project team will need to use fEC.

Table 10.1 is a useful reminder of what to do or avoid doing when drawing up a research proposal.

Table 10.1   Key dos and don'ts of research proposal development

Do	Don't
Look at the aims and objectives of the call closely.	Submit a proposal without addressing the aims and objectives of the call and funder.
Undertake background work, e.g. literature review, think about expertise and current or previous related work.	Bid in areas where previous expertise and experience is crucial if you and the bidding team have none.
Consider the best team to respond and have partners in place if appropriate.	Bid if partnerships are needed and these are not in place or are tenuous.
Follow the guidelines for submission closely and make sure any internal reviewers and support staff, e.g. research office staff, have access to these.	Ignore the guidelines for submission.
Follow any submission templates to structure the report.	Ignore the submission template.
Provide all of the information requested, e.g. CVs.	Leave out essential information requested by the funder.
Get expert support if available from colleagues with previous experience of the funder and from staff with expertise in costing and bidding.	Undertake proposal development alone without taking advice from those with more experience.
Include reference to ethical approvals as required and have these in place if needed.	Ignore the need for ethical approval if required and forget to obtain approval prior to submission if needed.
Make it clear in the bid who will be project manage and oversee the project to completion.	Submit a proposal without making clear who is the project manager taking responsibility for completion.
Include a clear dissemination strategy appropriate to the bid and funder.	Omit a dissemination strategy.

Chapter summary

- Nurse researchers are often required to submit a research proposal for a variety of audiences.
- When writing the proposal it is worth reviewing existing and available expertise and potential team membership.
- The proposal will need to include the research problem and background, aims and objectives, research methods, data collection, data analysis, ethical approval issues, project team and management, outputs and dissemination.
- The proposal will need to be costed for a funder.
- If sending the proposal from a university, it will need to include full economic costing (fEC) related to the costing and charging of the research.

References

Department of Health (2002) *Exploring Evaluating Roles for Health Service Users in Research Implementation.* Available at www.dh.gov.uk, accessed 29 January 2007.

Department of Health (2005) *Research Governance Framework for Health and Social Care*, 2nd edition. London: DoH.

Glen, S. and Moule, P. (2006) *E-learning in Nursing.* Basingstoke: Palgrave.

Goldblatt, D. (1998) 'How to get a grant funded', *British Medical Journal*, 317 (7173): 1647–8.

HM Treasury (2002a) *The Cross Cutting Review of Science and Research.* Available at www.hm-treasury.gov.uk/spending_review/spend_ccr/spend_ccr_science.cfm, accessed 29 January 2007.

HM Treasury (2002b) *Investing in Innovation.* Available at www.hm-treasury.gov.uk/spending_review/spend_sr02/spend_sr02_science.cfm, accessed 29 January 2007.

HMSO (1998) *Data Protection Act.* London: HMSO.

Locke, L., Spirduso, W. and Silverman, S. (1999) *Proposals that Work: Guide for Planning Dissertations and Grant Proposals*, 4th edition. London: Sage.

Miles, M. and Huberman, A. (1994) *Qualitative Data Analysis*, 2nd edition. Thousand Oaks, CA: Sage.

Robson, C. (2002) *Real World Research*, 2nd edition. Oxford: Blackwell.

Woods, L. (2000) 'Responding to calls for bids: process and preparation', *Nurse Researcher*, 8 (1): 19–27.

Yin, R. (1994) *Case Study Research: Design and Methods*, 2nd edition. Thousand Oaks, CA: Sage.

Suggested further reading

Chaplin, P. (2004) *Research Proposals: A Guide for Scientists Seeking Funding.* Cambridge: Cambridge University Press.

Glen, S. (1998) 'Guidelines for writing a research proposal', *Managing Clinical Nursing*, 2 (2): 61–3.

Punch, K. (2006) *Developing Effective Research Proposals*, 2nd edition. London: Sage.

Sandelowski, M. and Barroso, J. (2003) 'Writing the proposal for a qualitative research methodology project', *Qualitative Health Research*, 13 (6): 781–820.

Websites

Association of Medical Research Charities: www.amrc.org.uk
Department of Health: www.dh.gov.uk

Economic and Social Research Council: www.esrcsocietytoday.ac.uk
Higher Education Academy: www.health.heacademy.ac.uk
National Research Ethics Service: www.nres.npsa.nhs.uk
Resuscitation Council (UK): www.resus.org.uk
Royal College of Nursing Research Society: www.man.ac.uk/rcn
Wellcome Trust: www.wellcome.ac.uk

11

RESEARCH APPROACHES AND DESIGN

The development of the research design is an important part of the research process. The design is the plan of how the research aims, objectives, hypothesis and question(s) will be answered. The literature review can inform the development of the design. The researcher may be able to replicate a previous design or take elements of it into a new study. There are a number of designs available to the researcher in quantitative and qualitative research. Research questions may also require the researcher to work with a design that incorporates both quantitative and qualitative research, as a combination (triangulation) of both. The research design will include the approach, that can be seen as either quantitative, qualitative or both, though polarisation of the approaches isn't necessarily helpful as some research designs, such as case study research, can include what might be seen as qualitative and quantitative data collection methods.

The design is a map of the way in which the researcher will engage with the research subject(s) in order to achieve the outcomes needed to address the research aims and objectives. It also provides a representation of the researcher's beliefs about how knowledge is generated; for example, the researcher may believe that qualitative research is most valuable in informing the development of nursing practice. Therefore the selection of a design will depend on a number of factors such as the research question that needs addressing, the beliefs of the researcher, the resources available for the project, and will need to take account of data access and ethical approvals.

In this chapter we explore the research designs used by the nurse researcher to address those research questions, aims and objectives set out in research and we review the elements that compose research design.

Learning outcomes

This chapter is designed to enable the reader to:

- **Understand what is meant by the research design**
- **Identify the components of a research design**
- **Consider designs available within qualitative and quantitative approaches**

KEY TERMS

Deductive reasoning, Ethnography, Experimental design, Grounded theory, Inductive reasoning, Phenomenology, Qualitative approaches, Quantitative approaches, Quasi-experiments, Research design, Survey, Triangulation

---

Choosing a research design

In selecting the **research design** the nurse researcher needs to focus clearly on the research question and purpose of the study. The purpose of the research design is to ensure that the evidence collected is able to answer the research question. It is suggested that the researcher will need to review the data and information required to answer the questions set and identify the most effective research strategies in order to secure research data (LeCompte and Priessle, 1993). The design is therefore the plan of the research that will provide the evidence needed to answer the research question. It is likely to include the following:

1 Identification of the researcher's own beliefs about knowledge generation.
2 The research questions to be addressed.
3 The research approach – qualitative, quantitative or both.
4 The selection of sites and participants or source of data.
5 Ethical considerations for the study.
6 Timeline for the research.
7 Resources available for the research.
8 Methods of data collection.
9 Methods of data analysis.

The list above presents the processes to be completed in the research and includes the orientation of the researcher and the identification of the beliefs that guide the selection of research design. The nurse researcher may hold particular beliefs that means they prefer to work within a qualitative or quantitative research approach, though the differences between these are more blurred in reality. For example, it can be irrelevant to try to compartmentalise particular designs or methods into either qualitative or quantitative research. Marsh (1982) has long argued that what might be seen as quantitative surveys can often provide evidence of behaviour that might be seen as the domain of qualitative research. Yin reminds us that:

> some experiments (such as studies of psychological perceptions) and some survey questions ... rely on qualitative evidence and not quantitative evidence. Likewise, historical research can include enormous amounts of quantitative data. (1994: 14)

Different research designs and methods can be used within the research approach adopted. The selection of design will be affected by a number of practical factors. The research team will need to think about the time available for the research and the resources and costs of particular data collection methods. For example, if the researcher has a limited budget and timeframe for research, then a longitudinal study that includes observational techniques will not be practical.

The research design is also likely to reflect the skills and expertise of the researcher and research team. For example, if the researchers are not skilled in social interaction, then they are unlikely to choose a design that includes participatory observation for the research. There is also a need to ensure that the research complies with ethical requirements for a study in healthcare (see Chapters 4 and 5). A design that might cause unnecessary harm to the patients involved is unlikely to be approved.

The choice of research design is also dependent on access to participants or research subjects. There is little point designing a study to capture data from thousands of respondents if there are limited numbers available. Equally, there can be difficulties in designing studies involving particular vulnerable groups if they are difficult to access.

There isn't a perfect research design, and frequently decisions about aspects such as sampling and data collection methods will be guided by the practicalities of research endeavour, as discussed above. Our own research experiences have demonstrated that often decisions about data collection methods are taken based on availability of resources or participants. For example, individual face-to-face interviews may be preferable, yet telephone-based interviews may be conducted, as access to busy nursing staff spread across a range of clinical practice environments can be problematic. However, the researchers need to be confident that the methods of data collection used will not compromise the quality of the information accessed, as ultimately the research needs to be robust and collect data that will address the research questions. The focus of the research design has to be about whether it is appropriate to gain the evidence needed to answer the research question. There are issues of validity and reliability that need considering in the selection of a design. The design and methods of data collection used must be able to obtain the evidence needed in a robust way to address the research problem. For example, if we wanted to look at patients' views and experiences of service delivery there would be little point developing an **experimental design** that is more focused on testing cause-and-effect relationships. We would need to think about a design that allows the research team to explore patient views and experiences, taking a more qualitative approach and looking to explore experiences and views through data collection methods that could include interviews and recording of diaries or journals.

Prior to considering different research designs it is important to highlight the main aspects of **qualitative** and **quantitative research approaches**.

Research approaches

There are two approaches to research, qualitative and quantitative, which in the past have been presented as competing and divergent positions, but more recently there is recognition of the need to use a range of approaches to address the questions of nursing research. The contrasting elements of qualitative and quantitative research are described in Table 11.1. Qualitative research, in the crudest sense, is research that aims to generate data that comprises words and pictures. Qualitative research is most commonly part of an interpretivist approach and can be viewed as contructivist (Guba and Lincoln, 1982). Interpretivists in the broad sense simply believe that the social world needs to be interpreted to be understood. Qualitative researchers often tend to be focused on language, perceptions and experiences in order to understand and explain behaviour. In nursing research an interpretivist position would be used to describe and understand people's experiences of care, trying to understand the individual and their interactions with others. It acknowledges that there is no single truth or one understanding, but celebrates individual differences. For example, someone admitted to hospital may be anxious and upset, though the same person may not experience subsequent hospital admissions in the same way. Individuals can react to the same experience in different ways, and each of us can react to the same experiences in different ways.

Qualitative research may be used to look at issues such as the patient experience or the views of healthcare staff. To gain these insights the researcher needs to interact with the study participants. The researcher engages with the participant in a meaningful way to gain a holistic picture of life experiences and uses observation and interviews as the main methods of data collection to facilitate an interactive and subjective approach (Bryman, 1988). The results are not normally open to generalisation and wide application but describe the local context and can be open to transferability to other contexts.

The goal of quantitative research is to generate research data that can be analysed numerically using statistical techniques. Quantitative research tends to be driven by a positivist or scientific approach or by, more latterly, a post-positivist approach. Positivism emerged in the Enlightenment and was in part a reaction against the idea that knowledge was handed down by God and could only be interpreted theologically. Broadly, positivist approaches stress the importance of testing and measurement and believe scientific truths exist even in the social world. Positivists have tended to believe that through the controlled testing of variables, cause-and-effect relationships can be determined and the truth established. Positivists argue that the scientific method can also be used to study social phenomena, and that universal laws exist that can explain human behaviour in an objective way. They would suggest that there is one truth and objectivity.

Post-positivist beliefs, developed in the mid-20th century, recognise that social phenomena cannot be understood through uncovering universal laws, and that it is problematic to predict a cause-and-effect relationship that is true for all. For example, a universal law would suggest that our person admitted to hospital experiencing anxiety and upset would always feel this on every admission and everyone else would feel the same way. Post-positivist research seeks to look at relationships or correlations between variables being measured (see Chapter 22). The post-positivists maintain some of the processes of empiricism, answering hypothesis or research questions through a scientific approach. Numerical data is obtained through formal methods of data collection, which are objective and free from bias (Burns and Grove, 2005).

We can see that the nurse researcher occupying a positivist position can be drawn to quantitative research, whereas those favouring interpretivist philosophies may lean to qualitative. It should be remembered, however, that, as discussed earlier, other more practical factors influence the design selection, such as available funding, research skills, timeframe available, ethical approval and access to the research sample. Additionally, the researcher will need to give foremost consideration to the research problem and questions that need to be addressed. The research design selected needs to obtain the evidence required to address the research problem.

Induction and deduction

The production of knowledge through scientific method is often categorised as being through two approaches to generating knowledge, called 'induction' and 'deduction'. In practice, many research approaches cannot be categorised as purely inductive or purely deductive, but are rather a mixture of the two. However, the two terms are useful

Table 11.1 Contrasting elements of qualitative and quantitative approaches

	Qualitative	Quantitative
Philosophical origin	Interpretivist	Positivist
Researcher relationship with subject	Close	Distant
Researcher position in the research	Often insider	Outsider
Research strategy	Unstructured	Structured
Relationship with theory	Develops, interprets	Tests
Data collection	Observation, interviewing	Instruments
Type of data	Rich, individual	Hard, reliable
Data analysis	Interpretation	Statistical
Findings	Unique, transferable	Generalisable

Source: Bryman, 1988; Burns and Grove, 2005

tools in helping us to understand different approaches to producing knowledge through the research process.

Induction or **inductive reasoning** is a process of starting with the observations and details of an experience, our observations of something, that are used to develop a general understanding of phenomena. Specific observations and descriptions are made and used to develop a theory or hypothesis of a more general situation that can be tested or investigated further. For example, while on the ward our observations of patients may show a tendency for better sleep patterns if relaxation therapies are used before the ward lights are switched off for the night. These observations could be developed into a theory or a hypothesis. The hypothesis is a statement of predicted relationship (see Chapter 6), which if based on the initial observations would suggest that 'the use of relaxation therapies before night time will lead to patients having better patterns of night time sleep'. Typically, induction is seen as part of qualitative and quantitative research where the aim is to develop concepts and themes from the interpretation of observations and interviews.

Deduction or **deductive reasoning** starts with a general theory about something and moves to test the theory through undertaking further observations or by developing tests. Drawing on the example above, testing would look to measure whether there is a relationship between the use of relaxation therapies and the quality of patients' sleep. Researchers aim to deduce how the theory works and identify causal relationships through controlled testing or experimentation. Data obtained will be used to either verify the theory or discount it. Deduction is seen as being part of quantitative research as it looks to test theories or hypotheses for correlations and relationships. For example, the researchers would want to test the relationship between the use of relaxation therapies and patients' sleep.

Qualitative approaches

Qualitative approaches focus on understanding social settings; often in nursing this will be the ward or community environment. They facilitate exploration of relationships and human experience within the research setting and enable face-to-face, personal contact in data collection. Three qualitative approaches, **phenomenology**, **ethnography** and **grounded theory**, that are most frequently used in nursing research have their traditions in anthropology, sociology and psychology (Polit and Beck, 2006).

The researcher may be required to engage over a period of time with the research setting in order to collect data using methods where the researcher can become the research instrument. The researcher can work with a range of data collection methods. These can include observations, interviews, group discussions and the analysis of textual data, diaries, letters and other documents. These methods allow the researcher to gain insight into the social context of the research, to gain in-depth data from the participants, and to enable them to 'tell their story' and provide rich data about personal experiences, feelings and thoughts. The data are usually recorded on to audio, video or digital recording for verbatim transcription and analysis (see Chapter 23). A process of thematic analysis is used to identify key meaning and interpretations from the data. This involves a process of breaking the data into key units of meaning through a coding process, re-ordering data and drawing interpretations that are often verified by the participants (see Chapter 23). The process is described as data reduction, display, conclusion drawing and verification (Miles and Huberman, 1994).

The researcher may maintain a reflective diary or field notes recording the research events. These reflections are used in a similar way to our employment of reflective practice in nursing. The researcher uses the records to consider their role and influence in the research and in interpreting the data. A necessary emphasis is placed on this as the researcher is often immersed in the research setting and study and will need to take opportunities for reflexivity in which actions and analysis are critically reviewed. Diary recordings and field notes can form part of the data analysis which is usually prolonged and leads to the construction of narratives and validated interpretations of participant experiences.

The three approaches of phenomenology, ethnography and grounded theory are discussed in greater detail in Chapter 14, with a brief description provided here.

Phenomenology

Phenomenological approaches are grounded in philosophy and psychology and aim to explore the lived experience of humans within the context of that experience (Beck, 1994). A nurse researcher would employ such an approach if the research sought to find out how patients or staff experienced a particular phenomenon, to discover the meaning of the phenomenon. This approach can be selected if the nurse researcher wants to explore the experience of those caring for elderly relatives and consider their perception of the world as a carer and experiences of being a carer in today's society.

In phenomenological research a number of methods of data collection can be used; interviews that are in-depth and focus on the experience that is being explored are most common. Data can also be collected through diaries, autobiographies, written accounts and conversations. The example in Box 11.1 collected data through journals that recorded experiences, thoughts and feelings. These methods all allow the researcher to collect data about people's experiences that should provide an in-depth reflective account for analysis.

Box 11.1   Example of the use of phenomenology

Idczak (2007) sought to understand how student nurses in the USA make meaning of their interactions with patients.

Hermeneutic phenomenology, used when the research question seeks to understand the meaning of a phenomenon in order to comprehend the human experience (Crist and Tanner, 2003), was employed.

Twenty-eight volunteer students recorded electronic journals with their thoughts, feelings and emotional response to patient interactions.

Data were analysed through an interpretive process, coded by drawing on prior categories, and themes were extracted (see Chapter 14).

Five themes emerged to include: 1) fear of interacting with patients; 2) developing confidence; 3) becoming self-aware; 4) connecting with knowledge; and 5) connecting with the patient (Idczak, 2007: 69).

Ethnography

Coming from the tradition of anthropology, ethnography means a 'portrait of people' and involves writing about people and culture. Ethnographic approaches tend to be about using observational data collection methods, often over a long period. Ethnographers aim to gain an understanding of the culture and social norms of a particular group, such as nurses, by studying behaviours through fieldwork (Hammersley and Atkinson, 1993). Through ethnography the nurse researcher would attempt to learn from members of a particular cultural group and understand their world as it is lived and perceived (Polit and Beck, 2006). An example of this approach is given in Box 11.2. This approach can be used to answer questions about patients' experiences of a long-term treatment plan or student nurses' experiences of a pre-registration programme of study.

Box 11.2   Example of an ethnographic study

Simmons (2007) used ethnography to study the introduction of the nurse consultant role. She was an insider researcher, occupying the role of senior nurse manager. A purposive sample of nurse consultants was selected to take part in the study. Ethical approval was in place prior to data collection. The study commenced by describing organisational and policy contexts. The fieldwork was completed with six nurse consultants. This included five days of participant observation spilt across a two-year period. As a participant observer Simmons choose a passive role, where she was predominantly an observer, shadowing the nurse consultants in the main. Simmons also discussed her need to demonstrate reciprocity (a reciprocal relationship between the ethnographer and participants), which she felt was achieved through taking on the role of a critical friend to those nurses involved in the study.

Grounded theory

Developed in the 1960s by sociologists Glaser and Strauss (1967), grounded theory aims to develop hypotheses and theories from the data collected through observations and interviews with humans in their own environments. Grounded theory usually starts with specific observations and analysis of the data collected to generate a theory, therefore usually working in an inductive way, but can develop to use deductive reasoning.

The researchers initially develop themes and hypotheses from observations using an inductive approach. These hypotheses can be subjected to further observations to try to verify relationships and correlations, using a deductive approach. Induction, however, plays the greatest role in grounded theory. The researchers use the emergent themes from the analysis of observations or interviews to undertake theoretical sampling. The use of theoretical sampling is shown in research by Abid-Hajbaghery (2007), reported in Box 11.3. Analysis of initial data from registered nurses identified issues related to management. Abid-Hajbaghery explored these further by interviewing key managers. Grounded theory also attempts to compare similar findings in the data through a constant comparison method to try to gain a wider perspective of the issues arising in the study.

Box 11.3   Example of the use of grounded theory

Abid-Hajbaghery (2007) aimed to clarify the concept of evidence-based nursing and explore the factors influencing its use by Iranian nurses.

Grounded theory (see Chapter 14) was used as it allows the identification, description and explanation of interactional processes that occur between and amongst individuals and groups in a particular social context (Strauss and Corbin, 1998; Abid-Hajbaghery and Salsali, 2005).

Twenty-one registered nurses formed an initial purposive sample, selected because of their length of experience and full-time employment, followed by theoretical sampling. Initial interviews with staff nurses were coded to reveal management issues that were then explored with key staff. Observations were also conducted in clinical settings.

Data collection and analysis were simultaneous, and interview and observational data were reviewed concurrently to allow for constant comparisons.

Two main categories emerged from the data: 1) Nurses' perceptions of evidence-based nursing; and 2) factors affecting evidence-based nursing.

Quantitative research

Quantitative research seeks to generate numerical data that can be analysed using statistics. It emerged from a positivist position, which has developed more latterly into a post-positivist approach. Put crudely, positivism seeks to generate understanding from phenomena that are observable and generates scientific knowledge from verified facts (Bryman, 1988). Its approach seeks to be formal, objective, rigorous, controlled, and a systematic process is followed to generate knowledge. Post-positivists recognise that social phenomena cannot be understood through uncovering universal laws, and that it is problematic to predict a cause-and-effect relationship that is true for all. Post-positivists look at relationships or correlations between variables being measured (see Chapter 22) and maintain some of the processes of empiricism, answering hypotheses or research questions through a scientific approach.

Quantitative approaches are often used to describe new phenomena, such as whether a newly discovered drug treatment is better than existing prescriptions, or they can be used to test the effectiveness of alternative therapies on cardiac care patients.

The origins of quantitative research lie in the work of Fisher (1935), who developed the ideas of the hypothesis (a statement of predicted outcome tested by the researcher), research design and statistical analysis. This early work has developed into the experimental research used by nurse researchers today to measure cause-and-effect relationships (see Chapter 13) (Burns and Grove, 2007). The 'true experiment' has since been developed to include the quasi-experiment (Campbell and Stanley, 1963), used to test a cause-and-effect relationship where conditions are less controlled. **Quasi-experiments** are used in social science and healthcare research where it is often impossible to control and limit the effect of a number of variables, or to randomly allocate patients to groups (see Chapter 13). An experiment may be used to test the relationship between a particular treatment and its effect or outcome responses.

Correlation studies can be a precursor to experimental or quasi-experimental research, aiding the development of a hypothesis (Burns and Grove, 2007). Correlation research aims to identify the strength of a relationship between two variables, gauged through statistical testing that identifies results between a perfect positive ($+1$) to perfect negative (-1). Correlation may be used to measure the relationship between information provision and well-being.

Descriptive research is also used to generate nursing knowledge for practice. These approaches aim to describe phenomena, provide a description of what exists and present frequency measures that can be used to develop hypotheses for testing. These approaches can consider questions such as: What are the completion rates on particular nursing programmes?, How many hours a day do nurses spend in computer use?, What are patient's attitudes to physiotherapy services in rehabilitation?

Quantitative designs

Nurse researchers employing quantitative research will be addressing hypotheses that look to measure cause-and-effect relationships, seeking to measure the correlation relationship between two different phenomena or wanting to describe phenomena about which little is understood. Data collection will be structured with information being gathered from a representative sample (see Chapter 19); often the researcher may be detached from the process. Statistical analysis of collected data is aimed to accept or reject any predicted cause-and-effect relationship or describe a new phenomenon and generate a new hypothesis.

Though a number of different types of research design exist, those mainly used within nursing research include:

- Experimental
- Quasi-experimental
- Survey

These designs are discussed in detail in Chapter 13, with brief explanations provided here. Further designs include evaluative studies (see Chapter 15), case studies, action research (see Chapter 15) and Delphi technique (see Chapter 16).

Experimental research

A hypothesis will usually guide an experimental design that sets out to test a cause-and-effect relationship. The nurse researcher will include elements of control, randomisation and manipulation. Simply, the researcher will identify a specific research population, randomly allocate these to an experimental or treatment group and a control group. The researcher will introduce and manipulate particular variables with the treatment group and measure the effect on particular pre-defined outcome measures. The outcomes measures will be taken from the control group, who did not receive the intervention, and the data will be subjected to statistical comparison. An example is given in Box 11.4.

Box 11.4   Example of an experimental design

Eogan et al. (2007) compared two post partum laxative treatments with 147 women who had suffered anal sphincter injury at vaginal birth. The women were randomised into one of two groups. The control group received lactulose three times daily for the first three days following delivery and then daily for a further ten days. The experimental group took the lactulose and also had ispagula husk for the first ten days. All kept a diary of bowel movements.

Outcome measures included discomfort with first bowel movement, incidence of constipation and incontinence. The research found that the women receiving more than one treatment had a higher incidence of incontinence.

Quasi-experimental research

This approach mirrors that of the experimental design in many respects, with the use of a hypothesis to establish a cause-and-effect relationship. Often the design is employed when factors make one or more elements of control, manipulation or randomisation difficult to achieve.

Survey

Surveys can be used to gather data, through self-reporting, about an identified and specific population. This data is collected through postal, telephone, or online questionnaires, structured interviews or even observations (Burns and Grove, 2005). Thus, the survey can be used to collect data as part of quasi-experimental (Abramson and Abramson, 1999) descriptive and correlation studies. Box 11.5 provides an example.

Box 11.5   Example of a survey

Gilmour et al. (2008) used a questionnaire survey to identify the extent of postgraduate nursing students' information literacy skills in relation to electronic media and health information and to establish any barriers to access. A total of 223 postgraduate students were sent the postal questionnaire and replies were received from 123 (55.1 per cent).

The questionnaire included four sections. Section one collected biographical and demographic data. Section two asked about the nurses' knowledge of the Internet and opinions of patient use. Section three explored how nurses evaluated healthcare information and how difficult it was to find. Section four looked at the nurses' use of health information in practice and considered whether the nurses assessed patients' use of online health information and if they helped patients to make sense of this. The questionnaire was developed from previous literature and research and was piloted.

Triangulation in research

Triangulation in research draws on multiple methods, combining both qualitative and quantitative approaches in one research study to address the research questions, aims and objectives (Denzin, 1989). Nurse researchers may choose to triangulate research approaches in order to address complex nursing problems and combine study of relationships and human experience with measuring causality or correlation. For example, a combined approach may be used to explore questions about patients' ability and experiences of coping with living with a chronic condition, such as cardiac failure. It is suggested that operating with a triangulation of methods will require team expertise in each area and a commitment to maintain the philosophical underpinning of both approaches (Burns and Grove, 2005).

Chapter 20 highlights the different levels of possible triangulation and discusses the perceived benefits and issues associated with combining research approaches. It is suggested that through triangulation in data collection some of the concerns related to weaknesses of particular approaches can be lessened (Brewer and Hunter, 1989; Denzin, 1989). In contrast, there remain concerns that any such weaknesses may be compounded (Armitage and Hodgson, 2004) and that the difficulties of attempting to combine differing philosophical positions within one approach affect the trustworthiness of any claims. It is also suggested that the readers of research employing triangulation should be aware of the need to understand and review the strengths and weakness of a combined study considering issues of trustworthiness and rigour (see Chapter 12) in reviewing how a triangulated approach is used to answer specific research question(s).

Chapter summary

- The selection of the overall research approach must be appropriate to the study and can be described as quantitative, qualitative or a triangulation of both.
- Qualitative research is part of an interpretivist or constructivist position.
- Quantitative research is part of a positivist or scientific approach.
- The research design includes the approach, methods of data collection and analysis that will be used to address the research questions, aims and objectives.
- There isn't a perfect research design, and frequently decisions about aspects such as sampling and data collection methods will be guided by the practicalities of the research endeavour.
- The main qualitative designs include phenomenology, ethnography and grounded theory.
- The main designs used in quantitative research include experimental, quasi-experimental and survey.

References

Abid-Hajbaghery, M. (2007) 'Factors facilitating and inhibiting evidence-based nursing in Iran', *Journal of Advanced Nursing*, 58 (6): 566–75.

Abid-Hajbaghery, M. and Salsali, M. (2005) 'A model of empowerment of nursing in Iran', *Iranian Journal of Medical Education*, 10: 3–12.

Abramson, J. and Abramson, Z. (1999) *Survey Methods in Community Medicine*, 5th edition. Edinburgh: Churchill Livingstone.

Armitage, G. and Hodgson, I. (2004) 'Using ethnography (or qualitative methods) to investigate drug errors: a critique of a published study', *Nursing Times Research*, 9: 379–97.

Beck, C. (1994) 'Phenomenology: its use in nursing research', *International Journal of Nursing Studies*, 31 (6): 499–510.

Brewer, J. and Hunter, A. (1989) *Multi-method Research: A Synthesis of Styles*. Newbury Park, CA: Sage.

Bryman, A. (1988) *Quantity and Quality in Social Research*. London: Routledge.

Burns, N. and Grove, S. (2005) *The Practice of Nursing Research: Conduct, Critique and Utilization*, 5th edition. St Louis, MO: Elsevier/Saunders.

Burns, N. and Grove, S. (2007) *Study Guide for Understanding Nursing Research*, 4th edition. St Louis, MO: Saunders Elsevier.

Campbell, D. and Stanley, J. (1963) *Experimental and Quasi-experimental Designs for Research*. Chicago, IL: Rand McNally.

Crist, J. and Tanner, C. (2003) 'Interpretation/analysis methods in hermeneutic interpretive phenomenology', *Nursing Research*, 3: 202–6.

Denzin, N. (1989) *The Research Act: A Theoretical Introduction to Sociological Methods*, 3rd edition. Englewoods Cliffs, NJ: Prentice-Hall.

Eogan, M., Daly, L., Behan, M., O'Connell, P. and O'Herlihy, C. (2007) 'Randomised controlled trial of a laxative alone versus a laxative and a bulking agent after primary repair of obstetric anal sphincter injury', *BJOG: An International Journal of Obstetrics and Gynaecology*, 114 (6): 736–40.

Fisher, R. (1935) *The Designs of Experiments*, New York: Hafner.

Gilmour, J., Scott, S. and Huntington, N. (2008) 'Nurses and Internet health information: a questionnaire survey', *Journal of Advanced Nursing*, 61 (1): 19–28.

Glaser, B. and Strauss, A. (1967) *The Discovery of Grounded Theory: Strategies for Qualitative Research*. Chicago, IL: Aldine.

Guba, E. and Lincoln, Y. (1982) 'Epistemological and methodological bases of naturalistic enquiry', *Educational Communication and Technology*, 30 (4): 233–52.

Hammersley, M. and Atkinson, P. (1993) *Ethnography: Principles and Practice*, 2nd edition. London: Tavistock.

Idczak, S. (2007) 'I AM a NURSE: Nursing students LEARN the art and science of nursing', *Nursing Education Perspectives*, 28 (2): 66–71.

LeCompte, M. and Priessle, J. (with Tesch, R.) (1993) *Ethnography and Qualitative Design in Educational Research*, 2nd edition. New York: Academic Press.

Marsh, C. (1982) *The Survey Method: The Contribution of Surveys to Sociological Explanation*. London: Allen & Unwin.

Miles, M. and Huberman, A. (1994) *Qualitative Data Analysis*, 2nd edition. Thousand Oaks, CA: Sage.

Polit, D. and Beck, C. (2006) *Essentials of Nursing Research: Methods, Appraisal and Utilization*, 6th edition. Philadelphia, PA: Lippincott Williams & Wilkins.

Simmons, M. (2007) 'Insider ethnography: tinker, tailor, researcher or spy?', *Nurse Researcher*, 14 (4): 7–17.

Strauss, A. and Corbin, J. (1998) *Basics of Qualitative Research: Techniques and Procedures for Developing Grounded Theory*, 2nd edition. Newbury Park, CA: Sage.

Yin, R. (1994) *Case Study Research: Design and Methods*, 2nd edition. Thousand Oaks, CA: Sage.

Suggested further reading

Cresswell, J. (2003) *Research Design: Qualitative, Quantitative and Mixed Methods Approaches*. London: Sage.

deVaus, D. (2001) *Research Design in Social Research*. London: Sage.

McVicar, A. and Cann, W. (2005) 'Research capability in doctoral training: Evidence for increased diversity in skills of nursing research', *Journal of Research in Nursing*, 10 (6): 627–46.

Sim, J. and Wright, C. (2000) *Research in Health Care: Concepts, Designs and Methods*. Cheltenham: Nelson Thornes.

Wilkins, K. and Woodgate, R. (2008) 'Designing a mixed methods study in pediatric oncology nursing research', *Journal of Pediatric Oncology Nursing*, 25 (1): 24–33.

Website

Research methods tutorials: www.socialresearchmethods.net/tutorial/tutorial.htm

12

RIGOUR AND TRUSTWORTHINESS IN RESEARCH

Nursing research has its traditions in qualitative and quantitative methods, though is increasingly employing mixed method designs, combining both approaches in addressing research questions. A number of chapters in this book discuss the research approaches and methods that can be used (see Chapters 11, 13–17) and refer to the need for rigour, validity and reliability in their application. In this chapter we explain what these concepts mean and how they can be evaluated within nursing research.

Learning outcomes

This chapter is designed to enable the reader to:

- **Understand the terms 'reliability' and 'validity' in quantitative research**
- **Describe how reliability and validity can be assessed in quantitative research**
- **Understand how rigour and trustworthiness can be established in qualitative research**
- **Explain the four dimensions of trustworthiness**

KEY TERMS

Confirmability, Construct validity, Content validity, Credibility, Criterion-related validity, Dependability, Reliability, Rigour, Transferability, Trustworthiness, Validity

---

Rigour, validity and reliability in quantitative research

Nurse researchers working with quantitative methods have sought to ensure **validity** and **reliability** in their methods of data collection to maintain the **rigour** of the study. Validity and reliability are related to the data collection methods and tools employed in the research and to the extent that the researcher has been able to limit any bias in data collection processes. Having a valid and reliable data collection tool affords **credibility** to the instrument and subsequent research findings.

Validity

Validity is a measure of whether a data collection tool accurately measures what it is supposed to. In nursing practice we use validated measurement tools to record data on a daily basis. Such examples include the use of recording devices to measure a patient's blood pressure and pulse. Three types of validity measures are available to the researcher, with **content validity** being the most basic and others including **criterion–related** and **construct validity**.

Content validity

Content validity is concerned with the ability of the measure, say the questions in a questionnaire, to collect data about the phenomena under study. If we are interested in how much knowledge someone has on resuscitation, a pre-test can be developed to cover all aspects of the knowledge required. There is no one way of determining the content validity of this pre-test. One approach would be to get expert review. Experts in the field might be asked to look at the questions and comment on whether they represent the range of questions that might be asked in relation to resuscitation. They might also comment on any questions included that are irrelevant. Another way of validating the content of a questionnaire is through the calculation of a content validity index (CVI). To do this a panel of experts would review the questionnaire and rate the relevance of the questions to the subject. For example, a basic life support pre-test may include questions on maintaining safety, assessment for circulation and breathing, opening the airway and the delivery of breathing and chest compressions. The panel would decide which of these questions were 'very important', 'important', or 'not important'. The index is calculated to reflect the level of agreement seen across the panel member ratings. If all of the members felt a question was 'not important' it might be removed. An example is given in Box 12.1.

Box 12.1   Example of the generation of content validity

Wynd et al. (2003) employed expert review panels in determining the content validity of an Osteoporosis Risk Assessment Tool. Panel members were recruited as experts from the field of osteoporosis. In order to work out the content validity, the panel members were asked to look at the questions on the risk assessment tool and rate them using a scale of 'not relevant' to 'very relevant'. Those seen as very relevant were valid questions, whereas those viewed as not relevant would not necessarily be kept within the questionnaire.

The term 'face validity' can also be used. This implies that the measure appears to measure what it is intended to, 'on the face of it'. This judgement follows a review of the questionnaire, but not necessarily by a subject expert. The questionnaire could be given to one person, such as a colleague, to review. Alternatively, a number of participants might be asked to review the questionnaire and identify issues such as questions that don't make sense or those that might be difficult to interpret and answer.

Criterion-related validity

A second type of validity measure is criterion-related validity. In using this, the nurse researcher will attempt to measure the validity of the data collection tool by comparing its findings with those collected from another method. The results obtained by the measure to be validated might be compared with those obtained through another validated questionnaire. If the scores are closely correlated, then the tool can be described as having criterion-related validity. Two types of criterion-related validity exist: concurrent and predictive.

Concurrent validity describes the ability of two measures administered at the same time (concurrently) to achieve correlated outcomes. A survey measuring patients' nutrition whilst in hospital can have concurrent validity if the results identifying those patients who are undernourished correlate with nurses' observations of patients' dietary requests and feeding habits.

Predictive validity describes the ability of the measure to determine the possible difference between the current and future measures of the same criteria. For example, a tool that measures the attitudes of nurses to computer use in the workplace now, will have predictive validity if the findings are consistent with future behaviour and attitudes towards computer use. So if the tool finds that nurses have a negative attitude to computers, then it will have had predictive validity if nurses in the future react to computers in a negative way.

Construct validity

Polit and Beck (2006) suggest that establishing construct validity is more challenging than content or criterion-related validity as it involves making a judgement relating to what the instrument is measuring. In other words, how much is a questionnaire able to measure the criterion or constructs it is intending to measure, such as health, anxiety or empathy? These constructs are complex and therefore challenging to measure. The researcher would draw on the relevant literature to try to identify the different facets of the construct and use these to develop the questions in the questionnaire. For example, health might include facets of being free from disease, mentally and physically able, and in a state of well-being. The questions would need to identify the presence or absence of these facets to measure how healthy someone is.

Different techniques exist that allow researchers to measure construct validity. The use of 'known-groups technique' is one example (Polit and Beck, 2006). In this technique two groups that are known to differ in the attributes to be measured on the construct are asked to complete the questionnaire. For example, a measure of anxiety on hospitalisation for surgery can be validated by asking two groups of patients with different levels of experience to complete the questionnaire. One group would include those being admitted for a surgical procedure for the first time; the second group would be composed of patients who have had more than one previous operation. The two group scores would be compared to see if there was any difference in the group responses. We would expect that the patients being admitted for surgery for the first time would be more anxious than those with previous experience. If no difference was seen, then we might be concerned about the validity of the questionnaire.

Reliability

Reliability is the consistency with which a tool measures what it is intended to. Within nursing practice a number of tools have to be not only valid in what they measure, but also reliable. Therefore the instruments used to record blood pressure, pulse and temperature not only have to take accurate measures of these vital signs, but need to do so every time they are used. The nurse researcher is interested in three measures of reliability that include the stability of a measure, its internal consistency and equivalence.

Stability

Test–retest procedures enable researchers to establish whether a measure is stable, in other words, whether it obtains the same measurements when used on the same person at different times. Ward et al. (in press) applied the same attitude measure to a range of healthcare practitioners on two separate occasions. The scale measured attitudes towards information technology. In order for the tool to be deemed stable, the results when compared should be similar, or if different the change should be accounted for. If, for example, the staff involved in the study had completed computer training and become more involved in computer use in between the two measurements, that might account for a change in attitude, probably in a positive direction.

Internal consistency

The split-half technique is employed in measuring internal consistency. It is used with questionnaires that have a total score and measure a specific criterion. The questions are split into two groups and scored, then compared to see if they are similar. If this is the case, the questionnaire is said to have high internal consistency, as all questions are measuring the same criterion.

Equivalence

A test of equivalence is more usually applied in observational research when a number of researchers are collecting data using a schedule (see Chapter 21). Inter-rater reliability can be measured when two or more trained observers use the tool to record independent observations of the same event.

A reliability coefficient is calculated to show the strength of relationship between the observer recordings. This is illustrated in Box 12.2.

Box 12.2 Example of the use of inter-rater reliability measures

Odd et al. (2004) used two observers to independently review radiographs taken to identify the positioning of percutaneous central venous lines placed in neonates. The aim was to determine whether the addition of contrast media improved the identification of long line tips on radiographs.

The observers reviewed 106 radiographs taken without contrast and 96 with contrast. The interpretations drawn by the observers were subjected to reliability testing, to see how much agreement there was in their observations. A Kappa co-efficient was used to measure the level of agreement. This is a test designed to measure the degree to which two observers agree in their judgements.

The results showed that the observers were more likely to see the long line tip when contrast was used and were more likely to agree on its anatomical positioning. The research concluded that the use of contrast when placing long lines improves the likelihood that an

(Continued)

(Continued)

observer can see the tip of the long line and its position. There is more agreement between observers when contrast is used and therefore inter-observer variability is reduced. The research therefore recommended the use of contrast in long line placement to improve positioning.

Rigour and trustworthiness in qualitative research

In considering the maintenance of rigour within qualitative research, we can see that the validity and reliability measures employed in quantitative research are not transferable. Data collection in qualitative research can involve the research participants as part of co-enquiry methods (see Chapter 14) and the researcher is often involved with participants rather than remaining detached. Data is collected using a number of methods that are neither standardised nor necessarily structured. Qualitative researchers in nursing are hoping to present the 'truth' and describe the insider or 'emic' view and therefore need to use alternative approaches to support rigour in their research. For a number of years the research community has been challenged to find a way to meet these demands.

Lincoln and Guba (1985) have developed criteria for establishing the rigour and **trustworthiness** of qualitative research. The criteria aim to allow the researcher to demonstrate how the interpretations presented in the data, and conclusions drawn, reflect participants' experiences. Four key components are included: credibility, **dependability**, **confirmability** and **transferability**.

Credibility

The data presented in any qualitative research report or publication has to be seen to be credible, just as quantitative data needs to be seen as valid. Those reading the research must believe that the data presented is a 'true' representation of the participants' view, experience or belief. Readers must have confidence that the interpretations remain faithful to the insider view. A number of steps can be taken that support claims for credibility. These can include the use of triangulation in data collection and prolonged engagement in the field. Researchers can also employ expert review processes and member checking, asking the participants to review the analysis and interpretation.

Triangulation can be used to enhance credibility, as discussed in Chapter 21. This might involve obtaining more than one data source in a study about a particular phenomenon, using more than one researcher to collect data or drawing on multiple methods of data collection. For example, the research may be designed to study one phenomenon using data collected through both observations and interviews. See Box 12.3 for an example.

Box 12.3   Example of research that used triangulation in data collection

Moule (2006) examined whether healthcare students could develop an online community of practice as learners on an online module. The data was collected from nursing and radiography students about how they worked online. Three methods of data collection were used, including online diaries, interviews and discussion board data. The data showed different accounts from the students of their online working. The data were analysed to see if the different kinds of data showed the same conclusions. This adds strength to the conclusions.

Investing more time in the field and prolonging the length of engagement with participants will aid the development of trust with the researcher and enhance credibility. Immersion in the culture will facilitate the development of understandings that can be more readily corroborated over a prolonged period of observation.

Researchers can approach expert reviewers, such as fellow researchers, as objective peers to establish credibility. They can review the processes of sampling, data collection and analysis, and explore recordings of audio- or video-tape or field notes. What Maxwell (1992) refers to as 'descriptive' and 'interpretative' validity can only be provided by the participants themselves through a process of member checking. Descriptive validity refers to verifying the factual accuracy of the account. Interpretative validity refers to the emic account, to confirm what the participants meant in what they said or did. This involves returning the data and interpretations to the participants for their reactions and to confirm the credibility of the qualitative data.

A further measure of credibility relates to the researchers themselves and their ability to act as research instruments, as collectors and interpreters of the data. The reader of qualitative research might want to satisfy themselves of the researcher credibility referred to by Patton (2002), by reviewing the researcher's qualifications and research experience.

Dependability

Qualitative data cannot be seen as credible unless its dependability is known, its ability to stand the test of time. Establishing dependability can be seen as a parallel process to that of confirming reliability in quantitative data. Lincoln and Guba (1985) suggest that an audit trail of the research can assist in establishing the dependability and confirmability of the research. As audit trails are so closely linked to confirmability, a fuller discussion is provided below.

Confirmability

Confirmability is a measure of the objectivity of the data. To confirm the objectivity, the researcher presents an audit trail of the methods, presentation of data and analytical processes presented as a decision trail, which are subjected to external audit by a reviewer introduced towards the end of the study. The findings are then subjected to an audit to establish the trustworthiness of the data. This process has been criticised (Cutliffe and McKenna, 2004), though has been employed previously by a number of nurse researchers (Koch, 1994). The difficulties arise as it is deemed impossible to completely follow a decision trail. Data analysis is affected by researcher immersion in the field and data that bring uniqueness to the interpretation. It is suggested that the uniqueness of a study cannot be replicated by an independent auditor who may well form different conclusions when following an audit trial (Sandelowski, 1998). Yet Koch (2004) suggests that caution is needed in our criticisms, as more novice nurse researchers may need the framework of an audit trail to protect the rigour of a study.

Transferability

Researchers need to demonstrate the extent to which the research findings can be transferred from one context to another by providing a 'thick description' of the data, as well as identifying sampling and design details. Thick description is the thorough description of the research setting and research processes to enable the reader to establish how transferable the results are. This component is therefore similar to that of generalisability seen in quantitative research, though it should be remembered that in qualitative research there is interest in transferring rather than generalising the results.

Often it is beyond the scope of most publications to provide an in-depth discussion of the maintenance of rigour and trustworthiness in nursing research, though papers in the *Journal of Advanced Nursing* are asked to address this. One such paper provides a detailed example of the processes undertaken to maintain rigour in qualitative research (Mavundla, 2000; see Box 12.4).

Box 12.4   Example of the maintenance of rigour and trustworthiness

Mavundla (2000) discusses how the study achieved credibility, dependability, confirmability and transferability. Credibility was supported by the use of prolonged engagement in the field, triangulation of methods of data collection and member checking of the interpretations of the data. An external audit of the project supported measures of dependability and confirmability. Transferability was aided through the provision of a thick description of the research design and methods used. (For further information see Mavundla (2000)).

Chapter summary

- Maintaining rigour and trustworthiness is important to the quality of the overall study.
- Validity and reliability in methods of data collection are important to maintaining the rigour of quantitative studies.
- Validity is a measure of whether a data collection tool accurately measures what it is supposed to.
- Three types of validity measures are available to the researcher, with content validity being the most basic, others including criterion-related and construct validity.
- Reliability is the consistency with which a tool measures what it is intended to.
- The nurse researcher is interested in three measures of reliability that include the stability of a measure, its internal consistency and equivalence.
- Criteria have been developed to establish the rigour and trustworthiness of qualitative research to include the four key components of credibility, dependability, confirmability and transferability.

References

Cutliffe, J. and McKenna, H. (2004) 'Expert qualitative researchers and the use of audit trails', *Journal of Advanced Nursing*, 45 (2): 126–33.

Koch, T. (1994) 'Establishing rigour in qualitative research: the decision trail', *Journal of Advanced Nursing*, 19: 976–86.

Koch, T. (2004) 'Expert researchers and audit trails. Commentary', *Journal of Advanced Nursing*, 45 (2): 134–5.

Lincoln, Y. and Guba, Y. (1985) *Naturalistic Inquiry*. Newbury Park, CA: Sage.

Mavundla, T. (2000) 'Professional nurses' perceptions of nursing mentally ill people in a general hospital setting', *Journal of Advanced Nursing*, 32 (6): 1528–69.

Maxwell, J. (1992) 'Understanding and validity in qualitative research', *Harvard Educational Review*, 60: 415–42.

Moule, P. (2006) 'E-learning for healthcare students: developing the communities of practice framework', *Journal of Advanced Nursing*, 54 (3): 370–80.

Odd, D., Page, B., Battin, M. and Harding, J. (2004) 'Does radio-opaque contrast improve radiographic localisation of percutaneous central venous lines?', *British Medical Journal*, 89 (1): F41–3.

Patton, M. (2002) *Qualitative Evaluation and Research Methods*, 3rd edition. Thousand Oaks, CA: Sage.

Polit, D. and Beck, C. (2006) *Essentials of Nursing Research: Methods, Appraisal and Utilization*, 6th edition. Philadelphia, PA: Lippincott Williams & Wilkins.

Sandelowski, M. (1998) 'The call to experts in qualitative research', *Research in Nursing and Health*, 21: 467–71.

Ward, R., Glowgoska, M., Pollard, K. and Moule, P. (in press) 'Developing and testing attitude scales around IT', *Nurse Researcher*.

Wynd, C., Schmidt, B. and Schaefer, M. (2003) 'Two quantitative approaches for estimating content validity', *Western Journal of Nursing Research*, 25 (5): 508–18.

Suggested further reading

Lincoln, Y. and Guba, Y. (1985) *Naturalistic Inquiry*. Newbury Park, CA: Sage.

LoBiondo-Wood, G. and Haber, J. (2006) *Nursing Research: Methods and Critical Appraisal for Evidence-based Practice*, 6th edition. St Louis, MO: Mosby Elsevier. Chapter 15, pp. 335–56.

Polit, D. and Beck, C. (2006) *Essentials of Nursing Research: Methods, Appraisal and Utilization*, 6th edition. Philadelphia, PA: Lippincott Williams & Wilkins. Chapter 2, pp. 40–41.

Rolfe, G. (2006) 'Validity, trustworthiness and rigour: quality and the idea of qualitative research', *Journal of Advanced Nursing*, 53 (3): 304–10.

13

EXPERIMENTAL AND SURVEY RESEARCH

There is a long tradition of using experimental and survey research to support the development of nursing knowledge and practice. Experimental designs are employed to test the effectiveness of treatments and interventions, such as whether one drug treatment is more effective than a comparable product. Surveys are a form of social inquiry that has developed in recent years to take advantage of computerised technologies, but they can also be used more specifically to gather data through self-reporting about an identified and specific population. In this chapter we discuss these key research designs and consider the main experimental and survey approaches used to support healthcare practice. Additionally, we highlight the application of the designs in research practice and identify ethical considerations of use.

Learning outcomes

This chapter is designed to enable the reader to:

- **Understand the characteristics of experimental and quasi-experimental designs**
- **Appreciate the design of randomised controlled trials**
- **Describe the use of survey research in healthcare**
- **Discuss epidemiological research use in healthcare**
- **Explain the strengths and weaknesses of experimental and survey designs**
- **Show an awareness of the ethical considerations of experimental and survey research**

KEY TERMS

Epidemiological research, Experimental design, Follow-up studies, Longitudinal designs, Panel studies, Quasi-experimental design, Randomised controlled trial, Survey designs, Trend studies

Experimental design

Experiments can conjure up an image of people in white coats within laboratories, working with test tubes. These images fail to show the true extent of experimental research. Such research can take place in a number of settings, and **experimental designs** can be used to test either a research hypothesis or question (see Chapter 6). Commonly the research hypothesis is written as a statement that sets out the relationship between the independent (treatment or intervention) and dependent (outcome) variables and predicts an outcome. The hypothesis can be expressed as a 'null' hypothesis (H_o), suggesting there is no expected relationship. The hypothesis stated is never truly proven or not, but accepted or rejected through the research.

Experimental research could test the following hypothesis:

Relaxation therapy will slow the effects of cachexia in cancer patients (H_1)

this could be expressed as a null hypothesis:

Relaxation therapy is not effective in reducing the effects of cachexia in cancer patients (H_o)

In the above example, the independent variable and intervention is the use of relaxation therapy, with the dependent variable being the effects on cachexia. The study population is patients with cancer. In order to address the research hypothesis using an experimental design, certain characteristics will need to be in place. These include manipulation, control and randomisation.

Manipulation

The researcher will manipulate the independent variable, in this case the relaxation therapy, and then observe the effect on the dependent variable, the cachexia (condition of the late stages of cancer). The manipulation can involve delivering the intervention to one group of cancer patients (experimental group) whilst withholding it from another set of patients (control group). A pre-test–post-test design may be used to measure the effect of treatment, as discussed below. A pre-test–post-test design allows the researcher to record what changes were caused by the relaxation therapy, and compare these with data from the members of the control group.

Control group

The control group are research participants who are often selected because they possess similar characteristics to members of the experimental group. Data are collected from the control group and compared with findings from the experimental group. This allows the researchers to look at the effect of the independent variable on the experimental group. Thus, the level of cachexia will be measured in the cancer patients not receiving relaxation therapy and compared with those in the experimental group who were administered the treatment. This gives the researcher information about how effective the relaxation therapy (independent variable) is.

Randomisation

Researchers will use mechanisms, such as computer programmes and websites (www.randomisation.com), to randomise study participants from the population into either the experimental or control group. All participants should have an equal chance of inclusion in either group and will be comparable. This will limit systematic bias that could affect the dependent variable. In our example, if the patients in the control and experimental groups are very different, say in age or grade of cancer, then this could lead to differences in the measurement of cachexia (dependent variable) that need not necessarily be linked to the use of relaxation therapy, but to original differences between patients in the two groups.

Pre-test–post-test design

The pre-test–post-test design, sometimes known as the before-and-after design, is commonly used to measure change in experimental research. It includes randomisation of participants into either the experimental or the control groups. Using our example, the researcher will collect baseline data from the cancer patients prior to (pre-test) the intervention or relaxation therapy. Examples of baseline data may be recording of vital signs, hormonal levels, stress levels and others. The same measures are taken after the intervention as a post-test. Then the pre-test and post-test measures are compared. This gives a measure of the effect of the independent variable (relaxation) on the dependent variable (cachexia).

There are a number of other possible approaches that can be used. These include factorial design (two or more variables are simultaneously manipulated) and cross-over design (exposing participants to more than one treatment at different points of the research) (see Polit and Beck, 2006).

Limitations of experimental research

Though experiments offer the best approach to test a hypothesis and measure a cause–effect relationship, there are some limitations to their use in healthcare research. These limitations often relate to the need to manipulate variables, which may mean either the experimental or control group can be disadvantaged, something the ethical approval processes will scrutinise (see Chapters 4 and 5). The ethical standpoint taken will reflect the current evidence base, therefore if there was significant evidence to suggest that manipulation of relaxation therapy was potentially harmful, then testing of (H_1) or (H_0) above would be unlikely to secure ethical approval.

The Hawthorn effect (see Chapter 21) is the researcher impact on behaviour and performance (Roethlisberger and Dickson, 1939). This effect could have an impact on the research participants and subsequently on the dependent variable measures.

Internal and external validity

To establish the true relationship between the two variables being tested and nothing else, the researcher tries to limit the effect of any other variables that can be internal or external to the study. Internally, these can be biases or confounders. Biases may result at any stage of the study in the sample selection, data collection, analysis and interpretation of the results. The random allocation of matched participants aims to reduce sample bias. This, along with large sample sizes, also helps reduce confounding variables that may affect the dependent variable. In the example given above, a confounding variable may work in the same or a different way from the independent variable (the relaxation therapy), affecting the outcomes and dependent variable (the cachexia).

In order for the research findings to be generalisable to a wider population, external validity must be confirmed. This would enable the researcher to be confident in making recommendations for wider practice based on the research findings. To maximise external validity, the research participants must be selected and allocated randomly to either the experimental or the control group. The participants are not likely to be the same as the target population, but should be representative of them. For example, if the researcher is trying to look at patients' attitudes to rehabilitation therapy in cardiac care, then they may set inclusion and exclusion criteria to ensure that the initial population are cardiac care patients, and to ensure that the results can be generalised back to a cardiac care population.

Randomised controlled trials

The **randomised controlled trial (RCT)** is the 'gold standard' research design for use in evaluating the effectiveness of interventions (Centre for Reviews and Dissemination, 2001). It is used by healthcare professionals to develop an evidence-base for practice. Medicine has employed RCTs for some time (Whitehead, J., 1992), with drug trials often classified into the four stages shown in Table 13.1 (Pocock, 1983).

Within nursing there is the potential to employ RCTs to measure the effectiveness of practice delivery, comparing existing practices or evaluating new practices against those in existence, to provide an evidence base for practice. However, their use in nursing research has been limited. Literature reviews in the *Journal of Advanced Nursing* in 2002 identified 256 empirical papers, of which eight reported RCT use (Webb, 2004). This was felt to reflect a lack of understanding of RCT designs (Shuldham and Hiley, 1997), though reasons for late adoption are probably more complex. Whilst RCTs could support the development of a scientific base for nursing, it should also be acknowledged that the suggested criteria which must be met for a clinical trial in nursing, set out in 2005 (Burns and Grove, 2005), require the use of large patient samples, randomised into comparison groups to test a hypothesis. A number of nursing problems will not be open to hypothesis development and testing. Additionally, such trials require funding and support that may not be readily available to nursing researchers.

Table 13.1 Classification of clinical trials

Phases	Definition
Phase I	Initial drug testing, to establish safety and side effects, usually performed on human volunteers. Determine safe single dosage.
Phase II	Small-scale investigation with patients, with close monitoring.
Phase III	Compare drug treatment with standard treatments for a particular condition, often involving large number of patients. Rigorous, extensive investigation.
Phase IV	After regulatory approval the drug is subjected to monitoring for adverse effects; long-term effects on morbidity and mortality are conducted.

Source: Pocock, 1983

The RCT requires randomisation of the patients to the control and intervention groups through methods that are 'blinded', where those recruiting to the study are not involved in the process of allocation. This helps to reduce selection bias (Pocock, 1983). The control and intervention groups are from the same population, the only difference in treatment being that the intervention being tested is delivered to the intervention group only. In Box 13.1 the intervention group were repositioned on pressure-relieving mattresses more frequently than the control group.

Box 13.1   Example of a randomised controlled trial (RCT)

Vanderwee et al. (2007) measured the effectiveness of turning with unequal time intervals on the incidence of pressure sore lesions in Belgium. All eligible patients who gave informed consent (n = 235) were randomised into either the experimental (n = 122) or control group (n = 113). The intervention for the experimental group involved repositioning alternately, two hours in a lateral position and four hours in a supine position. The control group were repositioned every four hours, receiving normal practice. The European Advisory Panel grades were used to measure changes in pressure areas daily. They found no statistically significant difference in pressure sore severity between the two groups. They concluded that more frequent positioning on a pressure-relieving mattress would not necessarily provide more effective pressure sore prevention.

Given the importance of RCTs to the development of evidence-based practice, guidelines have been produced for authors to follow when presenting their findings. The CONSORT reporting of clinical trials (www.consort-statement.org/) is expected by a number of key nursing journals. These guidelines include headings and suggested content to support rigorous presentation. A range of critical review frameworks such as CASP (www.phru.nhs.uk/casp/casp.htm) (see Chapters 8 and 9) can be used to help those reading RCT papers to appraise the strengths of the trial, its validity and reliability.

Quasi-experiments

Having considered the characteristics necessary to conduct an experiment or RCT, it should be apparent that not all nursing research questions can be open to testing through such a rigorous true experimental design. When at least one of the three components of a true experiment (manipulation, control group, randomisation) is missing from a study, this is known as a **quasi-experimental design**. Researchers are not always able to randomly allocate participants or cases into either control or experimental groups to measure cause-and-effect relationships. There may be ethical or practical constraints that prevent an experimental or RCT design being used (Burns and Grove, 2007). For example, if nurses wanted to look at the effectiveness of

Table 13.2 Comparison design

Group type		Design stages	
Experimental group	pre-test	treatment	post-test
Comparison group	pre-test	no treatment	post-test

a new way of managing patient medication through self-administration, it would be difficult to research this within one setting, as having two systems running might cause confusion for patients and staff. It might be possible to organise the changes across two wards, introducing the new system within one whilst maintaining current practice in the other. In this example a new intervention is being introduced and compared with existing practice. There isn't true randomisation into control and experimental groups, but similar groups are being compared. This design doesn't allow the researcher to control for all of the extraneous variables, thus the cause-and-effect relationship measured isn't as certain, but strong. Thus, the researchers cannot be certain that any benefits to patient care seen in the intervention group are directly attributed to the change in medication administration.

There are a number of quasi-experimental designs available, such as the 'pre-test and post-test' sometimes known as the 'before-and-after'. Comparison group design with pre-test and post-test (see Table 13.2), as discussed above, is the most prevalent (Burns and Grove, 2007). In this design the participants are not randomly selected; the experimental group receives the intervention and the comparison group either receives no treatment or the treatment that is normally used.

If it is not possible to conduct a pre-test, such as when measuring the impact of a rehabilitation programme where there is no pre-test data, then a post-test measurement design is used that measures post-test data only. Such designs are limited by the lack of a comparison pre-test, which can threaten the studies' validity (Burns and Grove, 2007). See Box 13.2 for an example.

Box 13.2   Example of a before-and-after design in quasi-experimental research

Patterson et al. (2007) measured nurses' attitudes towards service users who self-harm repeatedly in a before-and-after design with two non-randomly allocated groups. Nurses' attitudes were collected on the first day of a 15-week accredited course on self-harm using a Self-harm Antipathy Scale. Further data were collected on the last day of the course and at least 18 months after completion. There was evidence of a 20 per cent reduction in antipathy towards patients who repeatedly self-harm. The educational intervention seemed to be effective in changing nurse attitudes to service users who self-harm.

Table 13.3   Dos and don'ts of experimental design

Dos	Don'ts
Do use to measure cause–effect.	Don't use when not trying to establish cause and effect.
In a pre-test and post-test design, do measure the outcome before and after intervention to allow comparison and measure effect.	In a pre-test and post-test design, comparisons cannot be made if pre-test and post-test data are not available.
Do include elements of randomisation, control and manipulation in an RCT.	Don't undertake an RCT without elements of randomisation, control and manipulation.
Do use a quasi-experimental design if unable to include all of the three components of an RCT.	Don't use a quasi-experimental design if all three components of an RCT are used.
Do seek ethical approval for experimental research.	Don't undertake experimental research without having gained ethical approval.

Ethical issues associated with experimental and quasi-experimental designs

Experimental and quasi-experimental designs are used to measure the effectiveness of a treatment or procedure, comparing this with existing practice in order to develop evidence-based care. Such research results in patients receiving treatments that have not been tried or tested and therefore there are possible disadvantages to being a member of either an experimental or a control group. It may be the case that patients will want to be part of the experimental group, in the hope that a new possible treatment may be more effective than those currently in use. This can lead to difficulties recruiting patients to the control group. To try to overcome these potential problems, researchers can obtain patient consent to take part in the research prior to allocation to either the control or the experimental group. However, as informed consent includes an option for patients to withdraw from the study at any time without prejudice, retention in the control group population may become an issue as the study progresses. Experimental and **survey designs** should be subjected to Ethical Committee Approval (see Chapters 4 and 5). The ethics committee members will want to ensure that the research will 'do the patient no harm' and that the benefits of the research are likely to outweigh any potential risks to the participants. Table 13.3 gives a list of dos and don'ts.

Survey designs

Surveys can be used to gather data through self-reporting about an identified and specific population. Data is collected through postal, telephone, online questionnaires or through interviews (Burns and Grove, 2005). Thus, the survey can collect important data as part of quasi-experimental, epidemiological (Abramson and Abramson, 1999) and other designs.

Descriptive surveys are not usually employed to provide information about a cause-and-effect relationship, but rather to describe a population, to study association between variables and establish trends and possible links between variables. Whilst they are easily completed, the findings may be questionable and are time-limited.

Correlation surveys aim to establish links between biographical data collected and behaviours or beliefs of the respondents. Comparative surveys measure the relationship between variables. Behaviours can be compared over time and related to age and class. Surveys can be conducted prospectively or retrospectively and over long periods. Prospective surveys explore what is likely to happen over a given period. Such a design could be used to explore how the lifestyle of those newly diagnosed with osteoporosis changes over time. Retrospective studies will, on the other hand, consider issues from the past. Here the researcher will draw on existing data. This can be a cost-effective approach, but has limitations related to the quality of the original data (Bowling, 2002). As the data was not originally collected for research purposes it may be incomplete and lack relevant information. Surveys may also be used in longitudinal, cross-sectional studies and **epidemiological research**, as described below.

Longitudinal and cross-section designs

Longitudinal designs are used to measure the effect of changes over time and include **trend, panel** and **follow-up** studies (Polit and Beck, 2006). They involve the collection of data at various points, sometimes from the same participants. Such a design leads to issues of attrition due to the longevity of interaction with the research, with the potential for large numbers of participants removing themselves from the study at various points in time (LoBiondo-Wood and Haber, 2006).

Trend studies explore how patterns change over time. They are used to try to predict future trends. This is achieved through sampling from a population over an extended period. One example might include research looking at the use of sun protection measures over time to forecast future development needs.

A panel study uses the same participants over a given time. Data are collected on two or more occasions. This design is useful to measure changes over time, such as identifying the characteristics of people who make healthy lifestyle changes following cardiac disease, as compared with those who don't.

The follow-up design involves seeing patients following a particular intervention or treatment to monitor progress. This design has been used in resuscitation research to monitor the long-term psychological effects of having witnessed resuscitation of a relative (Robinson et al., 1998).

Cross-sectional studies measure health outcomes or determinants of health in a population in either a short period or over a longer period. The design involves the collection of data from groups of people who are at different stages of their experience of a particular phenomenon. The design is limited as it relies on the collection of data from a number of groups rather than one group over time; this introduces the potential for difference between the groups.

Epidemiological research

Epidemiology is the study of disease occurrence, including where and why disease occurs amongst the population, and identification of the associated risk factors (Hennekens and Buring, 1987). It considers what the level of disease is, what factors place people at risk and the role of environmental factors in this (Bowling, 2002). This makes epidemiology important in maintaining a healthy population (Whitehead, 2000). Epidemiology can provide valuable information to support healthcare planning, through enabling the development of strategies that prevent disease occurrence and by supporting the implementation of management strategies for those with disease. Epidemiological research can, for example, support the development of immunisation programmes and changes in healthcare treatments.

Epidemiological research is often concerned with the collection of large data sets to support recommendations for healthcare practice and management. The approaches to data collection can include: case studies, surveys, case control studies, documentary analysis, cohort studies and RCTs or experiments (Bowling, 2002). Some of these are defined in Table 13.4. There is further discussion on these approaches to data collection in Chapter 21.

Table 13.4 Approaches to data collection in epidemiological research

Study type	Method
Case studies	Data from one or several cases is collected either prospectively or retrospectively. Often used to describe disease processes or treatment effects (Bowling, 2002).
Case control studies	Comparisons are made between the group who have been exposed to a risk factor or disease (case) and those without (control). Comparisons of existing or previous experiences can be made. Such studies are relatively cheap to conduct, though may have recall bias, inaccuracies and require large numbers of participants.
Documentary analysis	Epidemiologists can work with large official data sets where collected, such as registers of births and deaths, or morbidity data such as incidence of cancers. These documents provide current data for analysis, though there are limitations in data collection, with many countries worldwide unable to provide such detail.
Cohort studies	A group or cohort who have the same exposure to a condition or treatment are compared over a given period (often seen as longitudinal studies) with a group not exposed to the condition or treatment. Depending on the longevity of the study these can be time-consuming and costly.

Chapter summary

- Experimental research can take place in a number of settings and such designs are used to test either a research hypothesis or question.
- An experimental design includes characteristics of manipulation, control and randomisation.
- Experimental designs offer the best approach to test a hypothesis and measure a cause–effect relationship, though there are some limitations to their use in healthcare research.
- Randomised controlled trials are the 'gold standard' research design for use in evaluating the effectiveness of interventions.
- Usually at least one of the three components of a true experiment is missing from the quasi-experimental design (manipulation, control group, randomisation).
- Surveys can be used to gather data through self-reporting about an identified and specific population.
- Epidemiological research is often concerned with the collection of large data sets to support recommendations for healthcare practice and management.

References

Abramson, J. and Abramson, Z. (1999) *Survey Methods in Community Medicine*, 5th edition. Edinburgh: Churchill Livingstone.

Bowling, A. (2002) *Research Methods in Health: Investigating Health and Health Services*, 2nd edition. Buckingham: Open University Press.

Burns, N. and Grove, S. (2005) *The Practice of Nursing Research: Conduct, Critique and Utilisation*, 5th edition. St Louis, MO: Elsevier/Saunders.

Burns, N. and Grove, S. (2007) *Study Guide for Understanding Nursing Research: Building an Evidence-based Practice*. 4th edition. St Louis, MO: Saunders Elsevier.

Centre for Reviews and Dissemination (2001) *Undertaking Systematic Reviews of Research on Effectiveness*, 2nd edition. York: University of York, CRD.

Hennekens, C. and Buring, J. (1987) *Epidemiology in Medicine*. Boston, MA: Little, Brown.

LoBiondo-Wood, G. and Haber, J. (2006) *Nursing Research: Methods and Critical Appraisal for Evidence-based Practice*, 6th edition. St Louis, MO: Mosby Elsevier.

Patterson, P., Whittington, R. and Bogg, J. (2007) 'Testing the effectiveness of an educational intervention aimed at changing attitudes to self-harm', *Journal of Psychiatric and Mental Health Nursing,* 14: 100–105.

Pocock, J. (1983) *Clinical Trials: A Practical Approach*. Chichester: John Wiley.

Polit, D. and Beck, C. (2006) *Essentials of Nursing Research: Methods, Appraisal and Utilization*, 6th edition. Philadelphia, PA: Lippincott Williams & Wilkins.

Robinson, S., MacKenzie-Ross, S., Campbell-Henson, G., Egleston, C. and Prevost, A. (1998) 'Psychological effect of witnessed resuscitation on bereaved relatives', *Lancet*, 352 (9128): 614–17.

Roethlisberger, F. and Dickson, W. (1939) *Management and the Worker*. Cambridge, MA: Harvard University Press.

Shuldham, C. and Hiley, C. (1997) 'Randomised controlled trials in clinical practice: the continuing debate', *Nursing Times Research*, 2 (2): 128–34.

Vanderwee, K., Grypdonck, M., De Bacquer, D. and Defloor, T. (2007) 'Effectiveness of turning with unequal time intervals on the incidence of pressure ulcer lesions', *Journal of Advanced Nursing*, 57 (1): 59–68.

Webb, C. (2004) 'Editor's note. Analysis of papers published in JAN in 2002', *Journal of Advanced Nursing*, 45 (3): 229–31.

Whitehead, D. (2000) 'Is there a place for epidemiology in nursing?', *Nursing Standard*, 14 (42): 35–8.

Whitehead, J. (1992) *The Design and Analysis of Sequential Clinical Trials*. New York: Ellis Horwood.

Suggested further reading

Abramson, J. and Abramson, Z. (1999) *Survey Methods in Community Medicine*, 5th edition. Edinburgh: Churchill Livingstone.

Alreck, P. and Settle, R. (1995) '*The Survey Research Handbook: Guidelines and Strategies for Conducting a Survey*', 2nd edition. New York: McGraw-Hill.

Cook, T. and Campbell, D. (1979) *Quasi-experimental Design and Analysis Issues for Field Settings*. Chicago, IL: Rand McNally.

Mulhall, A. (1996) *Epidemiology, Nursing and Healthcare: A New Perspective*. Basingstoke: Palgrave Macmillan.

Pocock, J. (1983) *Clinical Trials: A Practical Approach*, Chichester: John Wiley.

Whitehead, J. (1992) *The Design and Analysis of Sequential Clinical Ttrials*, New York: Ellis Horwood.

Websites

CASP critical review framework: www.phru.nhs.uk/casp/casp.htm
CONSORT – reporting on clinical trials: www.consort-statement.org/
Website to use for randomisation: www.randomisation.com

14

QUALITATIVE RESEARCH APPROACHES

Nurse researchers tend to use qualitative research approaches to look at questions around life experiences, beliefs, motivations, actions and perceptions of patients and staff. Rather than aiming to test a hypothesis, as is often the case in quantitative research, qualitative approaches look to support the interpretation and understanding of human experience. They allow the researcher to focus on interpreting social settings, such as the ward or community environment.

Qualitative approaches facilitate the exploration of relationships and human experience within the research setting. Three main approaches are used: phenomenology, ethnography and grounded theory. Whilst all are qualitative research approaches they differ in many respects, including overall aim, data collection methods and analysis.

To enable understanding of individual experience and perception the researcher is close to the participants during the research, especially as part of the data collection, and may even be part of the research setting. Researchers use interactive methods of data collection, and often the participants are involved in verifying the interpretation of meaning drawn from analysis of the data. The findings can be presented as a set of descriptions, themes, theories and frameworks or models for practice.

In this chapter we discuss phenomenology, ethnography and grounded theory as the main qualitative approaches. We start by revisiting the characteristics of qualitative research (see Chapter 11) and the role it plays in developing nursing knowledge. For issues associated with maintaining rigour in qualitative research, see Chapter 12.

Learning outcomes

This chapter is designed to enable the reader to:

- **Understand the three main qualitative research approaches**
- **Identify the differences between the approaches**

KEY TERMS

Emic perspective, Ethnography, Etic perspective, Grounded theory, Hermeneutics, Phenomenology, Thick description

---

Qualitative approaches

There are a number of key characteristics shared by qualitative research approaches.

- Qualitative research is most commonly part of inductive reasoning, starting with a set of observations of a situation and moving to the generation of ideas and in some cases theory.
- The setting for the research is usually 'natural' and the researcher is immersed within it.
- The focus of the research is generally the views, experiences and perceptions of the participants.
- The researcher aims to take a holistic view, seeing the whole picture.
- Data collection and analysis may inter-relate and be flexible and reflexive.

Inductive reasoning

Typically, induction or inductive reasoning is seen as part of qualitative research where the aim is to develop concepts and themes from the interpretation of observations and interviews. Inductive reasoning is a process of starting with the details of an experience or our observations of something, and using these to develop a general understanding of phenomena. Specific observations and descriptions are made and used to develop a hypothesis and theory of a more general situation that can be tested. The researcher enters the research arena ready to learn and aims to gather a range of material, which is interrogated and open to scrutiny in order to draw understandings. The researcher will be trying to gain a clearer picture of the problems and issues through the analysis of data gathered through observations and discussions. This inductive approach to research is therefore helpful in exploring those areas of practice and care where there is currently limited understanding or where the current explanations are limited and fail to reflect individual experiences. Say, for example, a new practice role has been developed and implemented within cancer care. Using an inductive approach would allow the researcher to explore patient, manager and new practitioner perspectives and experiences of the role that might further inform its use and development. Through observations the researcher would be trying to identify what the issues and problems might be and what is happening as a result of implementing the role. The researcher would analyse data collected and reflect on the meaning of this, whilst also thinking about their own preconceptions in relation to the research.

A variety of data collection methods, such as observation, interviews, analysis of written data, is used to generate ideas, concepts and possibly theory. Often researchers work with participants, who verify or check interpretations. The researchers are keen to ensure impartiality in analysis and present interpretations that reflect the participant perspective.

Natural setting

Qualitative nurse researchers collect data in the natural or real world setting and may enter a number of different environments to study different phenomena. Denzin and Lincoln (2000) suggest that study in the natural setting allows researchers to make sense of and interpret phenomena. Depending on the qualitative approach, data collection may require the researcher to be present in the research setting for prolonged periods, for example to collect observational data of nurses working within a particular care environment. The researcher is aiming to follow the participants into their 'natural environment', which in healthcare could be a range of clinical or community care settings and home environments.

Participant perspective

Qualitative researchers believe the participants or research subjects are able to provide data on their experience of the social world that others can interpret and make sense of. The relationship between the researcher and participant is important to the achievement of the research. LoBiondo-Wood and Haber (2006) suggest that the research may influence the participants, but that the researcher is also affected and should be open to the participants, to avoid attaching their own meaning to the experience. The researcher needs to remain open to the ideas of the participants gained through listening and observing.

Holistic view

The nurse researcher is interested in the entire and whole human experience. The researcher will want to explore the complete experience, considering the context and inter-related factors affecting the participant. For example, when considering the user experience of a mental health condition, it could emerge that a number of situations are important components of the experience. The workplace, home situation, family relations, friends, healthcare staff and treatments can all impact on the overall experience. Through listening to the individual's complete story, these inter-related aspects will emerge.

Inter-related processes

A number of data collection methods are available that can be used flexibly. The researcher can collect data through interviewing, conducting focus group discussions, observing practice delivery and interactions or analysing video or digital recording, written diaries and text. Whilst there may be an initial suggested number of participants or observation episodes, the final sample total will be determined as the research progresses. The researcher has the scope to either increase or reduce the number of interactions involved depending on the quality of the data obtained during the data collection process, and provided any changes sit within the ethical approval obtained. For example, Huang et al. (2008) wanted to understand the coping experiences of carers living with a schizophrenic family member. Purposive sampling and in-depth, face-to-face interviews were used to collect data. The research team was unclear initially what the total sample size would be. As data collection and analysis progressed, they felt they had reached data saturation, and didn't need to collect any further data when the sample size comprised 10 carers (5 men and 5 women).

The process of data collection is flexible and can be guided by the participants. Open questioning, starting the interview with an overall question, allows the researcher to react to the interview situation and explore particular aspects or issues in more depth. The researcher will want to gain insight into the experiences and perceptions of the participant, so will use the data collection techniques to effectively achieve this. This process requires some skill and training and may require some innovation and creativity in approach, using the interaction to gain deeper insight into the main issues.

Phenomenology

Phenomenological approaches are rooted in philosophy (Beck, 1994). The origins can be traced to Immanuel Kant in the 18th century (Moran, 2000), though popular views site the origins with the work of German philosopher Husserl in the 20th century, who developed the philosophy that sought to describe human experience as legitimate without the need for external analysis (Baker et al., 1992). The work was subsequently adapted by a number of philosophers, notably Heidegger (Groenewald, 2004). Phenomenologists believe it is possible to understand human behaviour by describing and interpreting human experience within the context of that experience. They believe that meaning and truth can be drawn from people's lived experiences. In other words, through accessing and interpreting the experience of a patient with cancer, we can draw meaning and understanding of what it is like to live with cancer.

There are some important ideas underpinning **phenomenology**. First, phenomenological research seeks to gather life experiences, describe them and reflect on them.

Everyday experiences were described as 'lifeworld' by Husserl, though are more usually known as 'lived experiences'. These 'lived experiences' provide powerful data that can provide insights useful beyond the immediate case of research, described by Husserl as 'essences'. Common themes can be seen within the data that relate to the context and time of collection. These are presented in the data to show how themes identified in people's stories are linked and related. For example, Sweeney et al. (2007) explored the experiences of people living with a supra-pubic catheter. Data was collected through in-depth interviews with six adults living in the community who had a supra-pubic catheter for long-term urinary bladder drainage. Interpretation of the data occurred via thematic analysis of the participants' stories. They presented two distinct but interrelated themes: adjustment to life with a catheter and feelings of being unprepared or supported as they learned to live with a supra-pubic catheter. These two common themes were used to present the 'essences' of the six people living with a supra-pubic catheter.

The second concept seen in phenomenology is that of 'bracketing'. Husserl suggested researchers needed to remove their preconceptions from the field of data collection through 'phenomenological reduction'. This was meant to enable the researcher to enter the field with an open mind and be able to study phenomena without the burden of preconception. Often researchers will write down or record their preconceptions in some way and acknowledge them in order to be disciplined in data collection and to ensure they are aware of their own views and open to listening to the experiences of others.

As nursing works with a patient-centred approach to care delivery and attempts to keep the patient at the forefront, phenomenology can provide an important evidence base for practice. A number of researchers have used phenomenology to try to understand the experiences of patients and provide descriptions and reflections such as Sweeney et al. (2007) that can help nurses gain insight into the patient 'lived experience'. Having some understanding of 'what it is like' can support the development of empathy and patient-centred care.

Phenomenological research in nursing is usually described as having two main branches: descriptive and interpretive.

Descriptive phenomenology

The approach was conceived initially by Husserl (1962) and is also associated with Giorgi (1997). Descriptive phenomenology seeks to see researchers enter the field with an open mind, leaving preconceptions behind. Researchers should seek to complete descriptions that encompass a full range of everyday life experiences, which are gathered by the participants through what is heard, seen, felt, remembered, acted on and decided (Polit and Beck, 2006). Given the need to be open-minded, one of the main aspects of this approach includes the concept of 'bracketing'. The researcher identifies any preconceived ideas and beliefs about the phenomena under study, recognises and withholds these from the research. The researcher will record a reflexive journal or diary of the research to help maintain 'bracketing', recording their thinking and views. Despite this there can be difficulties in trying to 'remove' beliefs and preconceived thoughts from a research process.

The researchers are interested in identifying the 'essences', those themes that best describe the lived experience, what is common but also where the differences might be. For example, in looking at the lived experience of learning disabilities clients and a period of hospitalisation, we may find that there are common experiences of preparation for admission and poor discharge planning, though there may be differences in these experiences based on whether the admission was planned or an emergency.

Interpretive phenomenology

Heidegger, as a student of Husserl, developed interpretive phenomenology. He felt that understanding the lived experience was more important than merely describing it and termed **hermeneutics** as understanding the human experience. Interpretive phenomenologists do not 'bracket' themselves. Hermeneutic phenomenologists aim to be open to any new perspectives, but they may draw on preconceptions to enable them to appreciate what is new and different. Polit and Beck (2006) suggest the goal of the approach is to discover understanding, wisdom and possibilities from the study of another world. Hermeneutic phenomenologists are more likely to develop 'fusions of horizons' than 'essences'. The presentation is less concerned with providing a specific conclusion presented by descriptive phenomenologists, but offers a story or picture that allows the reader to draw interpretations and meaning for their own use.

Phenomenologists work with purposive samples (see Chapter 19), including participants who have the relevant 'lived experiences' to talk about in the study. For example, a study interested in parents' experiences of caring for children with leukaemia would seek to ensure that the participants had these experiences. They need not necessarily be current experiences, as stories can be accessed retrospectively, but often recent stories are drawn on. Data collection is generally through in-depth interviews (see Chapter 21) that are guided by the participants. Experiences can also be accessed through diaries and autobiographies. Data is analysed to identify interrelated themes and insights through processes of qualitative data analysis (see Chapter 23). The data is analysed to ensure that meanings are extracted, which requires reading the whole text. There are a number of different approaches used to support analysis; Van Manen (1994) presents a less systematic method, though approaches to analysis, such as that proposed by Giorgi and Giorgi (2004), can be used. This systematic approach involves reading the text, dividing it into meaning units, identifying meaning units in transferable and general ways, presenting common themes and experiences and illustrating these using quotations from the text to support their findings (see Giorgi and Giorgi, 2004). Sweeney et al. (2007) report a process of data analysis that includes being immersed in the data throughout the process of data collection and undertaking analysis by reading and re-reading the data:

> Immersion occurred at interview, during the transcription of the text, listening to the audio-tapes, and during the reading and re-reading of the data. Through thematic analysis of the textual data, interpretations were reconstructed to reveal common meanings and understanding of 'what it is like to live with a supra-pubic catheter. (Sweeney et al., 2007: 420)

In Box 14.1 an example is given of how hermeneutics is employed.

Box 14.1   Example of the use of hermeneutics

Mitchell (2007) aimed to describe the social and emotional effects of chemotherapy as experienced by patients. Hermeneutic phenomenology was employed to access patient's detailed stories of their experiences of chemotherapy. The researchers were expected to contribute to the data by acknowledging their own perspective and understanding of oncology treatment. They also worked in a reflexive way when collecting the data through individual interviews and in analysis where the researchers were able to look across and between the data obtained from the 19 participants and 98 interviews. The participants also recorded a diary of experience. The research team drew understanding for the data presented within themes that included the need to 'strive for normality', the 'role of significant others' including family and partners, 'feeling up/feeling down' and 'flagging', the feeling of fatigue.

Ethnography

Hammersley and Atkinson (1995) suggest there is some disagreement about the term **ethnography**, with diversity in definition and process. They go on to offer a definition that reflects the anthropological traditions (the study of human kind) of the approach, describing ethnography in this way:

> [I]t involves the ethnographer participating, either overtly or covertly, in people's daily lives for an extended period of time, watching what happens, listening to what is said, asking questions – in fact, collecting whatever data are available to throw light on issues that are the focus of the research. (Hammersley and Atkinson, 1995: 1)

Ethnography means a 'portrait of people' and involves writing about people and culture, providing descriptions of a group, such as intensive care nurses, and the culture they work in, the routines, rituals and customs of the intensive care unit and the roles of the people within it. An ethnographic approach is used to describe and interpret how the behaviour of people is influenced by the culture they live in. It is characterised by the researcher entering the 'natural' field to gather in-depth data. The researcher is described as 'going native', a phrase developed by the early studies of ethnographers such as Margaret Mead, who lived among the tribes of Papua New Guinea in the 1930s in order to understand them (Haralambos et al., 2004). As well as being characterised by the researcher entering the field and being immersed in the culture, the approach aims to gather the (emic) 'insider' perspective, so that a 'thick' and detailed analytical description can be provided of the people and culture. Ethnography would be seen as part of an inductive approach, where specific observations and details of an experience are used to develop a general understanding of phenomena.

Ethnographers use the term **emic perspective** to mean gaining the insider view, gathering data from those inside the culture, those who understand the rules, ways of working and are part of the culture. For example, if we were studying midwifery, practising midwives would have an emic perspective, being a member of the profession and practising as midwives either in hospital or community settings. The researcher going into the setting to gather data would have an **etic perspective**, entering the culture from the outside. The ethnographer, through their 'etic' position, presents the 'emic' perspective in a story that describes the culture and the positioning of the people within it.

The sample used is often purposive (see Chapter 19), in that a specific setting or population is selected for study. This might include maternity care, intensive care, student nurses studying mental health or patients' rehabilitation recovering from spinal injury. The selection is systematic (Hammersley and Atkinson, 1995), to ensure that the participants have the necessary experience and immersion with the culture to provide the 'emic' perspective.

As with other research approaches, the ethnographer needs to operate within ethical principles (see Chapters 5 and 6). It is less likely that ethical approval would be given for participant observation methods that included a covert observation role, where the researcher role is hidden. The researcher will be expected to operate with informed consent in place, allowing participants' scope to consent to take part in the research and with an option to withdraw from a study at any time without prejudice.

Data is predominantly collected through participant observation (see Chapter 18). Ethnographers will observe practice, interactions and behaviours, listen to conversations and ask questions. They may also gather data from documentation and through interviews. Ethnographers will maintain a fieldwork diary, recording their initial thoughts and interpretations of the culture. Ethnographic researchers may well operate from a position of reciprocity, where the intimacy of the relationship between the researcher and the participants is acknowledged and the researcher 'gives something back' to the participants. The development of reciprocity is advocated by Hammersley and Atkinson (1995), who believed the ethnographer should avoid merely exploiting the participant.

Data is analysed using the processes described in Chapter 23, which enable the researcher to interact with the data to develop key themes. The key stages include organisation of data such as a fieldwork diary, observational records and other data, reading and re-reading, reviewing observations, coding the data, reducing the codes to larger categories, looking for patterns across the categories and organising the data into themes and subthemes. The process may also include a process of verification of the analysis with the participants.

Fieldwork allows the researcher to produce a detailed account of the group culture and working, described as **thick description**. The thick description is an analysis of the group culture, a view of its patterns of working, member relationships, meanings and functions.

In presenting an ethnographic study, the nurse researcher will produce a rich and holistic description of the cultural setting. Interpretations of the culture are drawn, describing behaviour patterns seen. This is illustrated in Box 14.2.

Box 14.2   Example of an ethnographic study

Simmons (2007) used ethnography to study the introduction of the nurse consultant role. She was an insider researcher, occupying the role of senior nurse manager. A purposive sample of nurse consultants was selected to take part in the study. Ethical approval was in place prior to data collection. The study commenced by describing organisational and policy contexts. The fieldwork was completed with six nurse consultants. This included five days of participant observation split across a two-year period. As a participant observer Simmons chose a passive role, where she was predominantly an observer, shadowing the nurse consultants in the main. Simmons also discussed her need to demonstrate reciprocity (a reciprocal relationship between the ethnographer and participants), which she felt was achieved through taking on the role of a critical friend to those nurses involved in the study.

Grounded theory

Grounded theory was developed in the 1960s by sociologists Glaser and Strauss (1967). Grounded theory is a method that usually starts with specific observations and analysis of data collected to generate ideas or a theory, therefore usually working in an inductive way, but can develop to use deductive reasoning. Its whole purpose is to generate theories or hypotheses (see Chapter 6), and it is often used to study new research areas. The theory emerges from systematically collected and analysed research data. Once the hypotheses or theories are developed they can be tested through deductive research, an approach that tests a hypothesis through mainly quantitative designs, and the results will either support the predicted hypothesis or not.

Grounded theory has its foundations in 'symbolic interactionism' developed by Margaret Mead in the 1920s and 1930s, which focuses on explaining social processes, such as the way people make sense of social interactions and interpret them. It has the potential to support our understanding of human behaviour and how people interact. It is therefore important in supporting the study of nursing and healthcare where the understanding of human interaction and behaviours are important for improving care delivery and practice. For example, grounded theory may be used to develop an approach to managing the care of transgender patients in the hospital that supports them. Through data collection and analysis a theory can be developed about what happens when transgender patients are confronted with hospital admission for surgery and how the patients deal with it.

Grounded theory is very much 'grounded' in the field. For example, the research problem is often identified in the field. The types of research questions that might be explored include: What is happening in the research setting? What interactions occur in the setting? What are people's experiences and what do they mean? How is work organised? What is needed to improve things? Thinking of our example in Box 14.3, the questions may include 'How are Transgender (TG) patients identified by staff?' and 'How do staff react to TG patients?' The processes of sampling, data collection and analysis occur simultaneously. Nurse researchers will identify a sample, collect some data, analyse the data and identify categories, then describe the emerging issues before re-entering the process of sample, collection and analysis. Data collection employs in-depth interviews in the main, though observations and documentary analysis may also be used. It is suggested that up to 50 participants might be involved in in-depth interviewing (Polit and Beck, 2006).

A process of theoretical sampling is used, where the sample selection is guided by the emerging issues. The initial sample will be composed of key individuals in the research setting who will be able to talk about the research issue – perhaps in our example this would be the ward manager. Data is analysed, and as concepts and issues emerge the researcher will select further samples, either individuals or events, that they believe will provide further insight and contributions to developing the initial findings. So, for example, analysis of data may suggest that the researchers need to interview key staff involved in patient admissions. This can raise some challenges for the researcher as initial ethical approval processes may not account for the scope of the sample used and there may be a requirement to have ongoing dialogue with the ethics committee.

The researchers employ 'constant comparison' to identify the main problem and develop and refine the emerging categories. The categories identified from the new data collected are compared constantly with the initial identified categories. Researchers look for commonalities and differences in the data and use this process to collapse the number of categories. Data collection becomes more focused as time progresses and the researchers concentrate on the key emerging theoretical issues in data collection. The process of data analysis includes: constant comparison, data coding, reduction of codes and development of categories, developing links between the categories and developing a core category used to develop a theory. For example, research exploring TG patient experiences of hospitalisation could generate the following codes and core category: 'unsure how to care, lack of understanding, lack of experience' that might be linked to the code of 'unprepared for TG patients'.

More recently Strauss has published with Corbin an approach to grounded theory that challenges some of the earlier thinking presented in the 1960s (see Strauss and Corbin, 1990). You can read more on this debate in Boychuck Duchscher and Morgan (2004).

An example is given in Box 14.3.

Box 14.3   Example of the use of grounded theory

Mooney (2007) used a grounded theory approach when studying the insights of newly qualified nurses into their pre-registration preparation. In-depth interviews were used to collect data from 12 nurses working in one hospital location. Mooney used Strauss and Corbin's approach, with simultaneous collection, coding and analysis of data. After the initial interview, subsequent data collection was based on the emerging concepts identified previously. Data analysis began during the interviews and continued throughout transcription. Coding was used to identify subcategories from which categories were developed as analysis progressed, using what Strauss and Corbin (1998) call 'axial' coding. Two categories were finally identified as 'learning on the edge' and 'feeling like a shadow'.

Chapter summary

- The three main qualitative research approaches are: phenomenology, ethnography and grounded theory.
- Qualitative research can be described as 'inductive reasoning'.
- Inductive reasoning starts with a set of specific observations of a situation and moves to the generation of a general theory or hypothesis.
- The qualitative research setting is 'natural' and the researcher is immersed within it.
- The researcher gains the views, experiences and perceptions of the participants.
- The researcher aims to take a holistic view, seeing the whole picture.

- Data collection and analysis may inter-relate and be flexible and reflexive.
- Phenomenology aims to explore the life experience of individuals and explain what it means.
- Ethnography is used to describe and interpret how the behaviour of people is influenced by the culture they live in.
- Grounded theory starts with a set of observations of a situation and moves to the generation of ideas and theory. Its whole purpose is to generate hypotheses or a theory.

References

Baker, C., Wuest, J. and Stern, P. (1992) 'Method slurring: the grounded theory/phenomenology example', *Journal of Advanced Nursing*, 17: 1355–60.

Beck, C. (1994) 'Phenomenology: its use in nursing research', *International Journal of Nursing Studies*, 31 (6): 499–510.

Boychuck Duchscher, J. and Morgan, D. (2004) 'Grounded theory: reflections on the emergence vs. forcing debate', *Journal of Advanced Nursing*, 48 (6): 605–12.

Denzin, N. and Lincoln, Y. (2002) 'Introduction to the discipline and practice of qualitative research', in N. Denzin and Y. Lincoln (eds), *Handbook of Qualitative Research*. Thousand Oaks, CA: Sage. Chapter 1, pp. 1–28.

Giorgi, A. (1997) 'The theory, practice and evaluation of the phenomenological method as a qualitative research procedure', *Journal of Phenomenological Psychology*, 28: 235–60.

Giorgi, A. and Giorgi, B. (2004) 'The descriptive phenomenological psychology method', in P. Camic, J. Rhodes and L. Yardley (eds), *Qualitative Research in Psychology: Expanding Perspectives in Methodology and Design*. Washington, DC: American Psychology Association. pp. 243–74.

Glaser, B. and Strauss, A. (1967) *The Discovery of Grounded Theory*. Chicago, IL: Aldine.

Groenewald, T. (2004) 'A phenomenological research design illustrated', *International Journal of Qualitative Methods,* 3 (1): Article 4.

Hammersley, M. and Atkinson, P. (1995) *Ethnography: Principles in Practice*, 2nd edition. London: Routledge.

Haralambos, M., Holborn, M. and Heald, R. (2004) *Sociology, Themes and Perspectives*, 6th edition. London: Collins.

Huang, X., Sun, F., Yen, W. and Fu, C. (2008) 'The coping experiences of carers who live with someone who has schizophrenia', *Journal of Clinical Nursing*, 17 (6): 817–26.

Husserl, E. (1962) *Ideas: General Introduction to Pure Phenomenology*. New York: Macmillan.

LoBiondo-Wood, G. and Haber, J. (2006) *Nursing Research: Methods and Critical Appraisal for Evidence-based Practice*, 6th edition. St Louis, MO: Mosby Elsevier.

Mitchell, T. (2007) 'The social and emotional toll of chemotherapy – patients' perspective', *European Journal of Cancer Care*, 16 (1): 39–47.

Mooney, M. (2007) 'Newly qualified Irish nurses' interpretation of their preparation and experiences of registration', *Journal of Clinical Nursing*, 16 (9): 1610–17.

Moran, D. (2000) *Introduction to Phenomenology*. London: Routledge.

Polit, D. and Beck, C. (2006) *Essentials of Nursing Research: Methods, Appraisal and Utilization*, 6th edition. Philadelphia, PA: Lippincott Williams & Wilkins.

Simmons, M. (2007) 'Insider ethnography: tinker, tailor, researcher or spy', *Nurse Researcher*, 14 (4): 7–17.

Strauss, A. and Corbin, J. (1998) *Basics of Qualitative Research: Grounded Theory, Procedures and Techniques*. Thousand Oaks, CA: Sage.

Sweeney, A., Harrington, A. and Button, D. (2007) 'Supra-pubic catheters – a shared understanding, from the other side looking in', *The Journal of Wound, Ostomy and Continence Nursing*, 34 (4): 418–24.

Van Manen, M. (1994) *Researching Lived Experience: Human Science for an Action-sensitive Pedagogy*. London and Ontario: Althouse Press.

Suggested further reading

Hammersley, M. and Atkinson, P. (1995) *Ethnography: Principles in Practice*, 2nd edition. London: Routledge.

Silverman, D. (ed.) (2004) *Qualitative Research: Theory, Method and Practice*, 2nd edition. London: Sage.

Strauss, A. and Corbin, J. (1990) *Basics of Qualitative Research. Grounded Theory Procedures and Techniques*. Thousand Oaks, CA: Sage.

Websites

Association for Qualitative Research Journal, a dedicated resource for qualitative research in the human sciences: www.latrobe./edu.au/aqr/index.php?option=content&task=view&id=17&Itemid=35

Online journal for qualitative research, *The Qualitative Report*: www.nova.edu/ssss/QR/web.html

Peer reviewed *Qualitative Social Research Journal*: www.qualitative-research.net/fqs/fqs-eng.htm

15

EVALUATION AND OUTCOMES-BASED RESEARCH

The 1960s and 1970s saw the emergence of a distinct field of applied research known as evaluation research (Robbins, 1998). These decades were also characterised by an increasing concern about, and the need to assess, the quality, effectiveness and impact of large and more complex state-funded organisations such as the NHS.

Within UK healthcare services, and particularly in the NHS, the emphasis tends to be one of 'what counts is what works' (Rownsley, 2001). This is demonstrated by the National Institute for Clinical Excellence (NICE) and the National Service Frameworks which aim to promote a base for good quality and cost-effective clinical interventions. NICE even has a remit to consider the funding of interventions that are not effective (Brown et al., 2003). There are, therefore, pressures to demonstrate effectiveness not only of healthcare innovations but also of existing procedures and interventions as a way of confirming that available resources are used in the most effective and efficient way. One way of doing this is by undertaking formal evaluations. The usual aim of such evaluations or evaluation research is to investigate how well an intervention, practice or policy is working and, for nursing, the focus will often be on patient care and delivery systems.

This chapter explains what evaluation research is, why we do it and how to do it. Evaluation research in healthcare is frequently based on the collection of data about the structure, inputs, process, output and outcomes of a service, and these will provide the main guide for the chapter alongside discussion of the practicalities associated with undertaking evaluation research projects.

Learning outcomes

This chapter is designed to enable the reader to:

- Understand evaluation research and its role in healthcare and healthcare services
- Be able to identify the way different research designs can be utilised in evaluation research
- Describe some of the outcome measures that are used in evaluation research
- Appreciate the practicalities associated with the conduct of evaluation research in healthcare and healthcare services

---

KEY TERMS

Audit, Evaluation research, Outcomes, Process, Structure

Evaluation: what is it and why do it?

Evaluation research is a form of applied research that is designed to address current issues or questions about the way a service functions or the impact of services, care programmes or policies. Its practical orientation and direct links to care and healthcare practice is one of its distinguishing features (Clarke, 2001). Evaluation research and **audit** are often linked together in health services. However, it is important to remember that audit records that a change has or has not occurred, whereas evaluation is concerned with determining the reasons why, as well as what, change(s) have occurred.

In everyday use, evaluation refers to the making of judgements about the worth or value of something. This can be a subjective assessment, such as determining the literary merit of a new book. Evaluation can also refer to a more formalised or systematic process undertaken by researchers or professional evaluators. This formal evaluation is effectively a 'disciplined enquiry' in which scientific procedures are used to collect and analyse information or data about a planned intervention, such as a policy, practice or service (Lincoln and Guba, 1986).

Evaluation research makes use of the tools and techniques of basic research and applies them to research questions about need, efficiency, effectiveness, appropriateness and acceptability. It is, however, different from basic research because it does not aim to be value free and unbiased. Robbins (1998) suggests that evaluation research probably

219

works best when it embraces the values and norms of the service, programme or policy in order to be able to make judgements about that which is being investigated. For example, evaluation of a revised induction programme for newly qualified nurses will need to take into account the organisation's reasons for changing the induction programme and the context in which the programme is delivered.

The increasing prominence of evaluation research is associated with demands to ensure that healthcare delivery is of a consistently high quality, evidence-based, effective and efficient. It has been suggested (Gray, 1997) that decision making by healthcare practitioners, managers and policy makers (regardless of the way decisions are made or the level at which they are taken) is usually informed by three sets of factors:

1   Values held by the individuals making the decisions
2   Available resources
3   Evidence derived from research about what denotes good and effective practice.

A reliance on evidence to underpin the decision-making process has become more evident with increasing pressure on resources and a need to 'justify' the 'worth' of any intervention. These pressures are reinforced by an increasing awareness of what medicine can do on the part of potential users of healthcare services and of their rights to care. In the UK, the role of NICE in determining best practice, the development of National Service Frameworks (NSFs) (DoH, 1997), clinical governance (DoH, 1999) and a general call for the practice of evidence-based care (DoH, 1996) all serve to create a demand for evaluations of existing healthcare practices and services. Associated with this reliance on evidence-based practice is an expectation that new interventions and new ways of working are formally evaluated to ensure that they are actually delivering the care expected and meeting patients' needs in terms of quantity and quality as well as being cost-effective. This effectively means that in healthcare the focus tends to be on evaluation(s) of:

• the effectiveness of interventions
• the impact of new ways of working
• structured healthcare programmes targeted at specific patient groups
• the quality of care provision.
  (Clarke, 2001)

Are all evaluations the same?

Evaluation research can be divided into two types: formative and summative (Bowling, 2002). In formative evaluation the aim is to enable improvements or develop a programme, intervention or service by collecting data whilst it is still active. Summative evaluations involve the collection of data about a programme, intervention or service with the aim of deciding whether it should continue or be repeated. For example, deciding if a smoking cessation programme should be repeated or whether discharge co-ordinators improve discharge procedures. In summative evaluations the data collection can be active or inactive.

In healthcare and healthcare services the collection of data usually focuses on the structure, process and outcome (Donabedian, 1980).

- **Structure** refers to the organisational framework for an activity or care-giving environment. These will include facilities, healthcare professionals and ancillary workers and resources available, for example, number of qualified nurses available at any one time.
- **Process** refers to the activities themselves and how services are organised and delivered. This can include the collection of quantitative data, for example the number of patients being treated and waiting time to see a GP. It can also include the collection of qualitative data, such as details about the interactions between different professional groups and nurse–patient interactions.
- **Outcome** refers to the effectiveness or impact of any intervention in relation to the individuals and communities. For example, reduction in the number of teenage pregnancies following the introduction of a new advisory service in schools. Health outcome relates to the impact of the intervention on a patient, that is, the effectiveness on the health status of the individual (Bowling, 2002).

The structure and process can influence effectiveness, and outcomes are identified as an effectiveness criterion that can be confidently attributed to antecedent care (Donabedian, 1988). In other words, the reasons for a change in practice, policy or service are directly linked to the structures and/or processes relating to that practice, policy or service.

What approaches can be used?

There have been numerous attempts to categorise or make sense of the possible approaches that could be used for evaluation. The type of approach used will be dependent not only on what is being evaluated (intervention, practice or policy), but also on the types of measurement that it will be possible to make; whether it is possible, or desirable, to have firm goals and objectives for the evaluation; the setting where the evaluation will be conducted and the experience and, possibly, philosophical stance of the evaluator. Examples of some of the approaches that can be used are given below.

- Traditionally, a *goal-orientated approach* has been used in evaluation research. Here the aim is to measure the extent to which an intervention has achieved specific goals and objectives. The goals, therefore, need to be precise and measurable but will not necessarily be applicable to other services and so the evaluation may not give generalisable results.

Experimental methods tend to be used in the goal-orientated approach. They will often be large scale, with expert evaluators being used to reduce the possibility of bias that may arise if healthcare professionals collect their own data. It may, however, be possible to avoid some of the risk of bias by ensuring, wherever possible, that the outcome measures are objective. An example of this type of approach is given in Box 15.1.

Box 15.1   Examples of a goal-orientated and goal-free evaluation

A Clinical Nurse Specialist (CNS) running a nurse-led continence clinic wishes to evaluate the effectiveness of the advice she provides.

If she uses a *goal-orientated* approach she will need to set out precise and measurable outcomes of effectiveness from the outset of the evaluation process.

Effectiveness could be defined as whether attendance improves continence, and one intended outcome could be a 25 per cent reduction in the number of incontinent episodes for patients with stress-incontinence and measuring the number of incontinent episodes at the 1st and 5th advice sessions. She will need to ensure that improvement is the result of her advice and that it would not have been achieved by the usual advice/management. This could be done by randomly allocating patients to an intervention group (who get the CNS advice) or to a control group (who receive the usual advice/management).

The evaluation will need to include a sufficient number of patients to permit a statistical calculation of significance, and advice on the sample size should be sought. This demonstrates how like an experiment the goal-orientated approach is, and risk of bias is avoided or minimised by making the measure of effectiveness as objective as possible.

A *goal-free* approach to evaluating the nurse-led continence clinic would focus less on the impact of the CNS's advice on incontinence and consider the value of the clinic in terms of whether, or the extent to which, patients felt that their needs had been met. Patients' needs could be expressed in a number of ways, such as the impact incontinence has on different aspects of their life. They may, therefore, see a value in the opportunities to discuss specific problems with the CNS or share experiences and coping strategies with other sufferers. These aspects of clinic attendance may be very important to some individuals, especially if they are unlikely to be able to achieve full continence because of the cause of their incontinence.

Unintended consequences like these could not be obtained by using an analytical approach; what is needed is a way of discovering or eliciting the feelings or perceptions of patients about attending the clinic. This could be done by conducting interviews or even focus groups and demonstrates the non-experimental nature of this approach and reliance on qualitative methods for this type of evaluation.

- The *experimental approach* to evaluation applies the principles of scientific experimentation (Øvretveit, 2000). The aim is to be able to produce generalisable conclusions by controlling variables and simplifying the question being asked. The focus is on analytical methods and the data obtained will be quantifiable; for example, comparing outcomes of an intervention by random allocation to either the control group or intervention group (following procedures similar to those used for randomised controlled trials).

- *Goal-free approaches* to evaluation, according to Scriven (1972), assume that the focus on goals results in the possibility of missing important and unintended outcomes/consequences. A goal-free approach is similar to needs-based assessment where the actual needs being met are evaluated. This may mean that although an intervention does not achieve the specified goals, it is effective because it meets individual or local needs.

  Here, there is a desire and/or need to probe aspects of the intervention that are not precise or easily measured. Data, therefore, will be qualitative, and it is likely that the researcher will interact closely with participants whilst collecting data, for example when conducting interviews. One consequence of this is that it becomes difficult for service providers to collect data about their own practice or service without serious risk of bias. It is common, therefore, to use an external evaluator (that is, external to the specific service provision or practice but not necessarily to the organisation) when this approach is employed. An example of this type of approach is given in Box 15.1.

- A *utilisation-focused approach* to evaluation is suggested by Patton (1997) as being done for and with specific, intended primary users for specific, intended uses. Careful consideration of how every aspect of a project is used is central to a utilisation-focused approach. Therefore, the evaluator has to be involved from the outset and will assist users in deciding the exact nature and type of evaluation necessary. In other words, the evaluator will help users to define the questions they want answered about an intervention, practice or policy. An example of this type of approach is given in Box 15.2.

Box 15.2   Examples of utilisation-focused and economic evaluations

A team of education facilitators want to implement and evaluate a new programme for mentoring student nurses.

A *utilisation-focused evaluation* of the mentoring programme would involve everyone connected with mentoring. This would require mentors, student nurses, practice educators and, possibly, ward managers, to work together in order to frame the questions that they want answered. For example: a student nurse might ask how the new programme will benefit his or her acquisition of clinical skills; a practice educator might ask if the new programme enables student nurses to work regularly with their mentor; whereas a mentor might ask what impact the new programme had for enabling students to achieve the competencies specific to a placement.

An *economic evaluation* of the mentoring programme would involve the evaluator calculating the resources used and benefits arising from them. Thus the data collected would relate to things like: resources such as training of mentors and other members of the ward team who have a role in the mentorship programme, and any additional time spent on mentoring compared with the previous programme; and outputs, such as the impact of the programme on student nurses' clinical practice in relation to patient care.

- *Economic evaluations* essentially involve the calculation of all resources used and the benefits arising from them (Øvretveit, 2000; Stecher and Davies, 1987). The research process in this type of evaluation will involve trying to quantify the resources used and putting a cost to them. Further calculations are then necessary to assess or quantify the benefits that are accrued by the input of these resources, that is, perform a cost–benefit analysis. This may be an attractive form of evaluation for managers and service commissioners, but it will not always be possible to put a cost to the benefits of an intervention. For example, it will be relatively easy to evaluate a new dressing using a price comparison between the old and new dressing, time taken to apply the dressings, frequency of dressing changes needed and any change in healing time. However, a full evaluation should also include reference to patient comfort, and calculating the cost of this in terms of patient benefit will, inevitably, be difficult.

- *Mixed-method evaluations* are similar to any other mixed-method research and apply the same principles. In the example used above it is easy to see that an economic evaluation of a new dressing will not provide a complete picture of the value or merit of the product in terms of patient care. Here, the addition of a comfort assessment may be an appropriate addition to the evaluation. This could be done, for example, by developing a comfort scale from 1 to 10 and asking patients to indicate their level of comfort/discomfort during a dressing change and then compare responses for the old and new dressings. The addition of patients' perspectives may be particularly useful if there is minimal difference in the cost–benefit evaluation of the two dressings.

  The mixed-method approach highlights the fact that evaluation research makes use of a variety of research approaches and that it is important to use the approach that will best answer the question. This means that a good understanding of research designs and methods is necessary for anyone intending to undertake an evaluation research project.

What outcomes are used in evaluation research?

In healthcare, outcomes are the impacts healthcare interventions have on patients' health as well as patients' evaluations of their healthcare. Outcomes refer to the effectiveness of the activities in relation to the achievement of the intended goal (Bowling, 2002). They often focus on things like survival, urgency and seriousness of the healthcare needs, and measure 'health gains' and 'benefits' from specific interventions or programmes of care. These elements, however, are not usually the main prompts for nursing care where considerations of interventions or ways of working that will improve an individual's quality of life or the quality of care delivery tend to be the focus. Outcomes that can measure the effectiveness of nursing will be complex and are likely to incorporate indicators such as comfort, satisfaction, and sense of well-being alongside more readily measurable physical and social indicators, such as number of pressure ulcers and number of nurses with a specialist nursing qualification.

The outcome measures used in any evaluation have to be appropriate to the question being asked. They can be qualitative or quantitative or a mixture of both. Outcome indicators can be classified as patient, carer, staff and service based. For example, patient-based outcomes could relate to symptom severity and be measured using a structured self-completion symptom checklist. This will give quantitative data and may enable comparison between different patients or groups of patients. A staff-based outcome could refer to satisfaction with the nature of the care delivered and be assessed by the use of interviews and questionnaires. This would provide a mixture of quantitative and qualitative data and might assist in reducing bias that is inevitable when individuals are assessing their own practice. Qualitative outcomes, such as data from interviews or observations, are particularly useful when the evaluation approach used actively includes those likely to be affected by the results (Clarke, 2001).

Steps for conducting an evaluation research project

The steps to carrying out an evaluation are essentially the same as for any research project: setting and clarifying the aims and objectives, selecting an appropriate research design and dissemination of results. Evaluation research differs from a basic or 'pure' research project in that attention is directed towards practical problems or questions about an intervention, practice or policy rather than adding knowledge. It is characterised by a rigorous and systematic collection of evidence combined with an entering into a dialogue with those involved in order to identify with, and speak to, their different political interests and preoccupations (Room, 1986). The expectation for an evaluation research project is to use whichever research method is most appropriate, and it frequently uses a combination of methods rather than focusing on a single methodological framework.

Setting and clarifying the aims and objectives

The first step of any evaluation is to determine the overriding purpose or overall aim for the evaluation; for example, to assess the effectiveness of Breast Care Nurse Specialists (BCNS) in breast-screening clinics.

Once the overall aim has been clarified, then the objectives can be set. The objectives suggest how the evaluation can be realised; for example, to assess the effectiveness of the BCNS in relation to:

- patient support
- information giving
- quality of care.

This objective-setting process helps to establish, implicitly and explicitly, the criteria which will be used to judge whether the evaluation achieved its purpose. For example, a preoccupation with effectiveness and explicit outcomes rather than unintended outcomes/consequences may become apparent at this stage and will help influence the choice of research strategy. It is, therefore, important at this stage for the evaluator to confirm with the commissioners of the evaluation what type of effectiveness criteria they are interested in. For example, if the evaluation of the BCNS role is aimed at determining whether there is actually a role for BCNSs in screening clinics, the evaluation outcomes may include numbers of patients seen by the different professional groups working in breast-screening clinics. Alternatively, or in addition, the evaluation could investigate/identify the type of advice given by a BCNS and the benefit to patients' well-being compared with that given by other professionals. This later evaluation will have very different effectiveness outcomes from the former and may help the decision-making process if quality of care is the criterion for determining whether BCNSs should continue to have a role in screening clinics.

Selecting an appropriate research design

The choice of research design will be driven by the aims and objectives of the evaluation and the resources available to carry it out. In healthcare evaluations, the research strategies most commonly used have been the experimental (and quasi-experimental), survey and case-study methods (Robbins, 1998). However, as the complexity of healthcare has become more apparent, it has been recognised that a multi-method approach may provide more informative results from evaluations (Ong, 1994).

The selection of the most appropriate research design relies on having a good understanding of the aims of the evaluation and an awareness of the strengths and weaknesses of different research methods in being able to answer different types of question. For example, a survey which collects information in a standardised format (often via questionnaires) from groups of people could be used to evaluate the effectiveness of a healthy eating programme by asking participants to indicate what changes they have made in their eating habits. This type of approach may not, however, be appropriate if the evaluation focus was on the effectiveness of the healthy eating programme in reducing participants' weight or on reactions to the different elements of the programme.

Dissemination of results

All research results have to be reported, and this applies equally to evaluation research projects. The difference from other forms of research, however, is that the evaluations are undertaken in a social and political context with multiple stakeholders. There is also the possibility that service providers could be sensitive about their own performances and may feel strongly about the content of the report and how the results should be presented. For summative evaluations, in particular, where there is a risk of a service being terminated, then it is very important that the results are reported with due care and attention to those whom the report will have a direct impact upon.

There are, therefore, benefits of planning the dissemination strategy from the outset of the project. Similarly, developing a regular pattern of feedback and, where appropriate, interim reports will help maintain a rapport and ownership of the evaluation by those who are particularly involved with data collection and commissioners of the evaluation. This, according to Traylen (1994), will increase the likelihood of the results actually being used for reflection and practice.

It is common to see recommendations for future practice, policy and programme development as an integral part of an evaluation. Recommendations should be clearly derived from the data collected and presented in the report. They are also more likely to be acted upon and implemented if they are practicable. Good practice when developing the recommendations is to involve, wherever possible, those who will be making use of the results of the evaluation or the decision makers.

It is important to remember that evaluation research is not only concerned with the effectiveness of particular interventions that can be measured, but also with the processes that underpin the intervention, practice or policy.

Chapter summary

- Evaluation research is applied research that investigates the effectiveness of an intervention, practice or policy and, for nursing, the focus is often on patient care and delivery systems.
- Evaluation applies the scientific method of systematic and rigorous collection of research data.
- Evaluation research is different from audit because it aims to discover the reasons why changes have occurred as well as what changes have actually occurred.
- Evaluation in healthcare and healthcare services is characterised by the collection of data about the structure, process, outcomes and appropriateness of services.
- Outcomes will usually include measurement of the impact of an intervention, practice or policy.
- Evaluation uses a variety of research methods, and different methods will be appropriate for different questions.

References

Bowling, A. (2002) *Research Methods in Health: Investigating Health and Health Services*, 2nd edition. Buckingham: Open University Press.

Brown, B., Crawford, P. and Hicks, C. (2003) *Evidence-based Research: Dilemmas and Debates in Health Care.* Maidenhead: Open University Press.

Clarke, A. (2001) 'Evaluation research in nursing and healthcare', *Nurse Researcher*, 8: 4–14.

DoH (1996) *Towards an Evidence-based Health Service*. London: Department of Health.

DoH (1997) *The New NHS: Modern and Dependable*. London: Department of Health.

DoH (1999) *Making a Difference – Strengthening the Nursing, Midwifery and Health Visiting Contribution to Health and Healthcare*. London: Department of Health.

Donabedian, A. (1980) *Explorations in Quality Assessment and Monitoring: The Definition of Quality and Approaches to its Assessment*. Ann Arbor, MI: Health Administration Press.

Donabedian, A. (1988) 'Quality assessment and assurance: unity of purpose, diversity of means', *Inquiry*, 25: 173–92.

Gray, J. (1997) *Evidence-based Health Care: How to Make Health Policy and Management Decisions*. London: Churchill Livingstone.

Lincoln, Y. and Guba, E. (1986) 'Research evaluation and policy analysis: heuristics for disciplined enquiry', *Policy Studies Review*, 5: 546–65.

Ong, B. (1994) *The Practice of Health Services Research*. London: Chapman & Hall.

Øvretveit, J. (2000) *Evaluating Health Interventions*. Buckingham: Open University Press.

Patton, M. (1997) *Utilisation-focused Evaluation: The New Century Text*: London: Sage.

Robbins, M. (1998) *Evaluating Palliative Care: Establishing the Evidence Base*. Oxford: Oxford Medical Publications.

Room, G. (1986) *Cross-national Innovation in Social Policy*. London: Macmillan.

Rownsley, A. (2001) *Servants of the People: The Inside of New Labour*. London: Hamish Hamilton.

Scriven, M. (1972) 'Pros and cons about goal-free evaluation. Evaluation comment', *Journal of Educational Evaluation. Centre for Study of Evaluation, University of California*, 34: 1–7.

Stecher, B. and Davies, W. (1987) *How to Focus an Evaluation*. London: Sage.

Traylen, H. (1994) 'Confronting hidden agendas: co-operative inquiry with health visitors', in P. Reason (ed.), *Participation in Human Inquiry*. London: Sage.

Suggested further reading

Cornish, J. and Jones, A. (2007) 'Evaluation of moving and handling training for pre-registration nurses and its application to practice', *Nurse Education in Practice*, 7: 128–34.

Cunningham, T., Geller, E. and Clarke, S. (2008) 'Impact of electronic prescribing in a hospital setting: a process-focused evaluation', *International Journal of Medical Informatics*, 77 (8):546–54.

Hazra, A., Chanock, S., Giovannucci, E., Cox, D., Niu, T., Fuchs, C., Willett, W. and Hunter, D. (2008) 'Large-scale evaluation of genetic variants in candidate genes for colorectal cancer risk in the Nurses' Health Study and Health Professionals' follow-up study', *Cancer, Epidemiology, Biomarkers and Prevention*, 17: 311–9.

Hek, G. (2003) 'Developing self-evaluation skills: a pragmatic research-based approach for complex areas of nursing', *Nurse Researcher*, 11: 73–82.

Imhof, S., Kaskie, B. and Wyatt, M. (2007) 'Finding the way to a better death: an evaluation of palliative care referral tools', *Journal of Gerontological Nursing*, 33: 40–49.

Knowles, G., Hutchinson, C., Smith, G., Philip, I., McCormick, K. and Preston, E. (2008) 'Implementation and evaluation of a pilot education programme in colorectal cancer management for nurses in Scotland', *Nurse Education Today*, 28: 15–23.

Lee, L.-L., Hsu, N. and Chang, S.-C. (2007) 'An evaluation of the quality of nursing care in orthopaedic units', *Journal of Orthopaedic Nursing*, 11: 160–68.

Malin, N. (2000) 'Evaluation of clinical supervision in community homes and teams serving adults with learning disabilities', *Journal of Advanced Nursing*, 31: 548–57.

Manafi, M., McLeister, P., Cherry, A. and Wallis, M. (2008) 'Pilot process and outcome evaluation of the introduction of a clinical nutrition pathway in the care of in-hospital renal patients', *Journal of Renal Nutrition*, 18 (2): 223-9.

McClement, S., Care, D. and Dean, R. (2005) 'Evaluation of education in palliative care: determining the effects on nurses' knowledge and attitudes', *Journal of Palliative Care*, 21: 44–8.

Mor, V. (1998) 'The research design of the National Hospice Study', in V. Mor, D. Greer and R. Kastenbaum (eds), *The Hospice Experiment*. Baltimore, MD: Johns Hopkins University Press.

Website

Evaluation and the Health Professions: http://mmr.sagepub.com/

16

CONSENSUS METHODS

Consensus methods are used to try to establish common agreement in circumstances where there is a lack of understanding of a particular healthcare issue. The methods may be used, for example, when the healthcare team are trying to identify research priorities, are developing new roles or identifying competencies for practice. Consensus methods can be particularly helpful when the evidence base is lacking and the degree of effectiveness and appropriateness of care delivery is unknown. There are three main methods used in health: the Delphi technique, nominal group technique and consensus technique. Each is used to draw expert opinion together, collating the agreed views of those with experience for use in making care decisions and judgements. In this chapter we discuss the use of all three techniques.

Of the three techniques, the Delphi technique is more commonly used in healthcare. It is used to gain expert views on a range of issues, such as setting care and research priorities. Nominal group techniques combine aspects of the Delphi technique with that of focus groups (discussed in Chapter 21). Finally, consensus methods draw experts from a range of professions to review particular aspects of care or policy. These methods can be used to develop clinical guidelines for practice. All three techniques can include professionals and users (patients, carers, families) as experts and thus provide methods that can facilitate user involvement in healthcare development.

Learning outcomes

This chapter is designed to enable the reader to:

- **Understand Delphi, nominal group and consensus techniques**
- **Appreciate when these techniques might be employed in data collection**
- **Understand the advantages and disadvantages of using the techniques**

KEY TERMS

Consensus technique, Delphi technique, Nominal group technique

---

Delphi technique

The **Delphi technique** has increasingly been used in healthcare to gain consensus opinion from a group of experts on a specific area of enquiry. In healthcare settings the groups contributing to Delphi studies may include senior nurses, medical staff, members of the professions allied to medicine, and health service users. The Delphi technique involves trying to ascertain a consensus view amongst group members. The process of identifying consensus can involve returning to the group of experts at various stages of the research to draw agreement or obtain an overall view.

The Delphi technique starts with the research team identifying possible expert panel members. In some cases the nurse researcher may need to obtain ethical permission prior to approaching panel members. This can be the case if the research is to involve staff employed by the National Health Service (NHS) or users of healthcare services, when the research team will need ethical approval from the local NHS Research Committee and university ethics committee (See Chapters 4 and 5).

Once the panel members have been identified and consent to take part is obtained if necessary, the process of data collection can commence. This involves collecting data through a series of consecutive questionnaires. Using questionnaires can allow the researchers to collect data anonymously. These are usually posted to expert participants or can be emailed or made available for access on a password-protected website. Open-ended questions are used within the initial questionnaire to establish general ideas, views and attitudes of the expert group towards the research issue. The questionnaires are returned and feedback is collated. The initial findings are used by the researchers to develop a further, more targeted questionnaire. This second questionnaire will be focused on a number of specific issues. It is likely to be composed of a number of statements related to key topics. These are returned to the experts who are asked to rank their degree of agreement against the statements. Responses are again analysed before re-presenting a questionnaire that summarises the rankings. The experts are again asked to rank their level of agreement with the statements. Further analysis can establish the level of consensus or disagreement. If disparity remains, then the process of developing further statements in a questionnaire is re-visited and further questionnaires are sent to experts to rank.

The approach is particularly helpful when attempting to establish research or care priorities, defining new roles or ways of working, and can be used to agree on resource priorities. It is suggested that the success of the Delphi technique relies on four aspects of the process being administered effectively: the initial questions must be formulated and structured to support the process; individual responses must be accurately transcribed; the response rates through successive rounds should be maintained; and finally the meaning of consensus should be understood by the research team and participants (Crisp et al., 1997).

As a process of data collection, the Delphi technique has some advantages, including being less resource intensive than many other methods. Additionally, the experts can remain anonymous. Providing a degree of anonymity means that the individual view is more likely to be achieved. Experts have an opportunity to be involved with the research process without having to attend face-to-face data collection sessions, which can support a wide geographical input. The process of data collection is less time-consuming and can be managed more flexibly, which may be more appealing to the participants and less inconvenient.

Whilst there are a number of advantages to using the Delphi technique, there are some potential disadvantages. The initial selection of experts may be ill-conceived and bias may be evident amongst some experts. Those using this methodology can experience difficulties maintaining commitment to the project by the expert group. Reducing response rates can indicate difficulties in trying to maintain enthusiasm. Difficulties of maintaining the group may also reflect the problems some experts can have in agreeing with the statements as they are developed and focused, perhaps in a direction that isn't consistent with their views.

An example of using the Delphi technique is given in Box 16.1.

Box 16.1   Example of the Delphi technique

Hauck et al. (2007) used the Delphi technique to identify research priorities of clinical staff working with families in parenting and child health. The Delphi technique was used to gather anonymous replies and to achieve consensus. All clinicians were eligible to participate. The first-round questionnaire included five important research questions for participants to comment on. Content analysis of the 64 replies allowed the development of a second questionnaire. In this questionnaire respondents ranked research topics according to their views on which areas should be priorities. Following analysis, a third questionnaire was produced and sent to the group of experts. The experts were again asked to rank their top ten research topics from those identified in the questionnaire. The research team were able to achieve consistency in the number of responses received across the three questionnaire rounds.

Nominal group technique

The **nominal group technique (NGT)** was originally developed by Delbecq et al. (1975) for use in organisational planning. The technique uses some of the processes of the

Delphi technique and combines these with focus group methods (see Chapter 21). In contrast to the Delphi technique, the participants meet face-to-face to try to achieve a consensus through a process of ranking and refining responses to key issues. The participants are invited to join the nominal group because they have some experience of the topics under discussion. The NGT may include clinical staff and/or users. The groups are around five to nine in number and are used to discuss a range of care or education issues. Examples of the types of issues considered might include how best to involve users in developing education programmes or how to identify problems experienced by patients living with chronic heart failure in the community.

Experts can be asked to prepare for the focus group discussions by reading materials and thinking through their views before a face-to-face meeting, so that they come prepared to entered into discussion and to vote on available options (Bowling, 2002). The NGT is a facilitated, structured and formal meeting that aims to generate a ranked list of views. The meetings can continue for some time to allow for agreement amongst the experts. The facilitator tries to involve all the participants in the meeting, drawing their opinions into the discussion and requiring them to record their views through ranking the options available. The experts can be asked to rank or rate their expert opinion on a scale 0 (not important) to 9 (very important). These ratings are collated and presented to the group. During the meeting the experts are asked to review the rankings and discuss their differences. Relevant literature may also be sourced to inform the discussions before the ranking is revisited and ratings changed.

The process therefore includes: generation of ideas by the experts individually; recording of ideas from around the group; a facilitated and time-limited discussion on each idea; and ranking of ideas through voting.

As with the Delphi technique, NGT provides a resource-effective way of bringing experts together to achieve a consensus view. The approach is quicker and cheaper to administer than many other data collection techniques, especially individual interviewing. However, as with focus group techniques, NGT can be affected if there are dominant characters in the group who sway the general discussion. Further limitations arise from the face-to-face nature of the meeting that means anonymity cannot be guaranteed and participant views may therefore be tempered in an open discussion forum.

See Box 16.2 for an example of NGT in use.

Box 16.2   Example of the nominal group technique (NGT)

Tuffrey-Wijne et al. (2007) used the nominal group technique to elicit the views of users with intellectual disabilities on end-of-life care decisions. The study included a group of 14 people with intellectual disabilities, accessed from a theatre company. The data were

(Continued)

(Continued)

collected over a three-day period. Data collection included four stages. Initially the group was shown an image of a woman who was dying. The participants were asked what should be done to help her. Stage one involved the generation of ideas from all members of the group. All ideas were recorded on paper by the researchers. Stage two included the recording of all the ideas from individuals in the group. These were read out and written on flip charts. Stage three was a chance for clarification of the ideas, facilitated by the researchers. The final stage included a vote. The participants were given a collapsed list of ideas and asked to vote by identifying their top five ideas that were then ranked in importance. All votes were then counted.

Consensus techniques

Consensus techniques can be called 'consensus development panels' (Bowling, 2002) or 'consensus knowledge-building forums' (Burns and Grove, 2007). They work on the same principles as the NGT, bringing experts together in one face-to-face forum to gain either further understanding or consensus in a particular field. The consensus method involves a panel of experts invited to take part. They are often multi-disciplinary in nature and may be composed entirely of professionals, healthcare users or a mixture of both. The panels are often used to develop clinical guidelines for practice (Burns and Grove, 2007). The process of developing guidelines can require the experts to include reference support to ensure that the practice developed is evidence-based. This means that an initial search of the key literature may be undertaken to provide current evidence for the panel members to use. This can be given to panel members ahead of the meeting, providing the experts with current information to use in the discussions. The consensus panel will be able to draw on current knowledge in developing guidelines, and as part of the process of reviewing the existing evidence base they may identify gaps in knowledge. This means research priorities can also be identified as part of a consensus knowledge-building process.

Consensus techniques are facilitated by either an expert in the field or someone seen as credible in the eyes of the expert panel members. Though only one meeting is involved, this can continue over a number of days. The nature of the process can make this a more costly data collection method, as there are costs attached in gathering background materials and in paying experts.

The method can facilitate multi-disciplinary healthcare team discussions, involving nurses and other healthcare professionals, in the development of new clinical guidelines for practice. There is also scope to include healthcare users in the forums and enable their valuable input in the development of practice guidelines (see Box 16.3).

Box 16.3   Example of consensus methods

Barker and Burns (2001) used a consensus meeting to rate the strength of agreement amongst panel members when proposing a set of clinical guidelines developed through the Delphi technique. An expert panel of 12 physiotherapists reviewed the clinical guidelines and through facilitation a final version of the guidelines was agreed by the panel members and adopted for use by various professional groups.

Chapter summary

- Consensus techniques can be useful in cases where there is a lack of knowledge or understanding of a particular healthcare issue.
- Consensus techniques enable healthcare professionals to access the views of experts on aspects of practice, education and research.
- Consensus techniques can be used in developing clinical guidelines and in identifying agreement on health and research priorities.
- There are three main methods used in health: the Delphi technique, nominal group technique and consensus technique.
- The Delphi technique involves data collection via a series of consecutive questionnaires administered to the group of experts.
- One advantage is the anonymity provided to the participants, a second is the limited resources required to administer the technique.
- In the nominal group technique the participants meet face to face to try to achieve a consensus through a process of ranking and refining responses to key issues.
- The nominal group technique includes: generation of ideas by the experts individually, recording of ideas from around the group, discussion on each idea that is facilitated and time-limited, selection of group ideas and ranking of ideas through voting.
- Nurses and other healthcare professionals may be involved in consensus techniques as part of a multi-disciplinary healthcare team discussing the development of new clinical guidelines for practice.
- All three methods can include professionals and users (patients, carers, families) as experts and as such provide techniques that can facilitate user involvement in healthcare development.

References

Barker, K. and Burns, M. (2001) 'Using consensus techniques to produce clinical guidelines for patients treated with the Ilizarov fixator', *Physiotherapy*, 87 (6): 289–300.

Bowling, A. (2002) *Research Methods in Health: Investigating Health and Health Services*, 2nd edition. Buckingham: Open University Press.

Burns, N. and Grove, S. (2007) *Understanding Nursing Research*, 4th edition. St Louis, MO: Elsevier Saunders.

Crisp, J., Pelletier, D., Duffield, C., Adams, A. and Nagy, S. (1997) 'The Delphi method?', *Nursing Research*, 46 (2): 116–18.

Delbecq, A., Van de Ven, A. and Gustafson, D. (1975) *Group Techniques for Program Planning*. Glenview, IL: Scott, Foresman.

Hauck, Y., Kelly, R. and Fenwick, J. (2007) 'Research priorities for parenting and child health: a Delphi study', *Journal of Advanced Nursing*, 59 (2): 129–32.

Tuffrey-Wijne, I., Bernal, J., Butler, G., Hollins, S. and Curfs, L. (2007) 'Using nominal group technique to investigate the views of people with intellectual disabilities on end-of-life care provision', *Journal of Advanced Nursing*, 58 (1): 80–89.

Suggested further reading

Beattie, A., Hek, G., Ross, K. and Galvin, K. (2004) 'Future career pathways in nursing and midwifery. A Delphi survey of nurses and midwives in South West England', *Nursing Times Research*, 9 (5): 348–64.

Burns, T. (2000) 'A Delphi approach to characterising "relapse" as used in UK clinical practice', *International Journal of Social Psychiatry*, 46 (3): 220–30.

Fretheim, A., Schünemann, H. and Oxman, A. (2006) 'Improving the use of research evidence in guideline development: 5. Group processes', *Health Research Policy and Systems*, 4 (17): 1–4. Available at www.health-policy-systems.com/content/4/1/17, accessed 28 February 2008.

Jones, J. and Hunter, D. (1995) 'Nominal group technique (expert panel): consensus methods for medical and health services research', *British Medical Journal*, 311 (7001): 376–80.

Linstone, H. and Turoff, M. (eds) (1975) *The Delphi Method: Techniques and Applications*. Reading, MA: Addison-Wesley.

Tuffrey-Wijne, I., Bernal, J., Butler, G., Hollins, S. and Curfs, L. (2007) 'Using nominal group technique to investigate the views of people with intellectual disabilities on end-of-life care provision', *Journal of Advanced Nursing*, 58 (1): 80–89.

17

OTHER RESEARCH DESIGNS

In order to answer the research question or hypothesis the nurse researcher needs to identify an appropriate research design. In Chapter 11 we discussed the different qualitative and quantitative approaches available to researchers and related the selection of design to the need to address the research question. The research design includes methods of data collection and analysis that will be used to address the research questions, aims and objectives. In this chapter we discuss four research designs. Action research and feminist research can both encourage participant engagement in the research, attempt to empower users and ensure that the research is conducted with and for, rather than on, the participants. These designs can draw on a range of research methods. Historical research is drawing on data from the past and interpreting this to help understand and develop practice. Researchers may be working with different oral and documentary sources to inform knowledge development. Case study research is used to explore a particular practice or approach and can draw on both qualitative and quantitative methods of data collection. This design can help us to understand the particular and specific, but also to draw implications that can be more broadly applicable.

Learning outcomes

This chapter is designed to enable the reader to:

- **Understand action research, feminist, historical and case study research**
- **Appreciate when these designs might be employed**
- **Understand the issues of data collection and knowledge generation**

KEY TERMS

Action research, Case study research, Feminist research, Historical research

---

Action research

Action research tries to address the gap between theory generation and practice change. Researchers using this approach have moved away from a research process that runs from problem identification to knowledge generation, and aim to integrate the development of practice with the generation of knowledge as part of a cyclical process. The approach integrates research into the day-to-day working of the health-care environment and addresses implementation issues experienced in some research approaches, where the process of dissemination is lengthy and starts on completion of the research.

There are a number of definitions of action research; all identify concepts of change, participation and action, as seen in this quote from Reason and Bradbury:

> Action research is a participatory, democratic process concerned with developing practical knowing in the pursuit of worthwhile human purposes, grounded in a participatory world view.... It seeks to bring together action and reflection, theory and practice, in participation with others, in the pursuit of practical solutions to issues of pressing concern to people. (Reason and Bradbury, 2001: 1)

Holloway and Wheeler suggest action research is unique in that:

- The researchers collaborate with local participants or are themselves participants in the research setting.
- The research includes action.
- The approach includes research, intervention and change in the area of study.
- Change takes place in the research setting.
- Research findings are implemented in practice and the effect is assessed. (Adapted from Holloway and Wheeler, 2002: 189)

Action research was initially developed by Kurt Lewin (1946) and has been used in educational research, management and healthcare. The original approach adopted by Lewin included a number of stages: planning an initial change; implementation of the change; evaluation of the change impact; change actions to reflect the findings of the evaluation; and return to start the process. This initial action research process has developed and changed over the years and can now include a more participatory focus.

Whitelaw et al. (2003) identify three broad types of action research that span the methodological continuum for positivist to interpretivist (see Chapter 11). These are:

- Technical–scientific
- Mutual collaborative
- Critical and emancipatory

In the 'technical-scientific' approach the researcher occupies a position of expert, who plans the research, conducts the research with the professionals in the field and advises on the actions that should be taken. The researcher acts as the facilitator, taking the lead in the research. Often the research aims to 'test' an intervention and uses methods more akin to scientific research to do this, such as taking a quasi-experimental design with a control and experimental group.

In the 'mutual collaborative' approach the researcher and the professionals work together to identify the research problem. The researchers and professionals work more collaboratively together throughout and devise the intervention and change together. This approach to action research is more likely to involve other stakeholders in the research, such as service users. The design can be used to explore more practical problems and change can be rapid, but not necessarily sustained when the research team leave.

'Critical' or 'emancipatory' action research aims not only to improve outcomes for practice, but also to help professionals critique their work settings and the practices. There is a focus on helping professionals develop critical understanding of the situation they are in; the practice, practitioner and practice settings are considered. Kemmis suggests that:

> It aims to connect the personal and the political in the collaborative research and action aimed at transforming situations to overcome felt dissatisfactions, alienation, ideological distortion, and the injustices of oppression and domination. (2001: 92)

Through critical appraisal and self-reflection, local groups can take forward practice development and influence local policy. The types of data collection used can include reflection on practice, discussions with service users and staff and observation of practice.

The emphasis on participation in action research has led to it sometimes being known as 'participatory action research'. Kemmis and McTaggart (2000) suggest that though the two terms, action research and participatory action research, are used interchangeably, the later aims to undertake projects where there is shared ownership, and collaborators will analyse local problems and act on findings in their community. There is a focus on emancipation of the community members and empowerment of the participants in the research process.

The process usually involves a number of steps:

1 The researcher identifies issues or problems from observations of practice and discussions with service users and service providers. The researcher can use focus groups, question-naires and interviews to gain the views of the community. Analysis of the data provides a basis for discussion with a range of stakeholders, including managers. Through negotia-tion and consultation those in the research setting are encouraged to participate in iden-tifying the way forward and generating the research questions.

2 Once the areas for investigation are understood, the action research cycle commences, which includes: planning an initial change; implementation of the change; evaluation of the change impact; reflection on the findings; change actions to reflect the findings of the evaluation; and return to start the process. The process of change is monitored through a number of data collection processes. These may include participant observa-tion, reflective diaries and journals and field notes. Throughout this time there will be dis-cussions about the monitoring process with participants, so as to inform the continuing action. The researcher is likely to involve the participants in interpreting the data, as a col-laborative process to analysis is expected to draw more valid conclusions. Through analy-sis of the findings the participants are able to identify further ways forward, which are immediately implemented and then evaluated. This supports the cycles of action research where issues are identified, the way forward agreed and implemented, and the changes then evaluated and reviewed before further issues, ways to manage and so on are considered. This process is very much dependent on the participation of all those involved in the action research site.

3 A final evaluation phase occurs before the researcher leaves the field. Data are collected to see what the impact of the change has been. These are discussed with participants to allow reflection on what has been achieved.

Action research has gained much popularity in healthcare in recent years (Greenhaugh et al., 2004). This appeal may result from the strengths it holds as a research approach for the professions, particularly in its ability to support the introduction of change and involve professionals in the research and develop-ment process (see Box 17.1). However, according to Waterman et al. (2001), each potential strength has an equal and opposite potential weakness. For example, there is the potential for participation in the research process and the develop-ment of collaborative researcher–participant working. This has appeal as partici-pants can feel enabled and empowered in developing their practice, but can prove problematic if the participants feel coerced and are required to take part rather than desiring to do so. The research approach has real-world applicability and focus, supporting immediate change to a particular practice; however, the partic-ipants may not feel sufficiently engaged in the research process and can suspect political motives behind any change. Suspicions can be particularly aroused if the researcher is an outsider and it is perceived that they fail to understand the local issues sufficiently. Lack of trust can lead to difficulties with engagement in the change process leading to the impact of change being lessened.

> **Box 17.1   Example of action research**
>
> Jinks and Chalder (2007) used an action research approach to enable a group of mental health nurse consultants to map their roles and scope the dimension of their work. The first stage of the project refined the purpose of the study and involved fact finding. Focus group discussions were facilitated by a professor known to the nurses. The discussions were reflective and open and achieved some benchmarking of the nurse consultant role. The focus groups were attended by the nurse consultants, who discussed the major components of the role as suggested by the Nursing and Midwifery Council. The participants were involved in initiating and designing the study. Content analysis of the data revealed a number of categories and themes. To help verify data analysis, questionnaires were designed to identify consensus in views.

Feminist research

There are many variations in **feminist research**, though put simply it is research carried out for the benefit of women. Feminist research arose from a discontent with research studies that were thought to be male focused and hid the voice of women in society, as men conducted research on women, identifying topics for research that may have limited relevance for women. Kitzinger wrote:

> Feminist social scientists argued that men define reality on their own terms, to legitimate *their* experience, *their* own particular version of events, while women's experience, not fitting the male model, is trivialised and denied or distorted. (2004: 125)

Kitzinger (2004) identified the second wave of feminism in the 1970s as focusing on reclaiming and naming women's experiences and challenging the male dominance in establishing truth. Feminist researchers attempted to address the male monopoly on truth through undertaking research from a position that ensured women's views and experiences were researched and heard. The research methods used to access women's experiences were often qualitative, such as interviews or focus groups, which allow researchers to record and listen to women. The characteristics of feminist research were seen as women researching women, focusing on women's experiences, researching in a collaborative and non-exploitative way that focused on research with and for women rather than about them. The researcher and participant relationship aimed to create mutual knowledge as part of the research process and worked in a reciprocal way, so that both parties benefited from the research.

It is suggested that feminist research has gone beyond this 'qualitative' position and is using a wide range of research methods to conduct research for women (Olesen, 2000). For example, Oakley (1989) suggests that experimental research, such as randomised controlled trials, can be conducted in an emancipatory way to draw benefits for women. The variations in feminist research can consider the views and experiences of individual women through more qualitative approaches or can take a perspective of how policy and structures within society affect women more generally. Within nursing the large body of the profession are women, and therefore feminist studies have been able to explore the nature of women's work within healthcare and the experience of women patients, and to examine women's health. See Box 17.2 for an example.

Box 17.2   Example of feminist enquiry

Giddings (2005) used a life history methodology informed by feminist theory to collect stories of difference and fairness in nursing across New Zealand and the United States. Interviews were used to collect life histories that within a feminist approach captured women's voices as they gave their experience of being a nurse. Twenty-six female nurses were interviewed two or three times. The researchers provided information about their gender, age and identity as a nurse and midwife prior to the interviews, acknowledging the potential for unequal power relations to exist as a result of cultural and social differences. The women listened to, reflected on and commented about the first interview prior to the second, and were involved in creating the final interpretations, understandings and knowledge from the research.

Historical research

Historical researchers examine past events to increase understanding and gain new knowledge. They believe that by studying data and materials related to the past we can inform current and future practice. Until recently **historical research** received minimal attention, but the work of Teresa Christy (1975) has led to an increased interest in its use in nursing and health.

Those undertaking historical research need to identify research questions to address and consider the sources of material that may be available to answer them. A number of sources can be used including oral or documentary recordings. The types of sources available could include photographs, tape recordings, video and written documents such as letters, diaries, memoranda and formal written records. These might be held in libraries or private collections. In the future such sources could also include digitalised and web-based materials.

Many of the sources used will not have been collected for research purposes and therefore the quality could be questionable. The historical researcher will need to ensure the originality of materials used as they must be confident of reliability and validity of the source. External and internal criticism are used to determine the accuracy and authenticity of a source. The origins of the source need to be known to satisfy external criticism and establish validity. To review the validity of a source the researcher will need to establish who produced the material, when, where and how. These questions can be applied to any historical source, be it a written, visual or an oral account. Internal criticism seeks to establish the reliability of the material. In order to achieve this, a second piece of evidence related to the same event and recorded by an independent source is needed. This allows comparisons of materials to establish reliability. Thus the diary account of one person may be compared with that of another to establish reliability.

The sources available to historians are described as primary and secondary. A primary source is an eye-witness account, which may be recorded as visual, verbal or written data. For example, photographs and letters produced by nurses on a particular ward at a certain time provide primary data about the ward. This is seen as the most valid and reliable source. Secondary sources are produced by those who did not experience the event. Thus someone looking at a set of documents and photographs of a ward can produce their interpretation of it as a secondary source. Box 17.3 gives an illustration.

Box 17.3   Example of historical research

Kirby (2004) used documentary and oral evidence to compare the experiences of nurses as the subjects of research and as researchers. Documentary sources included government reports and professional journals. Oral evidence drew on interviews from survivors of the periods in history explored. In doing this Kirby has drawn on more than one source of evidence to allow comparisons and has obtained primary and secondary data.

Case studies

The **case study** approach allows the nurse researcher to conduct an investigation into single or multiple cases in their 'real life' context, though often just one case is researched to considerable depth. The case may be a patient, a family, a group, a hospital ward or an entire hospital or community. Though the amount of cases in the study is usually small, the number of variables considered by the researcher can be great, as all the factors thought to influence the case are included in the study. Researchers may be involved not just in collecting data about current behaviours and practices, but can also review the effect of the past, considering the history and previous behaviour patterns of the case subjects.

The researcher is interested in obtaining detailed information from the subjects and therefore may spend some time engaged with the case. Yin (1994) suggests that case study can be used to explore, describe or give explanation about the case. For example, case studies can be used to generate a hypothesis for testing, provide descriptive information about a group or give evidence to support theory or practice development. A case study design can allow researchers to demonstrate the effectiveness of a particular care approach or practice, looking at how an intervention impacts on the case. In order to provide description and/or explanation, case studies can include qualitative or quantitative research methods and often incorporate both. The range of data collection techniques used can include observations, interviewing, written data or physiological and psychological measurement (see Chapter 21). Data analysis may therefore include dealing with large amounts of qualitative material and quantitative results.

Case studies are being used more frequently in healthcare research despite the concerns expressed by some researchers that the method often relies on presenting data from a single case that may not be generalised more widely (Gomm et al., 2000). For example, a particular relationship may be peculiar to the group of patients studied as the case and may not be generally evident in other similar groups. Those involved in case study research work ensure rigour through the research process. The researchers clearly identify the initial identification of research questions, they explain the sampling of cases and collect multiple data, fusing different data collection methods. The researchers show how the data was analysed and discuss issues of generalisability to a wider audience (see Yin, 1994; Stake, 1995). In providing detailed description of the research process and findings, the researcher allows readers of the research to consider whether the results can be generalised to a wider population. An example is given in Box 17.4.

Box 17.4   Example of case study research

Moule (2006) collected data from a single case using multiple methods to explore whether healthcare students could develop as a community of practice of online learners. The case was formed from those students enrolled on an interprofessional module delivered online. Data was collected using a number of methods including the observation and analysis of online discussion boards, the analysis of online diaries held by participants and interviews with students. In total 15 students participated in the study. Rigour was enhanced through using multiple methods of data collection and involvement of the participants in reviewing the data interpretations. A full description of the case and its boundaries was provided in the publication to allow the readers of the research to consider generalisation through recognition and transfer.

Chapter summary

- The research design includes methods of data collection and analysis that will be used to address the research questions, aims and objectives.
- Action research can be a collaborative journey in research and development, with the researcher working within the research setting rather than on the research setting. The

action research process tries to facilitate change in health. The cycles of action research include the identification of issues, agreeing the way forward, implementing and evaluating the change before considering further issues and so on.

- There are many variations in feminist research which can be carried out by women, for women. Research problems considered are relevant for women and can be investigated through qualitative or quantitative methods.

- Historical researchers believe that by studying data and materials related to the past we can inform current and future practice. The historical researcher will need to ensure the originality of materials used as they need to be confident of reliability and validity of the source.

- The case study approach allows the nurse researcher to conduct an investigation into single or multiple cases in their 'real life' context. Case study design can be used to explore, describe or give explanation about a case, which might be a patient, ward or wider community. A case study design can allow researchers to demonstrate the effectiveness of a particular care approach or practice.

References

Christy, T. (1975) 'The methodology of historical research: a brief introduction', *Nursing Research*, 24 (3): 189–92.

Giddings, L. (2005) 'Health disparities, social injustice and the culture of nursing', *Nursing*, 54 (5): 304–12.

Gomm, R., Hammersley, M. and Foster, P. (2000) 'Case study and generalisation', in R. Gomm, M. Hammersley and P. Foster (eds), *Case Study Method*. London: Sage. pp. 98–116.

Greenhaugh, T., Robert, G., Bate, P., Kyriakidou, O., Macfarlane, F. and Peacock, R. (2004) 'How to spread good ideas: a systematic review of the literature on diffusion, dissemination and sustainability of innovations in health service delivery and organization'. Report for the National Co-ordinating Centre for NHS Service Delivery and Organisation R&D (NCCSDO). London: London School of Hygiene and Tropical Medicine.

Holloway, I. and Wheeler, S. (2002) *Qualitative Research in Nursing*, 2nd edition. Oxford: Blackwell Science.

Jinks, A. and Chalder, G. (2007) 'Consensus and diversity: an action research study designed to analyse the roles of a group of mental health consultant nurses', *Journal of Clinical Nursing*, 16 (7): 1323–32.

Kemmis, S. (2001) 'Exploring the relevance of critical theory for action research: emancipatory action research in the footsteps of Jurgen Habermas', in P. Reason and H. Bradbury (eds), *Handbook of Action Research: Participative Inquiry and Practice*. London: Sage. Chapter 8, pp. 91–102.

Kemmis, S. and McTaggart, R. (2000) 'Participatory action research', in N. Denzin and Y. Lincoln (eds), *Handbook of Qualitative Research*, 2nd edition. Thousand Oaks, CA: Sage. pp. 567–606.

Kirby, S. (2004) 'A historical perspective on the contrasting experiences of nurses as research subjects and research activists', *International Journal of Nursing Practice*, 10: 272–9.

Kitzinger, C. (2004) 'Feminist approaches', in C. Seale, G. Gobo, J. Gubrium and D. Silverman (eds), *Qualitative Research Practice*. London: Sage. Chapter 8, pp. 125–40.

Lewin, K. (1946) 'Action research and minority problems', *Journal of Social Issues*, 2: 34–46.

Moule, P. (2006) 'E-learning for healthcare students: developing the communities of practice framework', *Journal of Advanced Nursing*, 54 (3): 370–80.

Oakley, A. (1989) 'Who's afraid of the randomised controlled trial? Some dilemmas of the scientific method and "good" research', *Women & Health*, 15: 25.

Olesen, V. (2000) 'Feminisms and qualitative research at and into the millennium', in N. Denzin and Y. Lincoln (eds), *Handbook of Qualitative Research*, 2nd edition. Thousand Oaks, CA: Sage. Chapter 8, pp. 215–55.

Reason, P. and Bradbury, H. (eds), (2001) *Handbook of Action Research: Participative Inquiry and Practice*. London: Sage. Introduction, pp. 1–14.

Stake, R. (1995) *The Art of Case Study Research*. London: Sage.

Waterman, H., Tillen, D., Dickson, R. and de Koning, K. (2001) 'Action research: a systematic review and guidance for assessment', *Health Technology Assessment*, 5 (23): 1–166.

Whitelaw, S., Beattie, A., Balogh, R. and Watson, J. (2003) *A Review of the Nature of Action Research*. Cardiff: Welsh Assembly Government, Sustainable Health Action Research Programme.

Yin, R. (1994) *Case Study Research: Design and Methods*, 2nd edition. London: Sage.

Suggested further reading

Bridges, J. and Meyer, J. (2007) 'Exploring the effectiveness of action research as a tool for organizational change in health care', *Journal of Research in Nursing*, 12 (4): 389–99.

Gomm, R., Hammersley, M. and Foster, P. (eds) (2000) *Case Study Method*. London: Sage.

Olesen, V. (2000) 'Feminisms and qualitative research at and into the millennium', in N. Denzin and Y. Lincoln (eds), *Handbook of Qualitative Research*, 2nd edition. Thousand Oaks, CA: Sage. Chapter 8, pp. 215–55.

Reason, P. and Bradbury, H. (2001) *Handbook of Action Research: Participative Inquiry in Practice*. London: Sage.

Reitas, L. and Saarmann, L. (1989) 'The place for historical research', *Journal of Pediatric Oncology Nursing*, 6 (4): 143–4.

Spilsbury, K. and Meyer, J. (2005) 'Exploring the work of healthcare assistants and the implications for registered nurses' roles', *Journal of Research in Nursing*, 10 (1): 65–83.

Wilkinson, S. (2000) 'Feminist research traditions in health psychology: breast cancer research', *Journal of Health Psychology*, 5 (3): 359–72.

18

SYSTEMATIC LITERATURE REVIEWS

As nurses and researchers we bring expertise, clinical skills and past experiences to every clinical encounter. Patients bring their unique values, preferences, concerns and expectations. Nurses are expected to deliver, and patients expect care that is based on up-to-date clinically relevant knowledge, in other words, to practice evidence-based care. The notion underpinning evidence-based practice is that it closes the gap between clinical research and the real world and provides tools to interpret and apply research findings. There is, however, an increasing volume of research evidence in the nursing literature that is of variable quality and sometimes difficult to access. Systematic reviews can provide a means of summarising the literature on a specific topic that helps in assessing value for practice of some of this research evidence. They are, also, central to evidence-based practice because they synthesise the best evidence, can help to inform practice decisions by providing a quality-filter and synthesis of large amounts of evidence and provide a basis for clinical practice guidelines.

Literature reviews are usually referred to as systematic (with or without meta-analysis) or narrative. Narrative or traditional literature reviews are useful for providing a general perspective on a topic and are appropriate for describing the history of a problem or its management. They tend to be descriptive but do not necessarily answer a specific question nor comprehensively search the literature and are prone to subjectivity (Sim and Wright, 2000). Systematic reviews use explicit methods to systematically search, critically appraise and synthesise the evidence from clinical research. Effectively, systematic reviews provide an overview that summarises the world literature on a specific topic and are recognised as providing good quality research evidence.

This chapter discusses systematic reviews, meta-analysis and the techniques for undertaking a systematic review.

Learning outcomes

This chapter is designed to enable the reader to:

- Understand the nature and purpose of systematic reviews
- Recognise the processes involved in conducting a systematic review
- Have a basic understanding of meta-analysis and value in a systematic review
- Appreciate the value and role systematic reviews play in establishing an evidence base for practice

---

KEY TERMS

Evidence-based practice, Heterogeneity, Meta-analysis, Research hierarchies, Secondary analysis, Synthesis, Systematic review

---

Why are systematic reviews needed?

The imperative for all healthcare to be **evidence-based** has been one of the drivers for having good quality pre-appraised evidence in the form of **systematic reviews**. The idea of systematically reviewing the literature is not new but goes back to the earliest medical researchers. For example, Pearson, in 1904, synthesised the data from several studies on the efficacy of typhoid vaccination (Egger et al., 1998). He justified the aggregation of data because many of the studies were far too small to allow for any definitive opinion to be formed when note was taken of the probability of error involved.

Then the 1950s and 1960s saw rapid developments in healthcare that were not always supported by research evidence. Cochrane (1972) estimated that less than 10 per cent of medical interventions were supported by objective evidence that they actually did more good than harm. He also noted that many randomised controlled trials (RCTs) had been done but that the results were not readily accessible to practitioners:

> It is surely a great criticism of our profession that we have not organised a critical summary, by speciality or subspecialty, adapted periodically, of all relevant randomised controlled trials. (Cochrane: 1972: 1)

The challenge issued by Cochrane eventually led to the establishment of the Cochrane Collaboration. This is a worldwide network of healthcare professionals and research methodologists that has the aim of building up and maintaining a database of up-to-date systematic reviews that can be readily accessed by healthcare professionals and the general public. The Cochrane Collaboration is now just one of a number of organisations that exist to support the undertaking and dissemination of systematic reviews, and further demonstrates the role of systematic reviews in current healthcare practice.

What is a systematic review?

A systematic review is defined as:

> A review of the evidence on a clearly formulated question that uses systematic and explicit methods to identify, select and critically appraise relevant primary research, and to extract and analyse data from the studies that are included in the review. (CRD, 2001: 3)

The expectation is that a systematic review is undertaken with the same diligence as primary research, and when two or more study results can be combined statistically the review includes a **meta-analysis**. A systematic review is regarded as secondary research because it does not collect new data (primary research) but makes use of previous findings (Parahoo, 2006). The aim is to assess all of the available research on a particular topic. It is systematic because a rigorous approach to selection criteria, appraisal, synthesis and summary of findings is used.

Hierarchies of evidence (see Chapter 1)

The evidence from systematic reviews can be problematic because they tend to be linked with RCTs. This arises from the fact that systematic reviews originated from a positivist research paradigm. The positivist perspective proposes that the best way of finding out about the world is to use an approach that assumes data and its analysis are value-free and that data do not change because they are being observed (Krauss, 2005). Associated with this is an expectation that research aims to provide information that will help to predict what will happen in the future, for example research that demonstrates the effect of drug A on disease B or the impact of X on need for healthcare (Lindsay, 2007). This positivist viewpoint gives rise to the notion that it is possible to have a hierarchy or league table of research designs where some types of research are classed as being of better quality than others. These positivist **research hierarchies** vary, but they are all essentially in agreement; a suggested hierarchy is given in Figure 18.1.

It is worth noting that the notion of a hierarchy of research methodologies is not normally considered relevant by researchers who use a naturalistic approach where most of the data obtained will be qualitative. From this perspective the expectation is that the method chosen reflects the research question and as such a hierarchy is irrelevant and different methods are seen as being on a continuum.

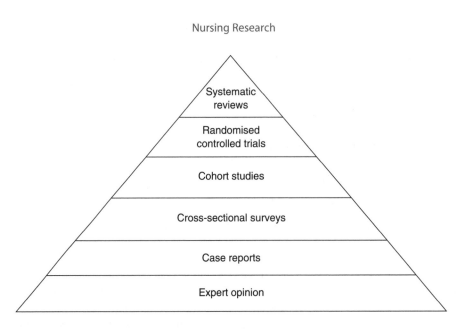

Figure 18.1   A positivist hierarchy of research evidence

An alternative approach is to combine a broad range of research designs to form a hierarchy that includes both quantitative and qualitative methodologies. This can be problematic because most published combined hierarchies place naturalistic research below experimental methodologies. For nurses this is an important point to note because a large proportion of nursing research yields qualitative data and there is thus a risk of their research being regarded as inferior to that conducted by researchers who use experimental methodologies. The value of systematic reviews for nursing practice requires that the role of systematic reviews and the type of research used in reviews are appropriate for nursing practice and will not necessarily follow the scientific, or positivist, approach which suggests that RCTs are the gold-standard for research evidence. More recently, however, there have been indications from organisations such as the NHS Centre for Reviews and Dissemination that qualitative research adds value to the assessment of evidence when making recommendations for best practice.

What are the advantages and disadvantages of systematic reviews?

There is a need to be wary of systematic reviews because outcomes and recommendations will depend on the amount of evidence (usually from RCTs and quasi-experimental studies) available. This highlights the fact that, although systematic reviews are often seen to provide the best possible evidence on which to base recommendations for practice, care must be taken to ensure that it has not been a case of 'garbage in, garbage out'. Remember that there has to be a sufficiency of research available for a review to be able to offer sensible and appropriate recommendations. This is quite apart from the need to ensure that other aspects important to the topic, such as quality of life and patient preference, are included if the evidence is to be used to guide practice.

Systematic reviews are regarded as beneficial in guiding practice because they use explicit methods that limit bias in the identification and rejection of studies included. This should also result in any conclusions and/or recommendations being reliable and accurate. One major advantage of systematic reviews is that healthcare providers, researchers and policy makers can assimilate large amounts of information quickly. Other advantages include the identification of studies that can be formally compared to establish generalisability of findings and consistency (lack of heterogeneity) and reasons for inconsistency in results across studies (heterogeneity). It has also been suggested that delay between research discoveries and implementation of effective diagnostic and therapeutic strategies may be reduced (Greenhalgh, 1997). Quantitative systematic reviews, that is, meta-analyses, are usually regarded as increasing the precision of the overall result.

Stages in the systematic review process

In this section the eight stages involved in a systematic review are explained, and Box 18.1 gives a list of some of the online resources available to help guide you through the process.

Box 18.1   Online resources for conducting systematic reviews

- NHS Centre for Reviews and Dissemination   www.york.ac.uk/inst/crd/crdreview.htm
- The Cochrane Collaboration – handbook for reviewers   www.cochrane.org/resources/handbook/index.htm
- Greenhalgh, T. (1997) 'How to read a paper: papers that summarise other papers (systematic reviews and meta analyses)', BMJ, 315: 672–5.   www.bmj.com
- Critical Appraisal Skills Programme (CASP)   www.phru.nhs.uk/casp

---

Stage 1: Determine the question

Just like any other type of research, a systematic review needs a well-formulated question or focus. The question needs to be stated very clearly so that there is no risk of misunderstanding the purpose of the review. Quite often, and particularly in Cochrane systematic reviews, the question is set out as a brief statement; for example, 'A review to compare the efficacy of two different interventions (A and B) in the management of a specific problem (X)'. The title of the review could be 'A or B in the treatment of X'. It is also not unusual for a review to answer more than one question. Although, as can be expected, the broader the question, the more difficult it can be to carry out the review and make recommendations (Parahoo, 2006). Greenhalgh (1997) suggests that the question must be very precise to facilitate the reviewers' ability to determine whether a paper should be included or rejected as being irrelevant, and this means that the question has to have clear objectives attached; for example, 'Laxatives for the management of constipation in palliative care patients' (Miles et al., 2006) had two clear objectives: (1) to determine the effectiveness of laxative administration for the management of constipation in palliative care patients, and (2) the differential efficacy of the laxatives used to manage constipation'.

In addition to the question guiding reviewers' assessments of the relevance of studies, a review's questions and objectives are used by readers in their initial assessment of the relevance of a review in their search for evidence (Cochrane Centre, 2008).

Stage 2: Define terms or concepts

The question and objectives are used to determine the key components for the initial searching strategies. It is, therefore, essential that the terms used are clearly defined and not ambiguous. For example, if you are reviewing studies on the management of constipation you need to decide, amongst other things, whether the focus is on acute or chronic constipation, as well as being clear what criteria define acute and chronic constipation and whether studies that simply refer to participants as being 'constipated' will be included. This process of defining the terms and concepts also assists in the development of the terms that will be used later to search for studies.

Stage 3: Set inclusion and exclusion criteria

Decisions about which studies to include in, and the scope of, a review often involve judgements. Therefore, inclusion and exclusion criteria are set to define the boundaries of the review (Cochrane Centre, 2008; Parahoo, 2006). These criteria have to be justified and able to withstand critical appraisal by experts and readers of the review. The expectation is that any limitations are relevant and appropriate for reducing the possibility of any significant evidence being missed. For example, in Parker et al.'s (2007) review of 'Prognostic/end-of-life communication with adults in the advanced stages of life-limiting illness: patient/caregiver preferences for the content, style, and timing of information' the exclusion criteria included studies where it was not possible to determine what percentage of the study group was being treated with palliative intent in articles published before 1985. This was because of changes in patient and community expectations and healthcare professionals' attitudes over time, and resulted in appropriate exclusion of studies prior to 1985. The types of study to be included in the review can also depend on reviewers' definitions of evidence, so that, for example, it is not uncommon for systematic reviews only to include RCTs because, as has already been discussed, RCTs can be regarded as providing the gold-standard of evidence. Reviewers' experience and understanding of the availability of certain types of evidence may also influence decisions about including other research designs.

Stage 4: Search for and collect studies that seem relevant to the focus/question of the review

A comprehensive, unbiased search is an essential requirement for any systematic review, and every attempt should be made to retrieve all relevant studies. Most research reports will be published in journals, but findings can also be presented at conferences (which may or may not be followed by publication) and in theses and dissertations. This requires a reviewer to make every effort to find unpublished works as well as searching all appropriate databases. It should also be anticipated and expected that studies with satisfactory statistical findings are more likely to be published before, or earlier than, those with non-significant findings (Sim and Wright, 2000). A checklist of data sources for systematic reviews is given in Box 18.2.

Box 18.2   Checklist of data sources for a systematic review

- CINAHL
- MEDLINE
- BNID
- Other medical and paramedical databases, e.g. AMED, CANCERLIT
- Cochrane controlled clinical trial register

(Continued)

(Continued)

- 'Grey literature' (theses, internal reports, non-peer-reviewed journals, pharmaceutical industry files)
- References (and references of references) listed in primary sources
- Other unpublished sources known to experts – find by personal communication
- Foreign language literature

Unfortunately, the success of a review will often be dependent on reviewers' abilities to locate articles. From a nursing perspective, perhaps the most relevant databases are the Cumulative Index of Nursing and Allied Health Literature (CINAHL), British Nursing Index (BNID) and MEDLINE – all of which can be accessed via the NHS National Library for Health. Although it is likely that most articles will be accessible via databases, there will be occasions when it is necessary to hand-search journals to locate relevant articles. For example, some nursing special interest journals may not be linked to the databases.

Actually searching successfully is a skill that requires training and experience and is considered in detail in Chapter 7. For a systematic review, the use of appropriate search terms is key to the successful identification of relevant material (Parahoo, 2006). The expectation is for the search strategy to be as comprehensive as possible. This means that the terms used in the search have to be as inclusive as possible but should be sufficiently exact to avoid the search locating large numbers of irrelevant articles. It is also very important to keep and record the search strategy so that the process could be repeated, as well as keeping a record of all the search results. There is now a variety of specially designed reference management software packages available to assist with this, such as Endnote, ProCite and Reference Manager. An example of a comprehensive search strategy and the search terms used in a review of 'Laxatives for the management of constipation in palliative care patients' from Miles et al. (2006) is given in Boxes 18.3 and 18.4.

Remember, though, that searching is only part of the process, and that it is just as important to review all of the articles found by the search to determine whether they are relevant to the research question (this is discussed in Chapter 9). Even the most appropriate search strategy is likely to identify irrelevant articles, such as discussion or opinion-based articles, rather than research reports.

Box 18.3   Search strategy for identification of studies for 'Laxatives for the management of constipation in palliative care patients (Review)'

The aim of the search strategy was to be as comprehensive as possible. The following search strategies were used to identify all relevant studies, irrespective of language and publication status. There have been three previously published systematic reviews look-ing at aspects of laxative use and constipation (Hurdon et al., 2000; Tramonte et al., 1997; Petticrew et al., 1997). The search strategies used in these reviews were considered and expanded. The following electronic databases were searched to identify all relevant studies, irrespective of language. Studies pre-dating 1966 were not sought. MEDLINE 1966 to 03/2001; EMBASE 1980 to 03/2001; CANCERLIT 1980 to 03/2001; SCIENCE CITA-TION INDEX 1981 to 03/2001; CINAHL 1982 to 03/2001; COCHRANE LIBRARY – Database of Systematic Reviews (CDSR), Database of Reviews of Effectiveness (DARE), Database of Controlled Trials Register (CCTR); Databases which provide information on grey litera-ture: SIGLE 1980 to 2001 (containing British Reports, Translations and Theses), NTIS, DHSS-DATA and DISSERTATION ABSTRACTS from 1961 to 2001; Conference proceedings from both International and National Conferences were hand searched, and databases on conference proceedings were accessed – BOSTON SPA CONFERENCES (containing Index of Conference Proceedings) and INSIDE CONFERENCES 1996 to 2001 and INDEX TO SCIENTIFIC AND TECHNICAL PROCEEDINGS from 1982 to 2001 and National Health Service National Research Register (containing Medical Research Council Directory).

Box 18.4 Search terms for 'Laxatives for the management of constipation in palliative care patients (Review)'

a. Constipation/laxative Studies

MeSH subject headings:
- Constipation
- Defaecation
- Diarrhoea
- Faecal incontinence
- Faeces, impacted

Textword terms/synonyms:
- bowel function$
- bowel habit$
- bowel movement$
- bowel symptom$
- colon adj. transit
- evacuation
- faecal adj. incontinence
- impaction
- impacted adj. faeces
- intestinal adj. motility
- irritable adj. bowel adj. syndrome

b. Laxatives

MeSH headings:
- Cathartics
- Dietary fibre
- Enema
- Fruit
- Glycerin
- Magnesium compounds
- Phenolphthaleins
- Phosphates
- Polyethylene glycols
- Sorbitol
- Plus BNF laxative terms and brand names.

Textwords/synonyms:
- names of drugs
- synonyms/related words (bulk, casantranol, cellulose, glucitol, glycerol, laxative$, purgative$, faecal adj. softener$, liquid paraffin,

(Continued)

(Continued)

- stool$
- stool with (hard or impacted)
- strain$
- void$

roughage, stool adj. softener$, suppositories)
- names of particular foods including: bran, fruit adj. juice, prune$, rhubarb

c. Patient Group

MeSH subject headings:
- Palliative care
- Terminal care
Textwords/synonyms:
- Care of the dying
- End-of-life care

Stage 5: Assess the quality, apply eligibility criteria and justify any exclusions

Before any **synthesis** of the retrieved relevant studies can be undertaken, the quality of them must be assessed. There are a number of tools available to help with this (see Box 18.1), and how to appraise studies is considered in detail in Chapter 8. Researchers can also grade the selected studies according to a predefined rating scale such as the Jadad scale (see Box 18.5) where the maximum score for any study is 5 (Jadad, 1998). This scale is not, however, appropriate for the rating of qualitative studies. Daly et al. (2007) suggest a hierarchy of evidence that can be applied in a similar way for qualitative studies but which gives levels of evidence rather than scores (see Box 18.6).

Box 18.5   Jadad scale

Question	*Score*
Is the study described as randomised?	• no or yes but inappropriate method = 0 • yes but no discussion of method = 1 • yes and appropriate method = 2
Is the study described as double blind?	• no or yes but inappropriate method = 0 • yes but no discussion of method = 1 • yes and appropriate method = 2
Is there a description of withdrawal/ dropouts?	• no = 0 • yes = 1

Box 18.6   Daly et al. (2007) hierarchy of evidence for qualitative studies

Level I – Generalisable studies	Sampling focused by theory and the literature, extended as a result of analysis to capture diversity of experience; analytic procedures comprehensive and clear.
Level II – Conceptual studies	Theoretical concepts guide sample selection, based on analysis of literature. Analysis recognises diversity in participants' views.
Level III – Descriptive studies	Sample selected to illustrate practical rather than theoretical issues. Record a range of illustrative quotes including themes from the accounts of 'many', 'most' or 'some'.
Level IV – Single care study	Provides rich data on the views or experiences of one person. Can provide insights in unexplored contexts.

The overall aim for the assessment of the quality of a study is to avoid subjectivity. One way of doing this is to get two or more researchers to undertake the assessment independently and to resolve any differences of opinion by discussion. To help with this process it is usual to develop a data extraction form specifically for the review. The information is then tabulated and gives researchers a quality assessment for each of the studies retrieved and ensures that only studies which meet the criteria set are included in the next stage of the review process. An example of an extraction data form is given in Table 18.1.

Stage 6: Synthesise the evidence – aggregate statistical results (meta-analysis) where appropriate

The aim of synthesis is to collate and summarise the data extracted from the primary studies included in the review (CRD, 2001). There are different ways in which this can be done, depending on the type of studies included in the review. Essentially, the reviewers are attempting to compare those study elements that are comparable in order to ensure that the results are valid. Sometimes the use of statistics can be a hindrance, and there is a risk that reviewers and users of reviews lose sight of the importance of reflection and judgement in the analysis (CRD, 2001). If, however, a statistical analysis or meta-analysis is possible (see below), the aim is to find out if there is a difference between the intervention groups and control groups in terms of the pre-selected outcome measures (Parahoo, 2006). Other elements of synthesis may focus on the **heterogeneity**

Table 18.1 'Laxatives for the management of constipation in palliative care patients (Review)', characteristics of included studies (Miles et al., 2006)

Study	Agra et al., 1998	Ramesh et al., 1998	Sykes, 1991
Methods	RCT	RCT	RCT Crossover
Participants	75 patients with terminal illness.	36 patients with advanced cancer.	51 hospice patients with cancer.
Interventions	Either 15ml (10g) lactulose or 0.4ml (12mg) senna daily for 27 days. Doses were increased if no BM for 3 days. Maximum doses were 60ml (40g) of lactulose and 1.6ml (48mg) of senna. Given as prophylactic when opioids started.	Either Misrakasneham (Ayurvedic herbal preparation starting at 2.5ml) or senna (starting at 24mg) in 3 steps of doses if previous level failed. Maximum doses were 72mg senna and 10ml Ayurvedic preparation. Given as prophylactic when opioids started.	Combination of senna liquid with lactulose (SL) in equal quantities or an equivalent volume of co-danthramer (CD) for 1 week and then switched to the alternative for a further week. Doses were modified according to response.
Outcomes	82% of recruited patients included in analysis. No significant difference noted between groups in efficacy, dropouts or adverse events. Trial authors recommend use of senna based on cost advantage. 37.5% of patients completing study required combined lactulose and senna to relieve constipation.	80% of Misrakasneham and 64% of senna patients completed the trial, 72% of all recruited were included in analysis. Of those completing the trial, 85% of the Misrakasneham group and 69% of the senna group reported satisfactory BMs – n.s.d. Trial authors recommend use of Misrakasneham based on favourable toxicity profile and cost advantage. This preparation may be difficult to obtain for use in the UK.	44% of recruited patients were included in analysis. Lactulose and senna was associated with significantly higher frequency of BM regardless of which laxative taken first ($p<0.01$) and required fewer rectal measures ($p=0.01$), although was more often stopped due to diarrhoea ($p=0.05$). Patient opinion split over favoured laxative. L+S 40% cheaper than CD.
Notes	Open randomisation necessary as substances different.	Open randomisation necessary as substances different.	Open randomisation necessary as substances different.
Allocation concealment	D	D	D

(variability in the characteristics) of the sample of individual studies. The synthesis of qualitative studies will be more descriptive, since findings are normally presented as themes which will often make comparisons difficult. In effect, analysis of qualitative studies in a systematic review follow a similar process to that undertaken for any qualitative study, that is, identification of themes (Daly et al., 2007). However, this can be difficult if the study characteristics are very diverse and will require considerable judgement and, according to the NHS Centre for Reviews and Dissemination (CRD, 2001), the synthesis of qualitative research within the context of a systematic review is exceptionally difficult and will be very subjective. It is, however, essential that the process is transparent, as would be expected of every other type of synthesis in a systematic review.

Stage 7: Compare analysis with other reviewers

One way of reducing the potential for subjectivity is for reviewers to compare their independent analyses and syntheses and then present a consensus. This will not completely avoid subjectivity and the possibility of bias, but it will add a level of transparency and increase the validity in a systematic review.

Stage 8: Prepare critical summary and make recommendations

The reason for undertaking a systematic review is to appraise and synthesise the evidence currently available to answer a specific question. It is expected that recommendations will be made on the basis of evidence appraised. The experience of collecting, appraising and synthesising the research that has been conducted means that the reviewers are also able to comment on the quality of that research and make recommendations for future research. For example, the conclusions from Miles et al. were that:

> The treatment of constipation in palliative care is based on inadequate experimental evidence, such that there are insufficient RCT data. Recommendations for laxative use can be related to costs as much as efficacy. There have been few comparative studies; equally there have been few direct comparisons between different classes of laxative and between different combinations of laxatives. There persists uncertainty about the 'best' management of constipation in this group of patients. (2006: 14)

Recommendations from a systematic review, however, may not be adequate for practical application, or sufficient guidance for practice, as seen in the example above. Data from systematic reviews can provide evidence for the development of clinical guidelines but in themselves are not likely to inform decision making unless they are based on a large body of good-quality research, and particularly from RCTs. Care has to be taken to ensure that findings from systematic reviews are used appropriately and that the evidence from research which takes into accounts things like quality of life and patient preferences are considered alongside that of 'scientific' research.

Meta-analysis

Any literature review will concentrate on appraising the evidence from primary sources, that is, research that has used original data or generated/collected its own data. This means that researchers will have carried out a primary analysis of the data. There are occasions when it is appropriate to undertake a **secondary analysis** of data or, more commonly, to synthesise a number of research studies and possibly aggregate the datasets within them (Sim and Wright, 2000); this is known as meta-analysis.

A meta-analysis is a statistical amalgam of the findings of a number of research studies that have been carried out on a specific topic. The term was first used by Glass (1976) and is sometime referred to as an 'analysis of analyses'. It is, however, really a synthesis or bringing together of the analysis of individual investigations of the same general topic. A systematic review that incorporates a meta-analysis does not simply incorporate the conclusions of the separate studies but amalgamates the data on which the results and conclusions were based (Sim and Wright, 2000). The data is analysed by the original investigators and will, where possible, be included in the systematic review and subjected to analysis by the reviewers. The aim is to provide a more precise and, therefore, a more trustworthy estimate of the true effect of an intervention (Beck, 1999). Meta-analysis can be a very useful tool when the findings from a number of individual studies have insufficient statistical power to provide credible information but where the aggregation of data enables more meaningful conclusions to be drawn (Sim and Wright, 2000). The amalgamation of findings may also facilitate the generalisability of findings which again would not be possible from the conclusion of individual studies. However, it must be remembered that studies can be very heterogeneous (inconsistent) in their design, quality and patient populations, and therefore it may not be valid to pool data from them.

There is a variety of ways of undertaking a meta-analysis. Most commonly, some sort of determination of 'average effect size' is made (Glass, 1976). It is expected that data from published RCTs can be extracted and pooled with those from other RCTs, providing that there is a minimum of commonality between the studies. The findings of the individual studies are not simply added up and averaged; weightings can be given according to the size and quality of individual studies, with larger studies and those with a good-quality rating being accorded a greater weighting.

Effectively, the summary statistics are combined, making a new analysis possible. The analysis appears to be valid but there are risks, such as inability to confirm that inclusion and exclusion criteria have been applied correctly; analysis of subgroups cannot be performed; additional variables cannot be used to adjust the relationship between the principal intervention variable(s) and outcome variables; and anomalies or inaccuracies in the data cannot normally be identified (Sim and Wright, 2000).

Chapter summary

- A systematic review is a mode of literature review that aims to summarise the world literature on a specific topic using explicit methods to systematically search, critically appraise and synthesise the evidence from clinical research.
- Systematic literature reviews are central to evidence-based practice because they synthesise the best evidence, can help to inform practice decisions by providing a quality-filter and synthesis of large amounts of evidence, and provide a basis for clinical practice guidelines.
- Meta-analysis is the use of statistical methods to summarise the results of individual studies with the aim of providing more precise estimates of the effects of healthcare interventions than those derived from the individual studies included in a review.
- A systematic review and meta-analysis are termed as secondary research because no new data is collected.
- A systematic review answers a specific question using a rigorous process of search, selection, appraisal, synthesis and summarisation of findings of primary research that is analogous to procedures that would be used in a randomised controlled trial.
- It is expected that all possible sources of literature are searched (electronically and by hand) in order to provide an as comprehensive as possible review of existing research to answer a specific question.
- Recommendations are made on the basis of the evidence appraised but may not be sufficient to guide practice and/or inform decision making unless they are based on a large body of good-quality research, and particularly from RCTs.
- Data from systematic reviews can provide evidence for the development of clinical guidelines.
- Care has to be taken to ensure that findings from systematic reviews are used appropriately, and that evidence from research that includes accounts of things like quality of life and patient preferences are considered alongside that of 'scientific' research.

References

Agra, Y., Sacristan, A., Gonzalez, M., Ferrari, M., Portugues, A. and Calvo, M.J. (1998) 'Efficacy of senna versus lactulose in terminal cancer patients treated with opioids', *Journal of Pain and Symptom Management*, 15 (1): 1–7.

Beck, C. (1999) 'Facilitating the work of a meta-analysist', *Research in Nursing and Health,* 22: 523–30.

Cochrane, A. (1972) *Effectiveness and Efficiency: Random Reflections on Health Services.* London: Nuffield Provincial Hospitals Trust.

Cochrane Centre (2008) *Cochrane Collaboration Handbook,* 5th edition. Oxford: Cochrane Collaboration.

CRD (2001) 'Undertaking systematic reviews of research and effectiveness: CRD guidelines for those carrying out or commissioning reviews', York: NHS Centre for Reviews and Dissemination, University of York.

Daly, J., Willis, K., Small, R., Green, J., Welch, N., Kealy, M. and Hughes, E. (2007) 'A hierarchy of evidence for assessing qualitative health research', *Journal of Clinical Epidemiology,* 60: 43–9.

Egger, M., Schneider, M. and Smith, G. (1998) 'Meta-analysis: spurious precision? Meta-analysis of observational studies', *British Medical Journal,* 316: 140–44.

Glass, G. (1976) 'Primary, secondary, and meta-analysis of research', *Educational Researcher,* 5: 3–8.

Greenhalgh, T. (1997) 'How to read a paper: papers that summarise other papers (systematic reviews and meta-analyses)', *British Medical Journal,* 315: 672–5.

Hurdon, V., Viola, R. and Schroder, C. (2000) 'How useful is Docusate in patients at risk for constipation? A systematic review of the evidence in the chronically ill', *Journal of Pain and Symptom Management,* 19: 130–36.

Jadad, A.R. (1998) *Randomised Controlled Trials: A User's Guide.* London: BMJ Books.

Krauss, S. (2005) 'Research paradigms and meaning making: a primer', *The Qualitative Report,* 10: 758–70.

Lindsay, B. (2007) *Understanding Research and Evidence-based Practice.* Tavistock: Reflect Press.

Miles, C., Fellowes, D., Goodman, M. and Wilkinson, S. (2006) 'Laxatives for the management of constipation in palliative care patients', *Cochrane Database of Systematic Reviews,* Issue 4. Art. No.: CD003448. DOI: 10.1002/14651858. CD003448.pub2.

Parahoo, K. (2006) *Nursing Research: Principles, Process and Issues.* Basingstoke: Palgrave Macmillan.

Parker, S., Clayton, J., Hancock, K., Walder, S., Butow, P., Carrick, S., Currow, D., Ghersi, D., Glare, P., Hagerty, R. and Tattersall, M. (2007) 'A systematic review of prognostic/end-of-life communication with adults in the advanced stages of life-limiting illness: patient/caregiver preferences for the content, style, and timing of information', *Journal of Pain and Symptom Management,* 34: 81–93.

Petticrew, M., Watt, I. and Sheldon, T. (1997) 'Systematic review of the effectiveness of laxatives in the elderly', *Health Technology Assessment,* 1: 13.

Ramesh, P., Suresh Kumar, K., Rajagopal, M., Balachandran, P. and Warrier, P. (1998) 'Managing morphine-induced constipation: a controlled comparison of the ayurvedic formulation and senna', *Journal of Pain and Symptom Management,* 16 (4): 240–44.

Sim, J. and Wright, C. (2000) *Research in Health Care: Concepts, Designs and Methods.* Cheltenham: Nelson Thornes.

Sykes, N. (1991) 'A clinical comparison of laxatives in a hospice', *Palliative Medicine*, 5: 307–14.

Tramonte, S.M., Mulrow, C.D. and O'Keefe, M.E. (1997) 'The treatment of chronic constipation in adults', *Journal of General International Medicine*, 12: 15–24.

19

SAMPLING TECHNIQUES

Nurse researchers will invariably need to employ sampling techniques in their research to make the project manageable. The time and expense involved in research projects prohibits data collection on the scale seen in the national census, involving the entire population. Therefore, researchers will want to ensure that the sample size and composition are appropriate to the study to strengthen the research outcomes and conclusion drawing. The process of sample selection is a crucial stage in the research process, with poor sampling techniques having the potential to compromise the research findings. A number of sampling strategies exist for use in both qualitative and quantitative or mixed-methods research, none being an exact science as each has individual strengths and weaknesses. In this chapter we consider the ways in which nurse researchers select populations and samples accessed to facilitate data collection. The discussion reviews a number of recognised sampling techniques that fall within probability and non-probability sampling strategies, identifying the strengths and weaknesses of the different approaches that can be employed.

Learning outcomes

This chapter is designed to enable the reader to:

- **Understand definitions of a research population and sample**
- **Appreciate the need for different approaches to identifying sample size within quantitative and qualitative research**
- **Appreciate the different sampling techniques used in qualitative and quantitative research**
- **Discuss the strengths and weaknesses of different sampling strategies available**
- **Appreciate the ethical issues involved in sample access**

KEY TERMS

Cluster/multi-stage random sampling, Convenience/accidental sampling, Network/snowball sampling, Non-probability sampling, Population, Probability sampling, Purposive sampling, Quota sampling, Sample, Sample size calculation, Sampling frames, Simple random sampling, Stratified random sampling, Systematic random sampling

---

Defining the population and sample

The researcher will be interested in collecting information or data from a particular **population** whose composition meets specific criteria. For example, nurse researchers might be asking research questions about undergraduate nursing students or service users suffering from particular mental health problems. These groups form the target population. Depending on the area of research interest, the population might be large, such as all nurses employed within the UK, or defined more narrowly as practising children's nurses within the UK. Populations need not always encompass human subjects, but may include documents, events or objects such as specimens.

Nurse researchers will often set specific parameters, limiting the study population through the use of inclusion or eligibility criteria that the population members must have or exclusion criteria that the population should not possess. These might include limitations on age, gender, professional qualifications or diagnosis. Those studies using quantitative methods will hope to sample from an accessible population in order to generalise the research findings to the target population. For example, the target population may include all patients recovering from a myocardial infarction in the UK, yet the researchers will work with an accessible population of (see Box 19.1) patients who meet the eligibility criteria.

Box 19.1   Example of an accessible population

Moule et al. (2008) sought to limit the potential population eligible to take part in research comparing e-learning and face-to-face study of basic life support. The eligible population needed to be employed within a mental health trust, to be members of the healthcare professions and have completed basic life support training within the previous year. Those holding automated external defibrillation qualifications were excluded.

A **sample** is a subset of the population, selected through sampling techniques. Polit and Beck (2006) suggest that the entities making up a sample are known as elements. Frequently nursing research will see individual patients or nurses as elements within a sample, though elements may be documents or biological specimens. Nurse researchers employ sampling strategies to enable them to work with a sample, as it is unrealistic and uneconomic to collect data from an entire population. As researchers are working with a sample it is important, particularly in quantitative research, that the sample selected is representative of the target population, being as similar as possible to the population to which the results will be generalised (LoBiondo-Wood and Haber, 2006). If there are major differences between the target and accessible population, these should be acknowledged by the researcher as a limitation of the study, as this can impact on the generalisability and transferability of the research outcomes. For example, differences between the target and accessible population would exist if a study was aiming to recruit children's nurses with more than ten years' oncology experience who were members of an ethnic minority group, but was unable to secure these criteria in an accessible sample. Though there is no guaranteed method of achieving a representative sample, the use of **sampling frames** and plans can assist the process.

Sampling frames

A sampling frame is developed to include all of the possible members of the population who might be eligible for inclusion in the final sample. It will be composed of a list of all of the patients, nurses, cases or events in the accessible population, established through the use of eligibility criteria. Those included in the sampling frame will therefore reflect as closely as possible the characteristics of the target population. The nurse researcher employs the sampling frame to identify the sample group. Many sampling frames are already in existence that can be used by researchers. Those wanting to study nurses and midwives could draw on the Nursing and Midwifery Council register, and universities hold lists of students enrolled on nursing courses that can be accessed. It should be noted, however, that the researcher may experience difficulties if the sampling frame is incomplete or inaccurate. In some cases it may not be possible to generate such a framework. Nurse researchers exploring questions with drug and alcohol users would not have access to a sampling frame and might find it difficult to construct one. Inaccuracies in a sampling frame may lead to errors in the generated sample. These systematic errors occur as the sampling frame is perhaps lacking particular elements of the population and cannot be remedied unless the frame is corrected.

It is also important to note that sampling frames have limited relevance to qualitative research, which does not seek generalise the findings of research to a wider population. The types of sampling approaches used in these cases are discussed later in the chapter.

Sample size calculation in quantitative research

Nurse researchers undertaking quantitative research will want to determine the size of the sample required so that the study can be powered to ensure any statistical differences between groups in intervention and comparison studies can be shown. The calculation of the sample size, a power calculation, is completed in the design stage, often by a statistician. For example, research by Moule et al. (2006) compared results from students who had completed nursing skill simulation training with those who hadn't. A power calculation suggested that the research should include a minimum of 62 participants in both the simulation and the control groups in order to demonstrate significant results at an 80 per cent confidence level. This meant that the significance level was set at 20 per cent and any significant results achieved would mean the researchers could be 80 per cent confident that the results were related to a real difference between the simulation and control groups. However, there was a 20 per cent chance that a real difference would not be detected. Usually the greater the power, such as increasing to a 95 per cent confidence level, the larger the sample size required.

The statistician will consider the outcomes being measured, tools of measurement and the expected differences between the groups in order to complete a power calculation. Those studies unable to achieve a sample size great enough to achieve the power required are seen as flawed. In some cases a pilot study may be completed and the results used to power a larger study. For further detail on power calculation, see Kidder and Judd (1987).

Sample size in qualitative research

We have seen that a specific **sample size calculation** is needed to support quantitative research where the final sample size is intrinsic to the data analysis. In contrast, qualitative researchers have no specific rules of sample size to work with. Morse (2000) suggests that researchers aiming to describe the experience of a population might use a sample of around ten. Where the researcher may want to look at variation across the group members, then the sample size should be larger (Polit and Beck, 2006). Ultimately, the size of the sample should be based on the need to obtain sufficient information to address the research questions. Often qualitative researchers will aim to achieve data saturation. This is achieved when the researcher fails to identify any new data from the participants, and at this stage sampling should cease.

Probability sampling

Probability sampling is characterised by the use of random selection to obtain sample members. The use of random selection occurs when the elements of a population, be that individuals, events or objects, have an equal chance of being included in the final sample. This approach to sampling allows the researcher to state the probability of an element of the population appearing in the sample. It reduces sampling errors and bias and increases sample representativeness, thus giving increased confidence in the sample. It is the preferable approach when a representative sample is required and is therefore often employed in quasi-experimental and experimental designs. However, bias can be present within random samples, resultant from random errors and systematic errors. Random errors are those occurring randomly within the final sample. For example, a randomly selected sample may have an over-representation of a particular ethnic group. Increasing the sample size used can reduce the chances of this type of sampling error. Systematic errors occur as a result of inaccuracies in the sampling frame and cannot be corrected through increasing the sample size. Correction would require changes to the sampling frame that remove inaccuracies. There are four commonly used probability sampling approaches: **simple random sampling, systematic random sampling, stratified random sampling and cluster or multi-stage sampling**.

Simple random sampling

A simple random sampling approach to identifying a sample is rigorous, but often time-consuming. The principles of simple random selection as described here are duplicated across the different random sampling approaches. There are a number of approaches that can be used to achieve randomisation, with the website www.randomisation.com providing an electronic resource for researchers. The nurse researcher will draw on the sampling frame to select a sample as a subset of the population. For example, if the researcher wanted to access patients recovering from resuscitation events, the sampling frame would include all patients meeting the eligibility criteria within a trust. The sampling frame might include a wider sample group of perhaps all those nurses working as emergency care practitioners across the UK. The simplest way of identifying a sample from the frame is through the use of a random number table. Often generated electronically, the list of random numbers from, say, 0 to 99 (see Table 19.1) or greater can be used to select pre-numbered elements from the sampling frame. Statistical packages such as Minitab or Statistical Packages for Social Scientists (SPSS) can generate random numbers to enable sample selection. If employing a random number table the researcher can either work horizontally or vertically though the table to select the sample, selecting, for example, numbers 03, 07, 84, 13 and so on as the sample group.

There are various advantages to this sampling approach. It removes the potential biases of the researcher from the selection process; any differences seen in the characteristics of the sample and population have occurred by chance, and as the sample size increases the probability of selecting a non-representation sample decreases. However, some disadvantages are also noted, including the time taken to use random number

Table 19.1   Random number table

03	35	11	98	74	20	23	61	32	30
07	09	15	22	21	88	94	90	50	71
84	10	02	91	24	35	47	63	99	04
13	82	31	44	70	65	38	80	92	01
23	33	18	76	97	06	64	53	70	98
17	21	09	05	14	30	31	82	54	56
77	62	02	19	27	48	59	92	71	25
66	04	12	55	42	60	83	24	37	22
05	90	08	69	33	93	57	74	29	10
30	44	74	28	09	67	24	18	99	81
45	89	12	75	65	22	48	21	08	55
78	26	72	03	28	91	36	42	10	89
88	56	23	14	73	54	22	07	52	39
25	78	65	91	63	45	71	01	86	49
67	04	30	05	73	29	96	39	24	49
14	71	27	18	46	28	34	97	24	12
16	48	73	92	45	29	37	19	28	10
13	85	49	37	40	16	72	95	41	08
17	39	73	37	19	91	65	28	76	95
45	42	97	28	02	36	73	95	46	99
77	54	28	16	34	07	16	94	73	54
65	48	27	04	62	48	37	19	21	45
24	91	54	38	18	35	42	87	06	72
06	12	21	26	29	44	79	13	19	46
12	05	43	05	51	10	78	36	58	25
18	25	37	19	54	28	75	53	24	82
96	14	52	75	62	01	99	53	24	42
45	68	24	02	15	73	57	28	27	25
56	81	72	24	04	38	26	78	15	29

Source: Hek and Moule, 2006: 66

tables, which persist despite the availability of computer software used to generate random number tables. The method also relies on access to a sampling frame. Those reviewing research using this sampling approach must recognise the limitations of the sampling strategy that can emerge if the researchers have been unable to list the target population. Box 19.2 gives or example of random number tables in use.

Box 19.2   Example of the use of random number tables

Halford et al. (2005) employed random number tables to identify their sample. Those in the sampling frame were allocated to one of three treatment groups as part of a randomised controlled trial (see Chapter 13). The sampling frame was composed of female partners of male problem drinkers. Sixty-one females were selected to receive either supportive counselling, or stress management, or alcohol-focused couples therapy.

Systematic random sampling

This approach to sampling can only be employed when a list is available that orders all the members of the population. For example, if researchers wanted to systematically sample qualified nurses in the UK, they could ask the Nursing and Midwifery Council to select the sample from the current database of qualified nurses. The sampling must start at a random point in the population, not necessarily with the first identified member. The researcher must know the total population size and the number of the sample required to allow calculation of the sampling gap (Burns and Grove, 2005). For example, if the population is 1,000 and 100 participants are required for the research, then every 10th member of the population will be sampled as $1,000/100 = 10$. The initial sample selection would occur between numbers 1 and 10, with the tenth person included thereafter. If number 8 were initially selected, then the sample would include numbers 18, 28, 38 and so on. See Box 19.3 for a further example. Whilst this approach should eliminate bias, it should be remembered that the approach relies on the original list being free from any bias in its generation.

Box 19.3   Example of systematic random sampling

Hsu (2005) used systematic sampling to select households within Taiwan. The research sought to examine consumers' preferences and information needs and problems encountered when using medical websites to access information. The sampling frame included 10,482 residents of Taipei. The sampling interval was calculated at 60, with every 60th household being selected, the first being taken from numbers 1 to 60.

Stratified random sampling

Nurse researchers might use a stratified random sampling technique when certain characteristics of the population are needed to address the research questions. It may be the case, for example, that particular age groups are required, grades of nursing staff, gender, ethnic groups or staff with particular levels of experience (see Box 19.4 for an example). A study might want to access surgical patients at different treatment stages arranged into four strata. It might include those patients currently receiving treatment and those six weeks, six months and one year following surgery. The participants are randomly selected to represent the four strata identified. Greater commonality in the sample is expected within each of the strata than across the four different strata.

The researcher can undertake proportionate sampling, ensuring that all the strata have the same total number of participants. If selecting a proportionate sample for the example above, each of the four strata would have 50 participants. Alternatively, there may be justification for selecting for a disproportionate sample. Research canvassing the views of nurses might want a sample stratified into males and females. A proportionate sample would see equal numbers of males and females included; however, this does not represent the total population of nursing, which employs more females than males. It might therefore be appropriate to select a disproportionate sample with a greater number of females than males in the strata. An alternative approach is to maintain strata of equal proportions and attach weighting to the findings of the strata to equalise the effect of the different strata sizes.

It is suggested that stratified sampling can challenge the researcher (LoBiondo-Wood and Haber, 2006). First, the sampling approach requires access to an initial list composed in a way that allows sampling in the strata required. Second, it can be difficult to ensure that the different sample proportions are achieved and, finally, the process can be time-consuming.

Box 19.4   Example of stratified random sampling

Zohar et al. (2004) examined the effect of structured, comprehensive nursing interventions administered over six months, with patients recovering from their first stroke. In total, 155 stroke survivors were stratified into either control or experimental groups by age, gender and ethnicity.

Cluster sampling

Cluster sampling is a term used interchangeably with multi-stage sampling. It is often employed when simple random sampling is too expensive and complex to organise and when the individual elements of a population are unknown. Cluster or multi-stage sampling involves a staged approach to sample selection that uses an initial sampling frame. Sample selection usually narrows from large to small clusters, such as selecting one strategic health authority from the initial sampling frame, then selecting one hospital from that strategic health authority and finally selecting to one or two wards within the hospital. From these wards individual patients or staff can be recruited.

This approach can enable the nurse researcher to access large samples at a small cost using a random sampling approach. Weaknesses in the approach can exist if the samples are closely associated and similar, as they originate in the same locality (Bowling, 2002).

This may mean that a larger sample size is required to increase precision (Burns and Grove, 2005).

Non-probability sampling

Non-random methods are used to select elements for inclusion in **non-probability sampling**. This means the researcher is unable to state the chances of elements of the population appearing in the final sample. Often non-probability sampling is employed by qualitative researchers who use different techniques from those seen in quantitative research to access their samples. Most qualitative researchers are not concerned with measuring specific attributes of a sample in order to generalise the findings to a wider population. Instead, the focus of qualitative research is to gain understanding, experience and meaning from the most appropriate sample. The main methods of sampling used include **convenience or accidental**, **quota** and **purposive sampling**. Samples can also be described as being generated through **network or snowball** techniques. It should be noted that though most commonly seen in qualitative research, these sampling approaches may be used in quantitative research if the researcher is unable to access data necessary to support random sampling techniques.

Convenience (accidental) sampling

Gathering information from those cases or people locally available is known as using a convenience or accidental sample. A market researcher who canvasses in the local supermarket or street corner will gather opinion and views from an accidental sample of shoppers and pedestrians who happen to be in the location at the time. This approach excludes all other members of the population who shop elsewhere or are using transport rather than walking. Nurse researchers often draw on the local community of staff and patients to form a sample of convenience (see Box 19.5). Conducting interviews with staff employed in the local hospital trust, student nurses at the local university or patients within a particular Accident and Emergency department would constitute the use of a convenience sample.

Often the sample is composed of those who volunteer or self-select, which can lead to concerns that those recruited have given their time because they have a particular view to present. A researcher accessing a convenience sample of healthcare staff to ask about the use of computers in the workplace may find that those volunteering are either keen to use computers or have a real dislike of information technology use in the workplace. The risk of introducing bias in this sampling approach is far greater, therefore, than in any other sampling technique (LoBiondo-Wood and Haber, 2006).

Box 19.5   Example of convenience sampling

Xia and McCutcheon (2006) completed a descriptive study that observed the actions of nurses at mealtimes. They were interested in how nurses mentored and assessed older patients' eating practices in acute care environments. Staff and patients on two medical wards were selected as a sample of convenience, with the actions of 50 nurses and the care delivered to 48 patients located on the wards being observed.

Quota sampling

In order to use quota sampling, the researcher must have some knowledge of the composition of the population of interest. The researcher will then be able to identify specific strata in the population and ensure that these are included in the sample. For example, if researching diabetic treatments, then the inclusion of patients from different age ranges may be important. Sample numbers would be selected to represent the proportions of patients in different age bands receiving treatment. If there are 1,000 patients receiving diabetic treatment and the final sample size is 100 or 10 per cent, then the proportion of each age group who should be included in the sample needs calculating. If 20 per cent, or 200 of the original 1,000 treated for diabetes are aged under ten years, then 20 per cent of the 200 will be selected, requiring the researcher to select 20 participants from the age group 0–10. See Box 19.6 for a further example.

The criteria for selection could include gender, ethnicity, socio-economic status, employment, educational level or diagnosis. The sampling technique should reduce the chances of over- or under-representation, but bias can still exist. This can occur as those included in the sample may not be typical of the population in relation to the variables being measured.

Box 19.6   Example of quota sampling

Pieper et al. (2006) used quota sampling to identify participants in research that sought to measure chronic venous insufficiency in human immunodeficiency virus (HIV). The strata of the population were identified as those HIV-positive persons with and without a history of injection drug use. The quota numbers were set at 46 for those with injection drug use and 27 for those without. Participants were enrolled until each quota was filled, achieving a final sample size of 73.

Purposive sampling

Often used in qualitative research, purposive sampling aims to sample a group of people or events with specific characteristics or set of experiences. The technique can also be referred to as 'judgement sampling', as the researcher is making a judgement about the composition of the sample, selecting participants who they believe have either experienced a particular episode or have a set of knowledge that relates to addressing the research question (see example in Box 19.7). Patton (2002) identifies several strategies that can be employed in purposive sampling, including extreme or deviant case sampling (extreme and unusual cases), typical case sampling (average or typical cases) and criterion sampling (cases where predetermined criteria exist).

A purposive sample has an over-representation of a particular group and is not representative of an entire population being studied. For example, if the research question is aiming to review emerging new roles in nursing, the researcher may select a purposive sample of modern matrons who are believed to operationalise the role in particular ways. The selection is based on the researcher's judgement to include those modern matrons practising in a variety of different ways.

It is suggested that purposive sampling can also be used to pilot questionnaires or develop hypotheses for further study (Bowling, 2002). Purposive sampling has also been employed within experimental designs to access patients receiving a particular treatment. Obviously the results from such a study could not be generalised as the sampling approach is non-randomised, though research outcomes could inform treatment development.

Box 19.7   Example of purposive sampling

Kealey and McIntyre (2005) employed purposive sampling in research that wanted to evaluate domiciliary occupational therapy services delivered to patients in the palliative care stages of cancer in a community trust. The criteria for purposive selection identified by the researcher included:

- referral to domiciliary occupational therapy services delivered by the community trust
- patients in the palliative stage of cancer care
- patients willing and able to participate
- aged 18 years or over
- understand written and spoken English
- have an informal carer.

A range of occupational therapists working in the trust provided cases from which the researcher selected patients according the predetermined criteria.

Network (snowball) sampling

Network or snowball sampling is the approach used when nurse researchers are aiming to select hidden samples. The researcher will need to draw on networks to identify the sample, often involving a third party in sample access (see Box 19.8). For example, researchers aiming to recruit the homeless, alcoholics, victims of abuse or other more hidden populations may access some participants through hostels or self-help groups, using convenience sampling methods. They then rely on the initial sample to draw on their networks to recruit further participants. Burns and Grove (2005) warn that such sampling techniques, whilst recruiting subjects with the knowledge and expertise to provide information for the study, have inherent biases because selection is not independent, as members of the sample are known to one another.

Box 19.8   Example of network sampling

Hughes et al. (2005) used network sampling to access a research population. The researchers identified an initial sample of those suffering from motor neurone disease, inviting them for interview. The research was exploring people's experiences of living with the disease and invited those interviewed to pass on introductory letters to family and friends, asking them to take part in the research.

Chapter summary

- An appropriate sample size and composition is crucial to strengthening the research outcomes and conclusion drawing.
- Nurse researchers will often set specific parameters, limiting the study population through the use of inclusion or eligibility criteria.
- A sample is a subset of the population, selected through sampling techniques.
- A number of sampling strategies exist for use in both qualitative, quantitative or mixed-methods research that fall within probability and non-probability sampling techniques.
- A sampling frame and specific sample size calculation can be used to support probability sampling for quantitative research.
- Probability sampling is characterised by the use of random selection to obtain sample members.
- There are four commonly used probability sampling approaches: simple random sampling, systematic random sampling, stratified random sampling and cluster sampling.
- Non-random methods are used to select elements for inclusion in non-probability sampling as qualitative researchers are concerned with gaining understanding, experience and meaning from the most appropriate sample.
- The main methods of sampling used include convenience or accidental, quota and purposive sampling. Samples can also be described as being generated through network or snowball techniques.

References

Bowling, A. (2002) *Research Methods in Health*, 2nd edition. Buckingham: Open University Press.

Burns, N. and Grove, S. (2005) *The Practice of Nursing Research: Conduct, Critique and Utilization*, 5th edition. St Louis, MO: Elsevier/Saunders.

Halford, K., Price, J., Kelly, A., Bouma, R. and Young, R. (2005) 'Helping the female partners of men abusing alcohol: a comparison of three treatments', *Addiction*, 96 (10): 1497–1508.

Hek, G. and Moule, P. (2006) *Making Sense of Research: An Introduction for Health and Social Care Practitioners*, 3rd edition. London: Sage.

Hsu, L. (2005) 'An exploratory study of Taiwanese consumers' experiences of using health-related websites', *Journal of Nursing Research*, 13 (2): 129–40.

Hughes, R., Sinha, A., Higginson, I., Down, K. and Leigh, N. (2005) 'Living with motor neurone disease: lives, experiences of service and suggestions for change', *Health and Social Care in the Community*, 13 (1): 64–74.

Kealey, P. and McIntyre, I. (2005) 'An evaluation of the domiciliary occupational therapy service in palliative cancer care in a community trust – a patient and carer perspective', *European Journal of Cancer Care*, 14 (3): 232–43.

Kidder, L. and Judd, C. (1987) *Research Methods in Social Relations*, 5th edition. New York: CBS Publishing.

LoBiondo-Wood, G. and Haber, J. (2006) *Nursing Research: Methods and Critical Appraisal for Evidence-based Practice*, 6th edition. St Louis, MO: Mosby Elsevier.

Morse, J. (2000) 'Determining sample size', *Qualitative Health Research*, 10: 3–5.

Moule, P., Albarran, J., Bessant, E., Pollock, J. and Brownfield, C. (2008) 'A comparison of e-learning and classroom delivery of basic life support with automated external defibrillator use: a pilot study', *International Journal of Nursing Practice*, 14: 427–34.

Moule, P., Wilford, A., Sales, R., Haycock, L. and Lockyer, L. (2006) 'Can the use of simulation support pre-registration nursing students in familiarising themselves with clinical skills before consolidating them in practice?', Faculty of Health and Social Care, University of the West of England, Bristol. http://hsc.uwe.ac.uk/net/research/Data/Sites/1/GalleryImages/Research/NMC%20Final%20Report%20UWE.pdf, accessed 28 February 2008.

Patton, M. (2002) *Qualitative Evaluation and Research Methods*, 3rd edition. Newbury Park, CA: Sage.

Pieper, B., Templin, T. and Ebright, J. (2006) 'Chronic venous insufficiency in HIV-positive persons with or without a history of injection drug use', *Advances in Skin and Wound Care*, 19 (1): 37–42.

Polit, D. and Beck, C. (2006) *Essentials of Nursing Research: Methods, Appraisal and Utilization*, 6th edition. Philadelphia, PA: Lippincott Williams & Wilkins.

Xia, C. and McCutcheon, H. (2006) 'Mealtimes in hospital – who does what?', *Journal of Clinical Nursing*, 15 (10): 1221–7.

Zohar, N., Zolotogorsky, Z. and Sugarman, H. (2004) 'Structured nursing intervention versus routine rehabilitation after stroke', *American Journal of Medicine and Rehabilitation*, 83 (7): 522–9.

Suggested further reading

Collins, K., Onwuegbuzie, A. and Jiao, O. (2007) 'A mixed methods investigation of mixed methods sampling designs in social and health science research', *Journal of Mixed Methods Research*, 1 (3): 267–94.

Field, L., Pruchno, R., Bewley, J., Lemay, E.P., Jr. and Levinsky, N. (2006) 'Using probability vs. nonprobability sampling to identify hard-to-access participants for health-related research: costs and contrasts', *Journal of Aging and Health*, 18 (4): 565–83.

Fulton Picot, S., Samonte, J., Tierney, J., Connor, J. and Powel, L. (2001) 'Effective sampling of rare population elements: black female caregivers and noncaregivers', *Research on Aging*, 23 (6): 694–712.

Oldfield, S. (2001) 'A critical review of the use of time sampling in observational research', *Nursing Times Research*, 6 (2): 597–608.

Websites

Directory of randomisation software and services: http://www–users.york.ac.uk/~mb55/guide/randsery.htm

Site that provides online randomisation: www.randomisation.com

Site on clinical trials by the National Cancer Institute that includes a discussion on randomisation: http://www.cancer.gov/clinicaltrials/understanding/what-is-randomization

20

MIXED METHODS

Nurse researchers are increasingly using a number of data collection methods in a single research project and combining both qualitative and quantitative approaches to address research questions. In this chapter we present a review of the reasons why a mixed method approach is proving popular in nursing research. The ways in which mixed methods can be applied within a research design are reviewed and the implications of combining research methods within one research project are considered.

Learning outcomes

This chapter is designed to enable the reader to:

- **Understand the rationale for using mixed methods in nursing research**
- **Appreciate when mixed methods might be employed**
- **Understand the implications of using mixed methods**

KEY TERMS

Hawthorne effect, Mixed methods, Qualitative research, Quantitative research, Triangulation

---

Table 20.1 Denzin's types of triangulation

Types of triangulation	Explanation
Data	Using a number of data sources with a similar focus to obtain a range of views about a question or topic, thus aiming to achieve validation through comparing diverse opinion.
Method	Combining more than one research method, such as qualitative and quantitative methods.
Researcher	Using researchers from diverse backgrounds, such as a psychologist, nurse and social scientist, who bring different viewpoints to a research team.
Theory	Comparing the usefulness of competing theories or hypotheses.

Rationale for the use of mixed methods

Denzin (1989) is a strong advocate of the use of **mixed methods** in social research. He suggests that researchers should seek to employ as many methodological perspectives as practical when investigating research problems. One of the main reasons for combining methods in research is the scope offered for **triangulation**, where the results of either a qualitative or quantitative method can be reviewed alongside the results generated by an alternative method (Robson, 2002). For example, the results of an attitude measure to, say, the use of computers in healthcare could be explored in interviews. Denzin (1989) suggests there are four possible types of triangulation that can be achieved in social research (see Table 20.1).

Accessing multiple data sources might involve interviewing student nurses and lecturers about curriculum design, or including healthcare professionals, patients and relatives as participants in research. Combining different research methods in one design can be achieved through perhaps using a survey tool with staff, followed by conducting interviews and possibly observations of practice.

Here we concentrate on the rationale for the use of mixed methods in nursing research. It should be remembered that nurses draw on a number of data sources in their daily practice in order to make judgements. For example, in the assessment of a patient the nurse will take quantitative measurements of blood pressure, pulse, temperature and respirations. Additionally, observational data will be used, gained from looking at the patients, and interviewing the patient will reveal further information about their health. Information will also be available through other physiological measures, such as the results of blood tests and from investigations including scans and invasive procedures. Given the range of information used in clinical practice it is unsurprising that researchers faced with the reported complex research problems of health (Barbour, 1999) should engage with a range of methods.

A review of the range of research methods available (see Chapter 21) highlights the strengths and weaknesses of each. Observations can introduce the **Hawthorne effect** through the intrusion of the researcher and can affect participant behaviour, whereas interview discussion can reflect power differences seen between the researcher and interviewee. No one method is perfect, though using a combination of methods can, it is argued, limit the potential deficits and biases of one particular method (Brewer and Hunter, 1989). Thus, combining methods from **qualitative** and **quantitative research** can enhance the reliability, validity and trustworthiness of a research study and its overall quality (see Chapter 12). See also Box 20.1 for an example.

Box 20.1   Example of methodological triangulation in midwifery education

Magnusson et al. (2005) drew on three different methods to limit the weaknesses of the individual methods, as the limitation of one method was addressed through the strength of another. They included individual interviews with student midwives and their mentors, collecting diaries from both and undertaking non-participant observations of care delivered by students and their mentors to investigate mentor–student relationships. They concluded that using methodological triangulation provided an effective approach, though obviously was more time- and resource-intensive than a single methodological approach design.

In using two or more methods of data collection to answer the same question, the nurse researcher can confirm the accuracy of the findings. For example, Magnusson et al. (2005) were able to analyse data from the interviews and diaries to gain the perspective of the students and midwives. This gave a view of how they felt the mentor–student relationship worked in practice. Through observations the research team were able to record the relationship in action, and through comparison of similar results drew greater validity from the findings, confirming the results and ensuring their appropriateness.

Having a range of results collected through different methods in one study allows the researcher to compare findings and make conclusions based on a variety of data. This reduces the likelihood of research making false claims based on results achieved through one method, when the research team can be convinced that they have achieved the only and correct answer.

Mixed methods are mainly used:

- To compare findings through triangulation.
- To research different perspectives of the same issue.
- To generate data from different approaches, often combining qualitative and quantitative methods.
- In the development, implementation and evaluation of interventions.

Figure 20.1   Use of mixed methods

Applications of mixed methods

Healthcare researchers use mixed methods to address a variety of research problems. Bryman (1988: 127) suggests eleven different ways in which mixed methods are employed in social research and challenges readers to identify more. These include use, at different stages of the research process, to access researcher and participant perspective in one design and to gain views of both macro and micro levels, reviewing the institution and the individual. In healthcare research mixed methods are also used in a number of different ways, as outlined in Figure 20.1, and can also be used to develop data collection tools.

Comparing research findings through triangulation

As mentioned earlier, there are various ways of achieving triangulation in a research study. In this section we will concentrate on the triangulation of research methods, the potential for combining qualitative and quantitative methods or triangulating different qualitative or quantitative methods in one research design (Barbour, 1999). More commonly, triangulation would involve the researcher using two or more different methods of data collection in a study (Denzin, 1989). Having obtained a range of data, the researchers would then compare the findings to try to present a more accurate or complete view.

It is suggested that triangulation of methods can either aim to improve the validity and accuracy of the findings and confirm results, or can add to the scope of the findings, enabling a broader understanding of the issues (Shih, 1998). There is the potential for mixed methods to achieve both increased accuracy and scope of a study. There are, however, concerns that employing triangulation of methods to achieve greater validity and accuracy can prove problematic (Sim and Sharp, 1998).

A number of researchers are using a mixed-methods approach to address complex research questions, employing a range of methods in the pursuit of knowledge. Whilst there are potential benefits to using mixed methods, it should be remembered that designs employing triangulation of methods would incur greater research costs and require additional resources. Triangulation should therefore be employed when a mixed-methods approach is thought necessary to answer the research question(s) posed (see Box 20.2).

Box 20.2   Example of the use of triangulation

Hyrkäs and Paunonen (2000) used triangulation of methods to measure patient satisfaction. Interview data were collected from 30 patients on three ward areas. Content analysis showed that the themes generated were equivalent to the item scales in a 'Quality of hospital care patients' viewpoint' questionnaire that was used in the same wards. Those patients interviewed had not seen or completed the questionnaire prior to the interview. The findings suggested that an interview supplemented the questionnaire data as a data collection method. The interview gave deeper information on the patients' views and experiences. The researchers concluded that triangulating methods provided an accurate view of patient satisfaction, though it was more resource intensive and the use of interviews could delay the processing of gathering patient views.

Using research methods to explore different perspectives of the same issue

Nursing practice can generate broad and complex research areas for study, often identifying several different approaches that can be taken to consider one area of practice. In these cases, mixed methods could be used to address different research questions or aspects of one issue.

For example, a number of research questions could be asked about cardiac rehabilitation services provided to patients following a myocardial infarction. In taking different perspectives on this issue, researchers might explore a variety of aspects that would require the use of different research methods, such as:

- patient experiences of the service
- relatives' views of the service
- to measure the effectiveness of cardiac rehabilitation programmes for those involved.

To address the first two issues in depth, interviews could be conducted with patients and relatives who have experience of the cardiac rehabilitation services. Data collected here would enable the research team to develop some understanding of patient and relative perspectives of cardiac rehabilitation services. A third component of the study centring on the effectiveness of cardiac rehabilitation programmes would measure, perhaps through a survey or physiological measures, the impact of the service on lifestyle and health. This could explore whether the service had any long-term benefit for the patient. In exploring different aspects of one area, a fuller picture can be gained to inform the further development of cardiac rehabilitation services.

Generating data from different approaches combining qualitative and quantitative methods

Given the complexity of nursing research questions and issues, there will be occasions when a research design will include both qualitative and quantitative methods, using one approach to support and enhance the other (see Box 20.3). Each research method has its limitations (see Chapter 21) and therefore combining methods within one study can achieve a more comprehensive view of the research subject.

A questionnaire survey can be used to obtain data from a large population on a particular subject. Analysis of the data will provide useful information, though may leave unanswered questions about context and a range of issues that could usefully be explored through conversation. Focus-group or individual interviews would give scope to explore understandings, experiences, interpretations and add a quality dimension to the research. Through a more in-depth discussion the researcher can explore the survey results more fully and has the potential to gain wider and deeper understanding. Alternatively, research collecting qualitative data initially through diaries or interviews could usefully gain a broader view of issues and employ a follow-up survey. The results of qualitative data may also enable researchers to generate a research hypothesis that can be tested through quantitative methods (see Chapter 6).

Box 20.3   Example of combining quantitative and qualitative research methods

Moule et al. (2007) used both quantitative and qualitative methods in research that explored the use and development of e-learning in health sciences and practice disciplines. The initial phase of the project included a survey of higher education institutes. Using a database from the funder (Higher Education Academy's Health Sciences and Practice Subject Centre), a survey tool was distributed. The results of the survey gave some information about the use of e-learning in the different disciplines across the higher education sector. The results of the survey were used to identify a sample for the second phase of the research. Four case study sites were used, including early and late adopters of e-learning. Within the case study sites, qualitative data were collected through interviews and a review of e-learning provision. This phase of the project enabled the researchers to explore in greater detail some of the aspects raised in the survey and to examine issues such as the barriers to e-learning and enabling factors.

Developing, implementing and evaluating interventions

Nursing and healthcare interventions are often guided by policy and practice guidance that are based on the best available evidence. Earlier chapters (see Chapters 1 and 2) have described the place of research in nursing and the hierarchy of evidence that informs practice and policy development. Often those developing practice guidance prefer to use the 'best' form of evidence, the 'gold-standard' being seen as research evidence developed through the randomised control trial method (see Chapter 13).

The current resuscitation guidelines (Resuscitation Council (UK), 2005) are based on different levels of evidence, some being developed through a systematic review of several randomised controlled trials (level 1), whilst other aspects of the guidance are developed from expert opinion (level 6) (Gray, 1997). These guidelines are based on the best current knowledge and are updated regularly as that evidence base is developed through research and practice. Resuscitation policy reflects a range of underpinning knowledge, from across the levels of evidence, though would ideally be developed from evidence positioned at level 1. There are other aspects of care delivery, however, that can be supported by evidence developed at level 6, from personal and professional expertise, including patient views and opinions. Thus, a range of research methods might be employed to develop, implement and evaluate the broad spectrum of care that nurses are involved with (see Box 20.4). What is of prime importance is the need to ensure that the methods used will enable the research team to address the research questions posed. Indeed, the Medical Research Council (2000) suggests that a range of methods might be used to address healthcare questions, with appropriate selection being paramount. Certain questions looking at patient satisfaction and experiences of interventions require a qualitative method.

Box 20.4   Example of research using mixed methods to develop, implement and evaluate a nursing intervention

Pagliari et al. (2004) used a mixed-method approach to evaluate the Electronic Clinical Communications Implementation in Scotland. This programme implemented electronic records in primary and secondary care, processing laboratory results, out-patient appointments and other clinical records online. A mixed-method approach, including quantitative and qualitative approaches, was used to try to capture a comprehensive evaluation of a complex intervention.

The team identified four main activities:

1   A survey of ECCI project managers.
2   In-depth studies of regional projects, document review, team member interviews.

3 Development of minimum dataset and implementation.
4 A survey of primary and secondary care ECCI users.

Though the benefits of using mixed methods are not made explicit, the research identifies the qualitative and survey methods as showing variation in the use of technologies. The survey of users in clinical practice gave greater understanding of behaviour and attitude to use of the system.

Implications of using mixed methods

It should be noted that not all researchers are advocates of combining qualitative and quantitative methods in one design, because they are based in different approaches (see Chapter 11) (LoBiondo-Wood and Haber, 2006). Indeed, Cresswell (1994) suggests there are three key positions in this debate. Against any form of multiple methods are the 'purists', whereas the 'situationalists' will apply certain methods to particular situations and the 'pragmatists' will employ a mixed-methods approach. The pragmatists take the view that provided the methods employed are appropriate to addressing the research question(s) and are well thought through, combining research methods within one study can be complementary and aid credibility.

Readers of research employing a mixed-methods approach to data collection should be aware of the need to understand the strengths and weakness of each individual method (see Chapter 21), as well as being able to review how the methods were used to answer specific research question(s). They should also be cognisant of the additional time and resource demands placed on a team employing a mixed methods approach.

Chapter summary

- Mixed methods are commonly used in nurse research.
- Triangulation can be achieved by using a number of data sources in one study, combining research methods and using researchers from diverse backgrounds.
- The percieved strengths of mixed methods offer the potential to increase the scope of the study and validity and accuracy of the findings.
- Mixed methods enable researchers to address complex research questions.
- Combining more than one method in the same study is not popular with 'purist' researchers.
- If different methods achieve conflicting results, this can be problematic.

References

Barbour, R. (1999) 'The case for combining qualitative and quantitative approaches in health services research', *Journal of Health Services Research and Policy*, 4 (1): 39–43.

Brewer, J. and Hunter, A. (1989) *Multi-Method Research: A Synthesis of Styles*. Newbury Park, CA: Sage.

Bryman, A. (1988) *Quantity and Quality in Social Research*. London: Routledge.

Cresswell, J. (1994) *Research Design*. Newbury Park, CA: Sage.

Denzin, N. (1989) *The Research Act: A Theoretical Introduction to Sociological Methods*, 3rd edition. Englewoods Cliffs, NJ: Prentice-Hall.

Gray, J. (1997) *Evidence-based Healthcare: How to Make Health Policy and Management Decisions*. London: Churchill Livingstone.

Hyrkäs, K. and Paunonen, M. (2000) 'Patient satisfaction and research-related problems (part 2). Is triangulation the answer?', *Journal of Nursing Management*, 8 (4): 237–45.

LoBiondo-Wood, G. and Haber, J. (2006) *Nursing Research: Methods and Critical Appraisal for Evidence-based Practice*, 6th edition. St Louis, MO: Mosby Elsevier.

Magnusson, C., Finnerty, G. and Pope, R. (2005) 'Methodological triangulation in midwifery education research', *Nurse Researcher*, 12 (4): 30–41.

Medical Research Council (2000) *A Framework for Development and Evaluation of RCTs for Complex Interventions to Improve Health*. London: Medical Research Council.

Moule, P., Ward, R., Shepherd, K., Lockyer, L. and Almeida, C. (2007) *Scoping e-learning in Health Sciences and Practice*. Bristol: Faculty of Health and Social Care, University of the West of England.

Pagliari, C., Gilmour, M. and Sullivan, F. (2004) 'Electronic Clinical Communications Implementation (ECCI) in Scotland: a mixed-methods programme evaluation', *Journal of Evaluation in Clinical Practice*, 10 (1): 11–20.

Resuscitation Council (UK) (2005) *Guidelines for Adult Basic Life Support*. Available at www.resus.org.uk/pages/bls.pdf, accessed 21 February 2008.

Robson, C. (2002) *Real World Research*, 2nd edition. Oxford: Blackwell.

Shih, F. (1998) 'Triangulation in nursing research: issues of conceptual clarity and purpose', *Journal of Advanced Nursing*, 28: 631–41.

Sim, J. and Sharp, K. (1998) 'A critical appraisal of the role of triangulation in nursing research', *International Journal of Nursing Studies*, 35: 23–31.

Suggested further reading

Brannen, J. (ed.) (1992) *Mixing Methods: Qualitative and Quantitative Research*. Aldershot: Avebury.

Burke Johnson, R. and Onwuegbuzie, A. (2004) 'Mixed methods research: a research paradigm whose time has come', *Educational Researcher*, 33 (7): 14–26.

Gilbert, T. (2006) 'Mixed methods and mixed methodologies: the practical, the technical and the political', *Journal of Research in Nursing*, 11 (3): 205–17.

Lynne Johnstone, P. (2004) 'Mixed methods, mixed methodology health services research in practice', *Qualitative Health Research*, 14 (2): 259–71.

Simons, L. (2007) 'Moving from collision to integration: reflecting on the experience of mixed methods', *Journal of Research in Nursing*, 12 (1): 73–83.

Wilkins, K. and Woodgate, R. (2008) 'Designing a mixed methods study in pediatric oncology nursing research', *Journal of Pediatric Oncology Nursing*, 25 (1): 24–33.

Website

Journal of Mixed Methods Research: http://mmr.sagepub.com/

21

METHODS OF DATA COLLECTION

Researchers must measure, observe or record data using specific techniques in order to answer their research questions. The selection of appropriate data collection tools is therefore a key part of the research process. In this chapter we discuss the main data collection tools available for nurse researchers. We give examples of their use in research studies, demonstrating the application of a variety of methods to the research setting.

Learning outcomes

This chapter is designed to enable the reader to:

- **Appreciate the differences between structured and unstructured observations**
- **Understand the participant observer role**
- **Appreciate the difference between quantitative and qualitative interviewing**
- **Explain the use of focus groups**
- **Understand the processes of questionnaire design and use**
- **Appreciate how tests, scales and measurements are used to collect data**
- **Understand the strengths and limitations of different methods of data collection**
- **Demonstrate the use of critical appraisal questions to review data collection methods**
- **Understand the ethical issues that arise from the use of different methods of data collection**

KEY TERMS

Critical incident technique, Focus group, Historical data, Interviews, In vitro, In vivo, Life history, Likert scale, Naturalistic observation, Observational methods, Questionnaires, Structured observations, Triangulation, Unstructured observations

---

Triangulation in data collection

Triangulation of data source and method is increasingly popular in research studies within nursing and healthcare, as researchers are often investigating complex issues that benefit from the use of multiple data sources or mixed methods. **Triangulation** is thought to improve the validity of a study, by drawing on multiple reference points to address research questions. Studies that employ triangulation in data collection are hoping to overcome potential biases of using a single data collection method, source or individual researcher. For further discussion on the use of mixed methods in research, see Chapter 20. It is worth highlighting here, however, that in reviewing methods of data collection it should be remembered that different combinations of approaches can be employed within one study.

Observational methods

Nursing practice includes the use of observation skills, drawing to different degrees on four senses – touch, sight, smell and sound – to formulate patient assessment. Though nurses will often base judgements on what they see and hear, data collection tools such as temperature-recording devices and blood-pressure recording machines can support assessment. Nurses therefore use observation skills and tools to collect patient data and support care delivery.

Used in research, observation is viewed as one of the most important methods of data collection (Jones and Somekh, 2005) which aims to provide a direct record of human behaviour. Observation methods can be used to examine phenomena such as communication, non-verbal interactions and activity. Researchers approach the use of observational methods in a systematic and purposeful way, as they are charged with collecting data in order to address research questions. Researchers have different **observational methods** available for use, often described as structured and unstructured approaches.

This section considers both structured and unstructured methods, giving examples of research that have employed each approach. It also identifies the limitations of observation methods and discusses the key issues to consider when critically reviewing papers presenting observational studies.

Structured observation

Research activity using a **structured observation** method will usually be guided by a predetermined data collection schedule. Prior to undertaking data collection, the researchers will have agreed the phenomena or subject of the observation and either obtained a suitable data collection tool that has been used previously or developed one for the purposes of the research. The data collection schedule can be constructed with a high level of structure that might include a checklist of tick boxes or rating scales. Though a more detailed discussion of rating scales is provided later in the chapter, it is worth highlighting here that a rating scale would usually provide a descriptive continuum with points along it, allowing the researcher to record between extremes. This requires the researcher to make a judgement about what is observed, such as recording a patient's mood as somewhere between depressed and elated. Whatever the composition, the researcher will use the schedule to guide observations made, and for data recording, therefore providing structure to the data collection activity.

There is scope to quantify structured observations, giving the ability to measure, for example, how many times a patient interacts with healthcare professionals in the course of a day. Consequently, Polit and Beck (2006) see this approach as supporting quantitative research designs (see Chapter 11), especially if a highly structured schedule is used where results can be readily quantified.

The use of structured data collection tools can aid reliability in observation recording, as the researcher is making judgements about particular behaviours or events within defined parameters. However, there can still be issues of inter-rater reliability, where two or more researchers may interpret the same situation differently and thus select different question responses. Research papers will often report pilot work that measured the degree of inter-rater reliability seen. Two or more observers would be asked to record their interpretations of the same event or behaviour. The findings would be subject to statistical analysis using, for example, a kappa test (see Landis and Koch, 1977). Achieving a score of 1.00 indicates total agreement between observers and a score of 0.60 or lower being less reliable than desired, as it suggests that only 6 out of every 10 events observed will be scored the same. For example, Whitfield et al. (2003) developed the Cardiff test of basic life support with automated external defibrillator use as a standardised checklist to evaluate performance in resuscitation skills with a manikin. Six observers were recruited to evaluate performance using the Cardiff test that has 42 variables, or different actions, that are observed. A kappa score showed inter–observer reliability was 0.70 or 70% (satisfactory), for 85% of the 42 variables. The Cardiff test used by Whitfield et al. (2003) provides an insight into the level of structure that can be seen in an observation schedule (see Box 21.1).

Box 21.1   Example of a tick-box observation schedule

Whitfield et al. (2003) undertook research to develop an up-to-date and reliable method of assessing the performance of basic life support with automated external defibrillator use. The observation schedule is a highly structured checklist and includes some measurements that are recorded through a computer package attached to a skillmeter manikin, thus removing all potential for observer differences.

The types of questions include:

Switch on automated external defibrillator	2. Performed	1. Not performed

Compressions: Average number of compressions of the chest delivered (obtained from the manikin data)	Insert number

---

Observation sampling

Structured observations are applied in relation to either time sampling (choosing a particular timeframe to record observations) or event sampling (selecting events to observe, which requires some knowledge of the patterns of events) (Polit and Beck, 2006). If a researcher was interested in observing patient interactions, they might use a time sampling frame, perhaps making observations at five-minute intervals across a certain time period. If the focus of the research was about interactions during ward rounds in a general ward environment, then the event of the ward round would provide the sampling timeframe.

Unstructured observation

In contrast to structured observations, **unstructured observations** are not guided by a predetermined checklist schedule; rather, researchers try to remain open to record events or behaviours that occur naturally. The researchers are guided by the research questions and will have a focus to their data collection, but are not tied to completing specific data collection tools. This approach is often referred to as **naturalistic observation**, with the researcher adopting the role of participant observer, taking part in the daily functioning of the setting under observation (Polit and Beck, 2006).

Box 21.2   Example of an unstructured observation schedule

Manias et al. (2005) created an observation schedule to support research that looked at how graduate nurses used protocols to manage patients' medications. Twelve graduate nurses employed in medical, surgical and speciality wards were observed during a 2-hour period when medications were being administered to patients. The observation schedule included six questions such as, 'State clearly the purpose of using the protocol, for example, to administer the medicine safely' (2005: 937). Nurses were asked about their medication management during the observation periods, and responses to these questions were recorded on audiotape.

The example in Box 21.2 demonstrates the use of an observation schedule composed of a list of questions for the researcher to consider whilst observing the behaviours of the nurses administering patient medication. Though structured, the questions are less restrictive than tick box responses seen in structured observation schedules.

Ethnographic research designs (see Chapter 14) have relied in part on participant observation, with its inclusion also seen in other qualitative designs such as case study research and grounded theory (also see Chapter 14). Early anthropological studies (Malinowski, 1922) describe the participant observer role used to study people in their natural environments, and Leininger (1985) suggests that there are four phases of observation participation:

- Phase one: primarily observation
- Phase two: primarily observation with some participation
- Phase three: primarily participation with some observation
- Phase four: reflective observation of impact

This model would see the researcher having a period of initiation to the research setting, getting to know the research environment and participants, with observation being the focus here. Gradually participation increases, as the researcher learns from the group and environment and then from their own experiences as participants in the group. Final reflections allow consideration of the entire observational period. Obviously the role of the participant observer may differ according to the context of the research; in some settings it may not be possible to adopt a role that involves participation in patient care delivery. See Box 21.3 for an example.

Classifications of the observer role were offered by Gold as long ago as 1958, when it was suggest an observer could operate as a complete participant, participant-as-observer, observer-as-participant or complete observer. This definition is problematic in today's research environment as the complete participant was described as acting without revealing a research interest, as a covert (hidden) observer. It is inconceivable that ethical approval would be granted today for any research design that included covert data collection, such as that described by Clark (1996), who used eavesdropping as part of secret participant observation to look at the concept of the therapeutic community in a mental health forensic unit. It is more probable that researchers would operate in an overt (open) role, using observations as one of a range of data collection methods within one study and undertaking the study for a limited period, given the costs of using prolonged observation methods.

Box 21.3 Example of research using participant observation

Kenen et al. (2004) investigated communication and interactions between healthy women from families with a history of breast/ovarian cancer and their friends, sisters, brothers, male partners and children, in order to understand how families cope with cancer genetics risk information. The researcher observed genetic counselling sessions conducted at a local clinic as part of the research design. The researcher involved held an honorary contract to allow admission to the hospital to collect data and talked of being treated as a member of the team, attending the clinic weekly for the duration of the research.

Data recording

The presence of researchers recording observations in a healthcare or any other environment will always have an impact on those being observed, affecting behaviour and possibly performance. Held up as the 'Hawthorne effect', the impact of the observer on the performance of the observed has been reported over many years. The phenomenon originates from management research conducted in the USA in the

1930s that considered the effect of increased lighting provision on productivity in the Hawthorne factory of Western Electric. The researchers concluded that increases in worker productivity were linked to the effect of observation rather than environmental changes (Roethlisberger and Dickson, 1939). Obviously the length of the observation period and the degree of intrusion brought about by the researcher role assumed would affect the extent to which the Hawthorne effect impacts on the research environment. The longer the period of observation, the more likely the researcher is to 'blend in' with the environment.

The advent of technology often replaces the need to take field notes and may enable researchers to capture data without having to physically locate themselves in the research environment. Tape, video (see Box 21.4) and digital recordings are available (see Jones and Somekh, 2005) and may help in achieving inter-observer reliability, though not necessarily as responsive and spontaneous as field-based researchers.

Box 21.4   Example of the use of video recording to collect observation data

Williams (2005) explored family member contributions to patients' care in intensive care environments. A range of data was collected including video recording of patient care episodes. These were discussed with the participants (the nurses responsible for care delivery) as part of a reflective discussion that elicited the participants' understanding and interpretation of patient care events.

Figure 21.1 lists the strengths and weaknesses of observational methods.

Interview techniques

Most people will have some experience of **interviews**, often as a participant answering interview questions. Interviews can be used formally to support applications for the workplace, but are also employed to access individual accounts and experiences; for example, when visiting the doctor, patients will be familiar with answering questions about their condition. Nurses will have experience of participating in and leading interviews, using interview techniques to gather information about patients as part of the initial assessment or admission process. Despite nurses being familiar with the processes of interviewing, it is suggested that some development is needed to employ interview techniques with the sophistication required to support measurement within research (Burns and Grove, 2005).

Potential strengths:

- Observation methods can be used to collect data from real-life situations and events.
- Real-time events/natural environments can be recorded.
- Used as one of a range of data collection tools, observation methods have the potential to verify individual perceptions of practice with actual conduct.

Potential limitations:

- Research using observation methods can be time-consuming.
- Potential difficulties can arise when accessing research environments.
- Inter-rater reliability scores need consideration.
- Observers can bias data collection by focusing on preferred issues.
- The Hawthorne effect can impact on the research outcomes.
- Observation methods are intrusive and require careful ethical consideration.

Figure 21.1   Potential strengths and weaknesses of observational methods

Interviews are used in a number of research designs; this said, the approach is seen more frequently in qualitative studies such as grounded theory (Taylor, 2005) and case study research (Ray and Street, 2005) (for further information on these research designs, see Chapter 17). The technique is used when the research is trying to address questions that relate to exploring personal experience, personal accounts, perceptions, beliefs, opinions and can be used to access attitudes. Interviewing often occurs in a face-to-face context, yet the use of telephone interviewing has seen an increase in popularity (Smith, E., 2005). This section will explore the interview techniques available, including the use of quantitative and qualitative interviewing, focus group and telephone interviews.

Quantitative interviews

Quantitative research designs can be supported through structured (see Box 21.5) and semi-structured (see Box 21.6) interviews. Such interview approaches will involve the use of a predetermined data collection tool, as seen with structured observations, often referred to as an 'interview schedule'. The interview may be conducted by telephone or in face-to-face contexts, and include interviews as part of survey research that might occur in the supermarket. The interviewer controls the speed of the interview and presents the same questions to participants in the same order. Frequently the questions used offer limited response options, though there can be occasional open response questions.

Box 21.5   Example of structured interview questions

1. How frequently to you visit your GP?
    daily ☐   weekly ☐   monthly ☐   yearly ☐
2. How do you travel to see your GP?
    car ☐   motorbike ☐   bus ☐   train ☐   bicycle ☐   walk ☐

Box 21.6   Example of a semi-structured interview

Rycroft-Malone et al. (2004) used semi-structured interviews in an exploration of the factors that influence the implementation of evidence into nursing practice. Seventeen nurses took part in the interviews, such lasting one hour. The interview questions used included those about the process of implementing evidence into practice and the barriers to implementation. The questions used were predetermined and ordered into an interview schedule, followed by the interviews.

In using predetermined interview tools it is hoped that the process of data collection will be standardised, minimising error. This assumes that the data collection tool is written in such a way that the content will be interpreted in the same way by all respondents. To support this, it is suggested that the questions are piloted, having participants completing them prior to the main study, to aid reliability and validity of the measure (Burns and Grove, 2005). It should be remembered, however, that the presence of the interviewer can aid the validity of the instrument by making sure it is measuring what it is expected to measure, through helping participants to understand the questions so that they are able to provide more relevant answers.

As the questions are all ideally asked in the same way, supported through providing training to the interviewers, reliability is increased. It may be desirable to ensure that inter-rater reliability of an acceptable standard is achieved (see 'Observational methods' above). The questions should yield consistency in responses, measuring what they were intended to measure across a number of participants.

Qualitative interviews

A range of terms may be used to describe qualitative interviews, including: open, unstructured, in-depth, ethnographic. Such interview approaches are often conversations, guided by an opening question. Generally, any interview conversation will have some structure to it, possibly with the researcher following up particular issues or areas of interest raised by the participant. The main purpose of the qualitative interview is to seek out the participant's perceptions, experiences and opinions, and to allow the participant to drive the interview direction. It is suggested that in taking this approach the researcher will gain an understanding of social life through interpreting the meaning individuals attach to their experiences (Fontana and Frey, 1998). The researcher will need to consider the most appropriate environment for data collection that will enable the participant to relax and facilitate engagement with the interview. The environment would ideally be quiet and afford a comfortable setting, yet if conducted in the participant's home the researcher will have little control over noise levels and disruptions.

Qualitative interviews may start with an open question that relates to the overall area of research enquiry, such as asking patients about care delivery: 'Can you tell me about the care you have received whilst in hospital?' The interviewer is in a position to listen to the participant's experiences of care, often recording the conversation to aid later analysis, following verbatim (word-for-word, including innuendo) transcription of the recording. An audio or video recording of the interview allows the researcher to concentrate on the conversation and focus on certain areas that arise in the discussion. Some qualitative interviews will want participants to talk about particular experiences, for example how they view the new modern matron role. In these cases the researcher will need to ensure that the discussions remain focused on this topic, perhaps requiring questions that re-focus the direction of the conversation. See Box 21.7 for an example of a qualitative interview.

Box 21.7   Example of a qualitative interview

McCabe (2004) used qualitative interviews to explore and produce statements relating to how patients experience nurse communication. Eight patients were involved in a tape-recorded, 30-minute interview. The interview began with an open question asking the patient to talk about their experiences of how nurses communicated with them during their in-patient stay. At certain times the researcher had to re-focus the interview direction and asked for clarification and elaboration on certain points.

Qualitative interview methods do not aim to achieve standardisation in the way the data is collected, as with quantitative approaches; rather, the quality is enhanced if the interview allows the expression of individual thoughts, feelings and experiences. To maintain rigour in qualitative interviewing, the participant's accounts are presented within any research report or paper, often as anonymous verbatim quotes. This reassures the reader that the data presented reflects the participant's 'voice', allowing the reader to 'hear' the participant's spoken word, a position which is seen to empower the participant by presenting their words in the research (Griffiths, 1998). Researchers often report seeking verification of the interpretations of data with participants. This might involve asking the participants to comment on draft transcripts of the interview and the analysis of this. Such presentation may also be supported by the researcher's reflexive account of the research journey (see Chapter 12), adding to the rigour of the design.

Group interviews

Group interviews are usually called **focus group** interviews. These are often held when the researcher wants to access the opinions and experiences of five to ten participants simultaneously (see Box 21.8). The approach can be a time-efficient way of obtaining the views of a number of participants at once and has the potential benefit of encouraging rich dialogue, as contributions may be increased as part of a group discussion. There are, however, some potential challenges for the researcher. Organising access to a number of participants at one time can prove difficult; Barbour and Schostak (2005) also report that problems with group dynamics can affect contributions with some individuals being more verbose than others, and maintaining confidentiality can be more problematic. Focus group interviews tend to form part of qualitative research designs and can form part of evaluative research, participatory action research and feminist approaches (see Chapter 17).

Box 21.8   Example of a focus group interview

Ward and Moule (2007) used focus groups to elicit the views of student nurses, midwives and allied health professionals. They explored how the students in practice settings used information and communication technology and how they felt this might be developed in the future.

Telephone interviews

Smith (2005) suggests that telephone interviewing in healthcare research is increasing. There are a number of perceived advantages to its use. These include reduced travel time and research costs, and access to participants who are widely dispersed. Participant rates can be higher as the approach is less intrusive, with most interviews lasting no more than 20 minutes. Despite the potential benefits, the use of the telephone interview needs some consideration. It is suggested that training in interview technique will be required, and there is some concern that the method may not produce the quality of data accessible in face-to-face interview settings (Baker, 1994; Thomas and Purdon, 1994). If a standardised data collection is used, this will need to be subjected to the same reliability and validity tests as those described in the design of quantitative interview methods, being piloted and subjected to inter-rater reliability testing. Use of telephone interviewing is illustrated in Box 21.9.

Box 21.9   Example of a telephone interview

Lauder et al. (2004) completed a social survey of loneliness in a community sample of 1,241 randomly selected participants. The telephone database was used to select the sample, and those meeting the eligibility criteria were asked to undertake a 30-minute interview. The interview followed a standardised format, including the same introduction, range of questions that included a loneliness scale and demographic questions. The tool was piloted prior to use.

Power issues

Interviews are often conducted between those of unequal status or position. For example, medical and nursing staff working as researchers in a mental health setting may interview vulnerable clients. There may also be issues arising from differences in race, culture, accent and other personal characteristics that affect the interview. Whilst such issues should be reviewed as part of the process of securing ethical approval, the effect of potential differences in power relations on the interview can be hidden or unknown. Feminist researchers have criticised unequal power relations within interviews that can relate to differences in status as well as in gender (Maynard and Purvis, 1994). Researchers suggest women can remain subordinate in interviews and that researchers should aim to achieve symmetry in an interview (Hollway and Jefferson, 2000).

Figure 21.2 lists the potential strengths and weaknesses of interviews.

Questionnaire design

Questionnaires often form the basis of data recording in healthcare, being used to collect data as part of assessment to support diagnosis. Used as a data collection tool in research studies, the questionnaire can be constructed to elicit facts about individuals, events or situations or to measure beliefs, attitudes, opinion and knowledge. In this section we examine the development and use of questionnaires as data collection tools within research and highlight the potential strengths and weaknesses of the questionnaire.

Potential strengths:

- Can be a flexible technique allowing the researcher to explore issues in depth.
- Potential to ensure that questions are understood, enhancing validity.
- Potential for the researcher to seek clarification of meaning from the participant.
- Focus groups can be time-saving and generate increased dialogue.
- Response rates can be high.
- Can be a more inclusive data collection method.

Potential limitations:

- Individual interviews can be time-consuming and costly.
- Power issues can affect data collection.
- Researchers need interview skills to collect quality data.

Figure 21.2   Potential strengths and weaknesses of interviews

Questionnaire development and use

The content of questionnaires is often predetermined by the researcher, who should look to the published literature to help formulate the questionnaire content, or possibly find a pre-validated tool. Questionnaires are developed for use as data collection instruments in a range of research designs, including surveys, descriptive studies and randomised controlled trials. The questionnaire is usually a standardised tool, with the same questions being presented to all respondents, and can be employed within quantitative research designs, though can also feature as part of a mixed-methods approach. Questionnaires are often seen as self-completion tools, being 'filled-in' by research participants without researcher input to the process. A self-completion process can support anonymity and be useful in overcoming power differences between participants and researchers. The approach to data collection can vary, however, and the questionnaire can form the basis of structured interviewing (see earlier section). Questionnaires are often developed to include closed questions, yet can be designed to include open-ended questions.

Closed questions

Closed response questionnaires can include a range of question types, including checklist response (such as the example in Box 21.5 above), multiple-choice questions, ranking questions and two-way questions which allow two possible responses. Different types of measurement scales, such as an attitude scale, can also be incorporated into question designs (see p. 306).

Multiple-choice questions (for an example, see Box 21.10) can often be used to measure knowledge, and may be employed as part of a research design that is looking for the effect of a particular learning package on knowledge attainment. In such a design, multiple-choice questions would be completed prior to using the package (pre-test), and following its use the participant would complete a second multiple-choice questionnaire (post-test).

Box 21.10   Example of a multiple-choice question

Question 1. (Tick one of the following)

In basic life support the breathing and compression ratio should be:

a) 2 breaths to 5 compressions   ☐

b) 2 breaths to 15 compressions   ☐

c) 2 breaths to 30 compressions   ☐

Two-way questions (see Box 21.11) can be used in designs that are exploring individual beliefs, where the researcher will ask participants to provide yes or no answers, agree or disagree, or confirm whether something is true or false.

Box 21.11   Example of the use of two-way questions

Tardy et al. (2003) asked patients over 65 years to complete a closed questionnaire to obtain their views of a deep-vein thrombosis treatment delivered as part of a randomised controlled trial. The questionnaire included 11 items related to feelings and reactions at the time of the proposed trial, quality of the information given and memories of the study and feelings at the study conclusion. The participants were to give yes or no answers to questions such as 'Reactions at the time of the trial – Did you feel shocked? (yes or no)' (2003: 151).

Researchers may want to know how individuals prioritise their needs and pose a question that requires the participant to rank in order of most to least important (see Box 21.12).

Box 21.12   Example of a ranking question

Question 1

What are the most important factors in choosing a dentist? Please rank from the list below by putting 1 to 4 in the boxes below (1 = most important, 4 = least important)

Distance from home   ☐

Parking spaces provided   ☐

Availability of appointments   ☐

Provides NHS service for children   ☐

Open-ended questions

Open-ended questions are used where the researcher wants to explore the participant's views, allowing the collection of textual data that might be written or recorded by the researcher in a structured interview (see above). Box 21.13 illustrates the use of such a questionnaire, and Box 21.14 gives an example of how an open-ended question might be phrased.

Box 21.13   Example of an open questionnaire

Bojtor (2003) used an open questionnaire to examine nursing staff workload. The questions related to increased demands at work, motivation factors and external force factors. It was administered to nurses on a self-completion basis.

Box 21.14   Example of an open question

Question 1
Please identify below the main reasons why you applied to start a physiotherapy degree:
....
....

Design considerations

There are several factors that need to be taken into consideration when designing and using a questionnaire. These factors may affect the clarity of the questionnaire and impact on the completion rates. The following points should be considered:

- Is there a supporting letter with a postal or electronic questionnaire, giving details of the research project and explaining what participation will involve?
- Are there clear instructions on how to complete the questionnaire?
- Is all terminology explained?
- Is the questionnaire presented in the languages needed?
- Are the questions unambiguous?
- Is one question being asked at a time?
- How long is the questionnaire (the shorter the better)?
- Does the questionnaire include questions that are relevant to the research question?
- Does the questionnaire have the appropriate question formats included?
- What is the proposed method of delivery?
- Is it clear how and to whom the questionnaire should be returned?

Establishing validity and reliability

The validity of the questionnaire relates to its ability to measure what it is expected to measure. Reliability relates to the consistency in that measurement, that the questionnaire always measures what it is supposed to measure and will identify similarities in answers across a number of participants, but will also measure differences (see Chapter 12). Prior to validity and reliability testing, the questionnaire can be subjected to a pilot test. Administering the questionnaire to a small number of individuals with similar characteristics to the final sample can identify errors in question design, problems with completion instructions and typographical mistakes.

To establish content or face validity, ensuring that the questionnaire measures what it is intended to measure, the researcher could submit the questionnaire to an expert panel for review. If researchers use an existing questionnaire, validated in previous research measuring the same phenomenon, the tool can be presented as pre-validated. Criterion-related validity can be established through comparing the results obtained from the questionnaire with other research data collected. For example, a questionnaire about confidence in computer use could be compared with observational data that recorded use.

Reliability is commonly tested through test–retest methods. This involves administering the questionnaire on two occasions and comparing the responses. Other tests might include testing the questions by presenting them in different forms, either through a slight change of wording (whilst maintaining the meaning) or through changing the order of the questions.

Administering questionnaires

Questionnaires can be administered to respondents in a number of ways, providing some flexibility to the researcher. The data collection technique also offers the potential to access nationally and internationally based participants. Questionnaires can be sent to participants through the postal system, via electronic mail or through Internet sites. They can be used to support a telephone or face-to-face structured interview. Questionnaires might be administered to a captive audience, such as patients attending a particular service, or student midwives within a teaching session. In these cases potential ethical issues will need consideration to ensure voluntary informed consent and to avoid coercion.

Whilst the questionnaire offers scope to access remote research participants via a number of presentation routes, one of the potential difficulties of use relates to poor completion rates. The return of self-completion questionnaires, particularly those sent in the post, can be low, often as little as 25–30 per cent of the initial sample return questionnaires (Burns and Grove, 2005). This can prove problematic for the researcher as it is suggested that a 50 per cent response rate is required to ensure representativeness of the sample (Burns and Grove, 2005). Completion rates can be improved by ensuring that questionnaire design is 'user friendly' and meets many of the design considerations set out above. Facilitating ease of return may also improve completion and return rates. Researchers often build reminder techniques into their research design, sometimes sending out reminder letters to the entire sample.

The design of questionnaires can exclude certain groups of participants, such as the elderly, those with learning disabilities and children. If the questionnaire is limited to the English language, this may prevent completion by ethnic minority groups. Researchers can consider providing questionnaires in different languages and use innovative ways to present the questionnaire (see Box 21.15). The mode of delivery may also exclude certain groups, especially if the telephone or Internet is used.

Box 21.15 Example of a video questionnaire

Saglani et al. (2005) used a video questionnaire to identify upper airway abnormalities in pre-school children with a reported wheeze. The researchers showed four video clips to parents, asking them to select the video resembling their child's symptoms.

Potential strengths:

- Can engage a large number of participants.
- Can enable data collection from a national and international sample.
- Anonymity can be supported.
- Can be a cost-effective method of collecting data.
- There is the potential for ease of administration and analysis.
- Potential for reduced researcher input, reducing the need for researcher training and possible researcher bias.
- Can be a useful way of collecting data if there are power differences between researcher and participants.

Potential limitations:

- Certain groups of potential participants can be excluded.
- The mode of distribution can exclude some participants, e.g. those without telephone or Internet access.
- Poor response rates.
- Return of incomplete or illegible questionnaires.
- Inability for the participant to clarify questions.
- Inability for the researcher to clarify responses.

Figure 21.3   Potential strengths and weaknesses of questionnaire use in research

Figure 21.3 lists the strengths and weaknesses of questionnaire use in research.

Using tests, scales and measurements

Tests and scales are often used in interviews or questionnaires forming part of data collection. It is suggested that when the data collected in this way can be measured mathematically to obtain an overall score, the measurement instrument is called a 'scale'. There are many scales available for use in healthcare research (see Oppenheim, 1992; Bowling, 2005). Physiological measures are employed to collect patient data on a daily basis. The most frequently used nursing measurements include recording temperature, pulse and blood pressure. This section will consider those tests, scales and measurements most commonly used in healthcare research.

Vignettes

Vignettes allow the researcher to present descriptions of incidents or situations, conjuring up images of real-life scenarios, to which the participants can respond. The scenarios can elicit information as to the participant's perceptions, opinions or knowledge about a particular situation (Polit and Beck, 2006). Though usually written, the vignette can be presented on a video or digital recording, or acted in real-life. Participants are usually asked either to respond to an open question about the scenario, such as 'What would you do now?' or are given a closed question to answer that relates to recording a measurement on a scale or selecting a multiple-choice response. See Box 21.16 for an example. The approach offers a way of exploring situations that may not be readily available in practice and a more resource effective way of capturing how individuals might behave in certain situations. It should be noted, however, that actual behaviour may vary from that recorded in response to a contrived event.

Box 21.16   Example of the use of a vignette

McGuigan and Moule (2006) used vignettes with nurses following their use of an online learning package about cancer care. The research wanted to find out whether nurses' learning had changed their practice delivery. They were asked to complete a vignette prior to the learning and following completion of the package. The vignettes were developed by specialist cancer-care nurses and reviewed by an expert panel. The scenarios offered closed-response options.

Rating scales

These form the most basic type of scale measurement. The researcher will compose statements that are 'rated' by the participant (see Box 21.17) and a score is then given to the assessment or judgement made (Oppenheim, 1992). The scales can be used to support observational measurement and can record measures of satisfaction, though caution should be exercised when constructing the statements, as extreme options are unlikely to be chosen (Burns and Grove, 2005).

Box 21.17   Example of a completed rating scale

Please rate from 1 (low) to 5 (high) the following satisfaction statements in relation to the library service:

1. Provision of electronic resources   (5)
2. Quiet working environment   (4)
3. Provision of inter-library loans   (1)
4. Range of text books   (3)
5. Opening hours   (2)

Likert scales

The most commonly used scale is that known as the **Likert scale**, composed of a number of statements on a topic, with participants being asked to identify to what extent they agree or disagree with the statement. Commonly, the statements will be both positively and negatively worded, with four or five possible responses being offered. These usually include strongly agree, agree, disagree and strongly disagree, with the fifth option being a neutral, neither agree nor disagree. The researcher scores the responses from 1 to 4 or 5, with a high score being achieved both for agreement with a positive statement and for disagreement with a negative statement. This reversal is required to ensure that a high score reflects a consistently positive attitude to the subject being measured (Polit and Beck, 2006). The scores for each statement are totalled to achieve a final score, with the higher scoring individuals having a more positive attitude to the subject. Box 21.18 gives an example of how a Likert scale can be used.

Box 21.18   Example of the use of a Likert scale

Colon-Emeric et al. (2004) undertook a 24-item survey using a 5-point scale (strongly agree, agree, neutral, disagree, strongly disagree). The study aimed to identify the barriers to the use of osteoporosis clinical practice guidelines perceived by medical directors and directors of nursing. The survey measured agreement to questions about a number of barriers to use, including environment and family-related issues.

Visual analogue scale

The visual analogue scale (VAS) is most often used to measure feelings and attitudes. The scale is a line, usually 100 mm in length with end points providing two extreme values. Frequently used as a measure of pain, the end points can be labelled as 'no pain' to 'pain unbearable'. The researcher asks the participant to mark their 'pain' on the scale, and the distance from the left end of the line to the mark is measured to provide the value. See Box 21.19 for a VAS in use.

Measuring reliability of the scale can be problematic, as a single measure is obtained for what is an individual feeling. Despite this, it is suggested that the scale provides a more sensitive measure than rating or numerical scales (Burns and Grove, 2005). There is a range of tests and scales available, yet there may be a need to develop a specific tool, which will require the researcher to implement a process of development and piloting to establish reliability and validity.

Box 21.19   Example of research using a visual analogue scale (VAS)

Meretoja et al. (2004) examined nurses' perceptions of competence in different hospital work environments. Participants were asked to assess their level of competence on a visual analogue scale (0–100 mm), with 0 being very low and 100 very high competence.

Physiological and biological measures

Physiological and biological measurement usually involves the use of specialist equipment, which can involve a cost to the research, and require training. Healthcare staff undertake a number of measurements as part of routine care. Radiographers complete anatomical measurement through examining radiographic images, and physical measurement is completed by nurses assessing pulse and blood pressure. Further measurements include chemical composition of blood and urine and microbiological measurements of cultures and specimens (see Box 21.20). Physiological measurements can be made away from the participant, for example **in vitro**, such as testing samples of blood in a laboratory, or **in vivo**, such as recording the pulse in the presence of the participant.

As the measurements are precise and sensitive, they are objective and seen as highly reliable. Provided the equipment used is functioning with accuracy and is used correctly, the data recorded with the instrument at the same time by different researchers will be consistent. This objectivity allows measurements to be used to look at individual reactions to events, such as response to stress, and to compare reactions between a control and experimental group. Though the instruments may be reliable, it is not necessarily the case that it will be valid. The researcher needs to have a tool that will facilitate the collection of data that is needed.

Box 21.20   Example of research using physiological measures

Bergeron et al. (2004) examined the effect of exercise on the heat and fluid intake on erythrocyte sickling and neutrophil activation (distorted red blood-cell shaping that reduces blood flow) in carriers of sickle cell. Core temperature and heart rate were measured. Venous blood was analysed for the percentage of erythrocyte sickling.

When using physiological measures, the researcher will need to consider the following:

- What factors might affect the measurement (the dependent and independent variables)? This might include age, diagnosis and effect of activity such as drinking hot fluids prior to temperature recording.
- How will data be collected? Are instruments calibrated, what is the procedure for use and has training been given?
- When will the measurements be taken (frequency and timing)?
- Can factors in the environment be controlled if needed (for example, consistency may be needed in room temperature or in physical surroundings)?

Figure 21.4 lists the potential strengths and weaknesses of uses scales, tests and measures in research

Potential strengths:

- Scales and tests are often used in interviews or as part of questionnaires.
- Scales can be used to translate responses into a numerical score.
- Vignettes allow the collection of data about perceived behaviour.
- Vignettes can be used to explore contrived practice situations with less intrusion.
- Physiological and biological measurements are seen as precise, sensitive and objective.

Potential limitations:

- Developing the reliability of a scale or test can be problematic.
- Measurements usually involve the use of equipment, bringing a cost to the researcher and training requirements.
- Measurements can be affected by a number of variables.

Figure 21.4   Potential strengths and weaknesses of using scales, tests and measures in research

Using documents

Documents are socially produced material that can include written records, photographs, video and audio recordings. The range of documents available for use in research is therefore vast, and includes official government statistics through to private diaries, letters and photographic records.

Types of documents

One of the main types of documents used is public records. These can include records of births, deaths and marriages, census material and the UK Electoral Register, political and judicial records such as records from court cases and budget or fiscal records, and documents from government departments including crime statistics or educational records. It is suggested that as the records include quantifiable data, they are perceived as being more objective. It should be remembered, however, that the records reflect the data the state sees fit to collate, and therefore the collection of data may indeed hold political or other biases (MacDonald and Tipton, 1993).

The media publish case law in the *Times Law Reports,* with the mass popular media presenting a view of social practices and values through broadsheets and tabloids, magazines, television and radio. These are often written or produced for mass audiences, appealing to readership and the viewing public. Literature and the arts can provide public material for analysis, though as documentary sources these are often under-used (Bowling, 2002).

Personal papers, diaries (see the section later in this chapter on diaries), letters and photographs or video recordings reconstruct events and tell individual stories. These are often private records, collected unofficially.

Within healthcare, researchers have access to a number of documents that fall into official and unofficial realms including patient case notes, nursing care plans, patient letters or diaries of treatment experiences. Researchers also draw on literature published online and in journals or textbooks (see Box 21.21). Some of the material collected in the health service over a number of years becomes archive data (see the section later in this chapter on archive material).

Box 21.21   Example of the use of a small-scale documentary analysis

Candlin and Stark (2005) selected a sample of documents for analysis, choosing 15 published papers referring to the actual practice of wearing plastic aprons during direct patient care delivery.

The analysis of documentary sources can be either quantitative, when extracting data from statistical records, or qualitative, in considering diary narratives. These documentary records can inform both quantitative and qualitative research designs (see Chapter 11).

Issues of document use

There are several advantages in the use of documents. The data is generally free from researcher bias, as documents are constructed without researcher input. Additionally, they can be convenient to access, there are fewer ethical issues involved and there can be resource savings. Databases often provide large databases with records reflecting information gathered over time.

Despite these benefits, researchers have criticised documentary research because those documents falling outside official statistics are seen as subjective and reflecting society's biases (Bowling, 2002). Researchers have to be convinced of the accuracy and representativeness of any documents used. MacDonald and Tipton (1993) suggest the researcher will need to ascertain the authenticity and credibility of the data before use, working as a detective. Additionally, availability of and access to the documents should be assured.

Figure 21.5 lists the potential strengths and weaknesses of using documents in research.

Potential strengths:

- Can remove the potential for researcher bias.
- Can be cost-effective.
- Can be an efficient approach to collecting data.

Potential limitations:

- Data may be incomplete and unusable as it was not originally collected for research purposes.
- There may be inaccuracies, bias or errors in the data.

Figure 21.5   Potential strengths and weaknesses of using documents in research

It is possible for documents to be falsified and they can provide an inaccurate account of events. Accounts in diaries, letters or literature may be exaggerated or distorted and be affected by the biases of the writer. The researcher will also need to consider whether the available documents constitute a representative sample of the scope of documents as they originally existed or whether particular documents are missing, which can be the case when materials are archived.

Life history and biographical material

Life histories and biographical material report individual life experiences often accessed through in-depth interviewing (see the section earlier in this chapter on interviewing). Denzin (1989) discusses the life-history approach as a methodology that emerged from anthropology. The approach reconstructs and interprets an individual life story. Interviews are taped and transcribed verbatim. Diaries, historical data and observations may also inform the development of a biography. Researchers may explore a patient's life history or that of staff.

Strengths and limitations of the technique

Life histories can provide rich data about an individual's experience of particular episodes or a complete life. Used to collect biographies from patients, histories can provide an understanding of life with particular illnesses and impairments. When considering staff, work experiences help us understand identity and roles in nursing. Though offering potentially rich data, collecting data through interview or written accounts relies on the participant having the ability to recall intimate detail from past events.

> **Box 21.22   Example of the use of life history technique**
>
> Smith (2004) used semi-structured in-depth interviewing to obtain life histories of clients experiencing the alcohol withdrawal process while voluntarily resident in a specialist facility.

Critical incident technique

Critical incident technique involves asking participants about key events they have experienced and collects observations of human behaviour in defined situations. The technique originates in the work of Flanagan (1954) and has been used to collect descriptions of specific events, either positive or negative, through observations, interviews and self-reporting. Using the technique, the researcher can explore actual activities that might relate to care delivery, management or education experiences.

Strengths and limitations of the technique

Critical incident technique draws on descriptions of actual events, capturing the real-life situation and acknowledging the context and pressures of the actual practice or education environment. An example is given in Box 21.23.

> **Box 21.23   Example of critical incident technique**
>
> Arvidsson and Fridlund (2005) used the critical incident technique to identify factors related to critical incidents that influence the competence of nurse supervisors. The critical incidents consisted of written self-reports of important events that occurred during supervision. These events could relate either to a successful work situation or to a difficult one where the supervisor experience was negative.

One potential weakness of this design is linked to the reliance on participants' recall and memory; participants will need to remember specific examples of effective and ineffective practice. There may also be reluctance among participants to report negative experiences or ineffective practice.

Diaries

Diaries have been used as part of historical research, looking at past recordings of individuals such as Samuel Pepys, who recorded diaries of 17th-century London.

Researchers also use diaries as part of qualitative research designs to ask participants to record current events, keeping a record over time of feelings, experiences, events, actions and reflections.

Use of diaries to collect data

Diaries are thought to offer greater accuracy in collecting data about events than interviews, as recall is more likely to be precise at the time of the experience than some time after the event. Burns and Grove (2005) suggest diaries allow researchers access to data that is difficult to collect through other methods. Diaries can be used to collect data about behaviours at home (eating patterns, exercise patterns) and symptom experience (pain, medication needed, mobility issues).

Box 21.24   Example of research using a diary

Corrigan and Bogner (2004) used diaries to record help needed at home by previous patients of a Traumatic Brain Injury Unit. A stopwatch was used to record the actual periods when assistance was required over a 7-day period. This included time taken for daily activities of living such as eating and dressing.

Diary recording can be very structured (see Box 21.24), recording time taken to achieve something or ticking a checklist. A participant might be required to complete a health diary, recording symptom experience by answering structured questions such as 'Did you experience pain? Yes/No'. The degree of structure can vary, often with questions acting as a prompt for more open responses (see Box 21.25).

Box 21.25   Example of a set of diary questions

Please complete the following diary questions about your experiences of learning online as part of a student group looking at interprofessional working:

What were the main reasons for you going online this week?
What have been the main benefits to going online this week?
Were there any problems with your online activities this week?
Briefly outline any personal learning from the online discussions this week.
Feel free to comment on any other aspect of your online learning.

Moule (2006: 153)

Conversely, it is suggested that diaries can be completely unstructured, asking individuals to record their day, providing sensitive descriptions of their daily life (Polit and Beck, 2006). See Box 21.26 for an example.

Box 21.26   Example of diary use to record intimate daily life

Broussard (2005) completed research that sought to interpret and understand women's experiences of bulimia nervosa. Thirteen women kept a personal diary of daily life, recording their experiences of living with an eating disorder.

Aspects to consider when using diaries for data collection

Burns and Grove (2005) report acceptable validity and reliability in the use of health diaries when compared with interviews and point to guidance given by Burman (1995) in the use of health diaries. To try to improve validity and reliability, the researcher must consider whether a diary gives scope to collect data of interest, determine the degree of structure required of the diary, and pilot-test the tool. A pilot test will enable the researcher to review the clarity of completion instructions and ensure that any structured questions are robust. The period of data collection should be determined. Daily diaries may be completed over a short period, such as the seven days suggested by Corrigan and Bogner (2004). Weekly diaries, however, might be collated over a longer period, such as the 7-week completion time adhered to by students reporting online learning experiences (Moule, 2006).

Participant fatigue can be an issue in diary collection, with incomplete diaries returned or non-completion being problematic. Researchers can employ a system of reminders to encourage completion and it is suggested that diary completion rates can be high (80–88 per cent) (Burns and Grove, 2005). It is also thought that the completion of health diaries in particular can affect the participants' behaviour as they become more aware of their behaviours and implement change (Burns and Grove, 2005).

Figure 21.6 lists the potential strengths and limitations of diary use in research.

Using archive material

Researchers using archive material draw on data from the past rather than the present. The use of archive material may form part of historical or retrospective

> Potential strengths:
>
> - Diaries can offer historical insight.
> - There is the potential to provide an intimate description of everyday life.
> - Diaries can access data not readily recorded by other tools.
>
> Potential limitations:
>
> - Participant co-operation can be an issue.
> - The quality of recording can be variable.
> - Diary completion can lead to a change in participant behaviour.

Figure 21.6   Potential strengths and weaknesses of diary use in research

studies (see Chapter 17). Historical studies will draw on data from the past, such as photographs or records, to understand events at a particular time in history. Such analysis may draw new knowledge that can inform current practice, but may not necessarily seek to do so. For example, analysis of student nurse training data archived some 35 years ago will allow a description of the student nurse population at that time which could be contrasted to the current student population, though it has a primary aim of describing previous nursing cohorts. Burns and Grove (2005) suggest that as part of the process of completing historical research an inventory of sources will be needed, as the researcher may be drawing on a number of different materials.

Retrospective studies will take a current issue, such as the implementation of the new modern matron role, and explore past events that may have impacted on the development of the new role. The aim is therefore to use archived material to try to understand and inform present practice.

Sources of archive data used may include written or audio documents, diaries, interview data or photographs (see Box 21.27). As discussed in the earlier section on using documents, the researcher drawing on these data sets will need to consider issues of accessing archived material and confirm the authenticity and completeness of the data.

Box 21.27   Example of the use of archived documents

Sweet (2004) used a range of historical documents to research the histories of mission hospitals in rural South African communities. These included medical and nursing journals, archives of a number of medical missionary societies and of the Overseas Nursing Association. Research was also informed by oral histories of healthcare professionals.

Strengths and limitations of use

There are a number of concerns associated with the use of archive material in research that are consistent with those identified earlier when discussing the use of documents. The researcher is relying on previously collected data that was not collated for research purposes. There may therefore be inaccuracies and instances of missing data. The data can present biases and be subjective, though this will depend on the type of data used.

Generally, the researcher is drawing on existing materials with the benefits this brings. The researcher will not have been involved in data collection and is not expecting individuals to recall events or experiences. Provided access to materials can be negotiated, data collection can be less time-consuming and readily achieved.

Figure 21.7 lists the potential strengths and weaknesses of using historical and archive materials in research

---

Potential strengths:

- Draws on existing and historical material.
- Removes the potential for researcher bias in data collection.
- Can be cost effective.
- Can be an efficient approach to collecting data.

Potential limitations:

- There may be issues with data access.
- Data may be incomplete and unusable as it was not originally collected for research purposes.
- There may be inaccuracies, bias or errors in the data.

Figure 21.7   Potential strengths and weaknesses of using historical and archive materials in research

Internet and web-based techniques

The Internet has been one of the fastest growing phenomena in recent years. Within healthcare it is being used to access information and to support expert discussion forums. The World Wide Web, originally developed for research use, offers scope for educational provision across international healthcare environments. There is no wonder that its use within research is also increasing. The Internet can be used to access information that can aid in the development of research, sourcing background literature or information, research design and statistical procedures. It is also used to aid data collection, often through the use of email or through providing online data collection sites, accessed through a web address. These sites are secure and provide flexibility in data collection, allowing the participants to upload information or complete online data collection tools when they choose.

Whilst there remain some limitations of use, the Internet/web can support the completion of questionnaires, diaries or blogs (web-based logs), focus groups (see Box 21.28), discussion forums or can use the email system to collect text data. There is even scope to undertake observational research online, recording observations of interactions and conversations taking place within chat rooms, wiki (development of a paper/document online) and virtual classrooms.

Box 21.28   Example of the use of virtual focus groups

Alder and Zarchin (2002) used the Internet to collect data from a sample of seven women over a period of four weeks. The women were on home bed rest for the treatment of pre-term labour. Focus groups were held online to explore their lived experience of being pregnant and confined home bed rest.

Issues of use

There are many potential benefits in the use of email, the Internet and the Web to collect research data. These include being able to access international participants; having scope to access large numbers of participants at a low cost; flexibility for the participants in the completion of data collection material; and the potential to generate qualitative and quantitative data. There can also be benefits in resource savings, reducing the data collection period and facilitating ease of online analysis. Additionally, there is flexibility to use data collection methods that are either asynchronous (not real-time) or synchronous (real-time).

The possible limitations of online use relate to the need for participants to have access to computer hardware with Internet connection. Though the numbers with Internet access are increasing at home and in the work place, a number of participants may be excluded from online data collection for a number of reasons, including lack of information technology (IT) skills, inability to access computer hardware and limits set by employers to Internet connections. There are additionally issues to overcome in ensuring that participants have the necessary Web addresses and passwords to enable access to data collection sites or tools. A number of healthcare staff may also be reluctant to engage in online data collection processes, preferring either paper-based tools or a more personal approach.

Researchers using Internet or web-based data collection techniques will need to ensure that they have the technological support to develop data collection materials and support their use, including addressing any emergent technical issues. Development costs may be incurred, though these need to be offset against likely resource savings in researcher data collection time, travel costs and photocopying.

Figure 21.8 lists the potential strengths and weaknesses of using the Internet for data collection

---

Potential strengths:

- Can offer flexibility to the participant.
- Scope to reach dispersed samples of large numbers.
- Can be used to collect qualitative and quantitative data.
- Can reach some sample groups, i.e. elderly and disabled who may otherwise be unable to take part in research.
- Can be cost-effective and save researcher time.

Potential limitations:

- May exclude those without computer and Internet access.
- Can exclude those with limited or no IT skills.
- Will incur some set-up costs.
- Computer-based data collection techniques will not appeal to everyone.

Figure 21.8 Potential strengths and weaknesses of using the Internet for data collection

Chapter summary

- There are a number of data collection tools available to the nurse researcher.
- The main techniques in use include observations, interviews, questionnaires.
- Each data collection technique has its own strengths and weaknesses when used in research.
- Researchers need training in the different approaches to data collection.
- The Internet is providing a new approach to data collection that can enable ease of access to world-wide research participants.

References

Alder, C. and Zarchin, Y. (2002) 'The "virtual focus group": using the Internet to reach pregnant women on home bed rest', *Journal of Obstetric, Gynecologic and Neonatal Nursing*, 31 (4): 418–27.

Arvidsson, B. and Fridlund, B. (2005) 'Factors influencing nurse supervisor competence: a critical incident analysis study', *Journal of Nursing Management*, 13 (3): 231–7.

Baker, T. (1994) *Doing Social Research*, 2nd edition. New York: McGraw-Hill.

Barbour, R. and Schostak, J. (2005) 'Interviewing and focus groups', in B. Somekh and C. Lewin (eds), *Research Methods in the Social Sciences*. London: Sage. pp. 41–8.

Bergeron, M., Cannon, J., Hal, E. and Kutlar, A. (2004) 'Erythrocyte sickling during exercise and thermal stress', *Clinical Journal of Sports Medicine*, 14 (6): 354–6.

Bojtor, A. (2003) 'The importance of social and cultural factors to nursing status', *International Journal of Nursing Practice*, 9 (5): 328–35.

Bowling, A. (2002) *Research Methods in Health: Investigating Health and Health Services*, 2nd edition. Buckingham: Open University Press.

Bowling, A. (2005) *Measuring Health: A Review of Quality of Life Measurement Scales*, 3rd edition. Maidenhead: Open University Press.

Broussard, B. (2005) 'Women's experiences of bulimia nervosa', *Journal of Advanced Nursing*, 49 (1): 43–50.

Burman, M. (1995) 'Health diaries in nursing research and practice', *Image – Journal of Nursing Scholarship*, 27 (2): 147–52.

Burns, N. and Grove, S. (2005) *The Practice of Nursing Research: Conduct, Critique and Utilization*, 5th edition. St Louis, MO: Elsevier/Saunders.

Candlin, J. and Stark, S. (2005) 'Plastic apron wear during direct patient care', *Nursing Standard*, 20 (2): 41–6.

Clark, L. (1996) 'Participant observation in a secure unit: care, conflict and control', *Nursing Times Research*, 1 (6): 431–40.

Colon-Emeric, C., Casebeer, L., Saag, K., Allison, J., Levine, D., Theodore, S. and Lyles, K. (2004) 'Barriers to providing osteoporosis care in skilled nursing directors and directors of nursing', *American Journal of Medical Directors*, 5 (6): 361–6.

Corrigan, J. and Bogner, J. (2004) 'Latent factors in measures of rehabilitation outcomes after traumatic brain injury', *Journal of Head Trauma Rehabilitation*, 19 (4): 445–58.

Denzin, N. (1989) *The Research Act: A Theoretical Introduction to Sociological Methods,* 3rd edition. Englewoods Cliff, NJ: Prentice-Hall.

Flanagan, J. (1954) 'The critical incident technique', *Psychological Bulletin*, 51 (4): 327–58.

Fontana, A. and Frey, J. (1998) 'Interviewing', in N. Denzin and Y. Lincoln (eds), *Collecting and Interpreting Qualitative Materials*. Thousand Oaks, CA: Sage. pp. 47–78.

Gold, R. (1958) 'Roles in sociological field observations, *Social Forces*, 36: 217–23.

Griffiths, M. (1998) *Educational Research for Social Justice: Getting off the Fence*. Buckingham: Open University Press.

Hollway, W. and Jefferson, T. (2000) *Doing Qualitative Research Differently*. London: Sage.

Jones, L. and Somekh, B. (2005) 'Observation', in B. Somekh and C. Lewin (eds), *Research Methods in the Social Sciences*. London: Sage. pp. 138–45.

Kenen, R., Arden-Jones, A. and Eelles, R. (2004) 'Healthy women from suspected hereditary breast and ovarian cancer families: the significant others in their lives', *European Journal of Cancer Care*, 13 (2): 169–79.

Landis, J. and Koch, T. (1977) 'The measurement of observation agreement', *Biometrics*, 33: 159–74.

Lauder, W., Sharkey, S. and Mummery, K. (2004) 'A community survey of loneliness', *Journal of Advanced Nursing*, 46 (1): 88–94.

Leininger, M. (1985) *Qualitative Research Methods in Nursing*. Philadelphia, PA: W.B. Saunders.

MacDonald, K. and Tipton, C. (1993) 'Using documents', in N. Gilbert (ed.), *Researching Social Life*. London: Sage. pp. 187–200.

Malinowski, B. (1922) *Argonauts of the Western Pacific*. London: Routledge & Keagan Paul.

Manias, E., Aitken, R. and Dunning, T. (2005) 'How graduate nurses use protocols to manage patients' medication', *Journal of Clinical Nursing*, 14 (8): 935–44.

Maynard, M. and Purvis, J. (eds) (1994) *Researching Women's Lives from a Feminist Perspective*. London: Taylor & Francis.

McCabe, C. (2004) 'Nurse–patient communication: an exploration of patients' experiences', *Journal of Clinical Nursing*, 13 (1): 41–9.

McGuigan, D. and Moule, P. (2006) *A Multi-method Approach to Explore Nurses' Experiences of Using a Web-based Learning Package in Cancer Care and its Impact on Patient Care Delivery*. Bristol: University of the West of England. http://hsc.uwe.ac.uk/net/research/Data/Sites/1/GalleryImages/ Research/ last%20and%20final%20draft%20E-learning%20project.PDF, accessed 29 February 2008.

Meretoja, R., Leino-Kilpi, H. and Kaira, A.-M. (2004) 'Comparison of nurse competence in different hospital work environments', *Journal of Nursing Management*, 12 (5): 329–36.

Moule, P. (2006) 'E-learning for healthcare students: developing the communities of practice framework', *Journal of Advanced Nursing*, 53 (3): 370–80.

Oppenheim, A. (1992) *Questionnaire Design, Interviewing and Attitude Measurement*, 2nd edition. London: Pinter.

Polit, D. and Beck, C. (2006) *Essentials of Nursing Research: Methods, Appraisal and Utilization*, 6th edition. Philadelphia, PA: Lippincott Williams & Wilkins.

Ray, R. and Street, A. (2005) 'Who's there and who cares: age as an indicator of social support networks for care givers among people living with motor neurone disease', *Health and Social Care in the Community*, 13 (6): 542–52.

Roethlisberger, F. and Dickinson, W. (1939) *Management and the Worker*. Cambridge, MA: Harvard University Press.

Rycroft-Malone, J., Harvey, G., Seers, K., Kitson, A., McCormack, D. and Titchen, A. (2004) 'An exploration of the factors that influence the implementation of evidence into practice', *Journal of Clinical Nursing*, 13 (8): 913–24.

Saglani, S., McKenzie, S., Bush, A. and Payne, D. (2005) 'A video questionnaire identifies upper airway abnormalities in preschool children with reported wheeze', *Archives of Disease in Childhood*, 90 (9): 961–4.

Smith, E. (2005) 'Telephone interviewing in healthcare research: a summary of the evidence', *Nurse Researcher*, 12 (3): 32–41.

Smith, M. (2004) 'The search for insight: clients' psychological experiences of alcohol withdrawal in a voluntary, residential, health care setting', *International Journal of Nursing Practice*, 10 (2): 80–85.

Sweet, H. (2004) '"Wanted: 16 nurses of better educated type": provision of nurses to South Africa in the late nineteenth and early twentieth centuries', *Nursing Inquiry*, 11 (3): 176–84.

Tardy, B., Lafond, P., Viallon, A., Buchmuller, A., Zeni, F. and Decousus, H. (2003) 'Older people included in a venous thrombo-embolism clinical trial: a patients' viewpoint', *Age and Ageing*, 32 (2): 149–53.

Taylor, R. (2005) 'Can the social model explain all of disability experience?', *American Journal of Occupational Therapy*, 59 (5): 497–506.

Thomas, R. and Purdon, S. (1994) *Telephone Methods for Social Surveys. Social Research Update. Issue 8*. Guildford: University of Surrey. Available at www.soc.surrey.ac.uk/sru/SRU8.html, accessed 29 February 2008.

Ward, R. and Moule, P. (2007) 'Supporting pre-registration students in practice. current ICT use', *Nurse Education Today*, 27: 60–67.

Whitfield, R., Newcombe, R. and Woollard, M. (2003) 'Reliability of the Cardiff test of basic life support and automated external defibrillation', *Resuscitation*, 59 (3): 291–314.

Williams, C. (2005) 'The identification of family members' contribution to patients' care in the intensive care unit: a naturalistic inquiry', *Nursing in Critical Care*, 10 (1): 6.

Suggested further reading

Allan, H. (2006) 'The relevance and importance of ethnography for illuminating the role of emotions in nursing practice', *Journal of Research in Nursing*, 11 (5): 397–407.

Bowling, A. (2002) *Research Methods in Health: Investigating Health and Health Services*, 2nd edition. Buckingham: Open University Press.

Bowling, A. (2005) *Measuring Health: A Review of Quality of Life Measurement Scales*, 3rd edition. Maidenhead: Open University Press.

Gould, D. and Fontenla, M. (2006) 'Strategies to recruit and retain the nursing workforce in England: A telephone interview study', *Journal of Research in Nursing*, 11 (1): 3–17.

Han, B., Tiggle, R. and Remsburg, R. (2008) 'Characteristics of patients receiving hospice care at home versus in nursing homes: results from the National Home and Hospice Care Survey and the National Nursing Home Survey', *American Journal of Hospice and Palliative Medicine*, 24 (6): 479–86.

Oppenheim, A. (1992) *Questionnaire Design, Interviewing and Attitude Measurement*, 2nd edition. London: Pinter.

Websites

Social Research Update, University of Surrey: www.soc.surrey.ac.uk/sru/SRU19.html
Surveys of all key areas of the human world, such as social and economic life: www.worldvaluessurvey.org/
UK Medicines Information provides information on questionnaire design: www.ukmi.nhs.uk/Research/ResSkillsQDesign.asp

22

ANALYSIS OF QUANTITATIVE DATA

Mollie Gilchrist and Chris Wright

Previous chapters (13–17, 20–21) have discussed a range of methods that nurse researchers use to collect data for the primary purpose of addressing their research questions or hypotheses. Data analysis is the process through which researchers manage the collected data to identify key patterns or features that are important when answering (or attempting to answer) research questions. To the novice researcher, the literature contains a bewildering variety of methods for data analysis. The objective is to choose appropriate methods so that results from a research study are valid and can be used to inform practice and guide future research.

This chapter provides an introduction to some fundamental principles and concepts for the analysis of quantitative (or numerical) data. It explores ways of summarising and presenting data, and introduce inferential statistical methods. It also considers different meanings and implications of statistics and related ethical issues. Details of specific methods can be found in texts such as those listed at the end of the chapter.

Learning outcomes

This chapter is designed to enable the reader to:

- **Understand different meanings of the word 'statistics', and discuss the role of statistics in relation to research**
- **Understand different types of data, and their measurement**
- **Discuss key features of graphical and numerical summaries**
- **Discuss basic concepts of hypothesis testing, interpretation of ensuing results and their practical importance**

- **Appreciate the use of computers for data analysis**
- **Consider ethical issues in regard to the analysis of quantitative data**

KEY TERMS

Averages, Charts, Correlation coefficient, Interval level, Measures of central tendency, Measures of dispersion, Nominal data, Ordinal data, Parametric methods, Ratio level, Statistical hypothesis testing, Statistics

---

Statistical methods

The word **statistics** has several meanings (Wright, 2002). We are all familiar, in everyday life, with official statistics such as numbers of births and deaths. Nurses routinely meet statistics in their everyday practice; for example, bed occupancy in a ward, number of daily admissions or discharges. The term also refers to quantities that summarise various characteristics of numerical data; for example, 'mean' waiting time for a colonoscopy, 'range' of weight loss in patients with cancer. Such statistics are useful for administrative purposes, for example scheduling routine procedures in hospital day units. A broader use of the term encompasses methods that are used to collect, analyse and interpret quantitative data to inform decision making when accounting for variation in, for example, human behaviour or response to treatment.

In the context of this chapter, the phrase 'statistical methods' is used to refer to procedures that have been developed specifically for the analysis of quantitative data. An understanding of basic principles will enable nurses to read and critique articles or reports in which such techniques have been employed, and to identify:

- use of appropriate and inappropriate methods to analyse data
- well-reported results, as well as misreported or misleading results
- valid and incorrect interpretation of results
- overstated generalisation of findings.

In general, statistical methods are categorised as descriptive or inferential. Descriptive statistics are employed in all studies in which quantitative data are collected, whereas inferential statistics are applicable when seeking to generalise findings from the study sample to a wider population. These are discussed in later sections.

Choice of method depends on the type of data collected which, in turn, is dependent upon the methods employed for their collection. Appropriate selection is also influenced by the research question and research design. This inter-relationship means that methods for data analysis must be planned at the outset, alongside development of the research question, design and data collection methods. Failure to pre-plan the method of analysis could result in the collection of data that cannot be analysed to address the research question.

Types of data

A research study will include the collection of data on several attributes (also termed 'variables'); for example, gender, blood group, degree of pain, satisfaction with treatment, temperature, weight, size of leg ulcers, and volume of urine. Data collected on these attributes might take different values for different participants and, broadly speaking, are labelled as one of two types: categorical or quantitative.

Categorical data

Gender and blood group are examples of 'categorical' variables, where each participant in a study belongs in only one of the categories. Data would comprise the labels associated with each category; for example, male or female in the case of gender. This type of data is said to be at a **nominal** level of measurement, which is classed as the lowest level.

Sometimes, a meaningful order is apparent in the possible responses associated with a variable. For example, when questioned about satisfaction with the outcome of treatment, a Likert scale might ask for responses from 'strongly disagree' through to 'strongly agree'; or responses to a question on the degree of pain experienced before treatment might range from 'none', 'mild', 'moderate', 'severe' to 'intolerable'. Data measured at this level are termed **ordinal**; they belong to named and ordered categories. It could be said that someone who responded that they had 'moderate' pain before treatment reported a higher degree of pain than a person who responded using the 'mild' category and lower than a person who reported pain in the 'intolerable' category.

For ease of handling, categorical data are often coded or scored prior to data analysis, especially when using computer software. For the variable gender, for example, 'male' might be represented by 0 and 'female' by 1. Degree of pain might be coded as 0 for 'none' through to 4 for 'intolerable' pain. Care needs to be taken to distinguish these coded numbers from the measured numbers outlined below. Numbers that denote different responses at a nominal level of measurement are purely labels reflecting distinct categories or responses. At an ordinal level, however, larger numbers represent more of some attribute (or less, depending on the coding) compared with lower numbers.

Quantitative data

Quantitative data comprise numerical information, expressed in terms of basic dimensions such as distance, time, pressure, temperature and weight. Measurement of most physical or physiological attributes (for example, body temperature, blood pressure, body weight) produces quantitative data. Other examples include: years since diagnosis of a disease; time (days) since discharge from hospital; number of asthma attacks per week. Here, the numerical values are said to be measured at an **interval** or **ratio level** of measurement.

An interval level of measurement is named, ordered and measured on a scale marked in equal intervals. For example, a body temperature of 40°C is higher than one at 37°C which, in turn, is higher than one at 34°C (that is, the scale is ordered). In addition, the difference between 40°C and 37°C is equal in some sense to the difference between 37°C and 34°C (that is, equal intervals have the same meaning). However, 0°C is not an absolute zero, so we could not say that a room at 40°C was twice as hot as a room at 20°C.

A ratio level of measurement is named, ordered and measured on a scale marked in equal intervals and has an absolute zero. This absolute zero enables us to compare relative sizes of scores as well as differences in scores and order of scores and makes ratio the highest level of measurement (that is, portrays the most detailed information about attributes). For example, considering a situation of three people who weigh 80 kg, 60 kg and 40 kg, we can report that the first person is heavier than the second, who is heavier than the third, and that the difference in weight between the first and second persons is the same as that between the second and third persons. In addition, it could be reported that the first person is twice the weight of the third person. For the purposes of the statistical analyses presented in this chapter, there is no need to make a distinction between interval and ratio levels of measurement. They are termed 'scale' in some data-handling software packages, for example, Statistical Package for the Social Sciences (SPSS).

The examples above relate to the objective measurement of attributes to produce quantitative data. However, the nurse researcher will be interested in many attributes that might be considered more subjective; for example, pain intensity, general health status, physical disability and handicap, psychological well-being and quality of life. Researchers have expended much effort, over many years, developing standard tools to quantify subjective estimates of attributes that cannot be measured directly. Two popular types of tool are the visual analogue scale (VAS) and rating scales. Use of VAS Pain is an attempt to record subjective estimates of pain intensity (McDowell and Newell, 1996). Participants translate assessment of their pain onto a line (10 cm in length) and their pain is scored 0 to 100, with 0 indicating no pain and 100 indicating 'pain as bad as could be'. Theoretically, the resultant scores are recorded at an ordinal level of measurement, although some research has demonstrated that a ratio

A paper by Gask et al. (2006) reports a study that evaluates skills training for managing people at risk of suicide. The paper contains data collected from variables at each of the levels of measurement discussed above. Some of these are listed below:

Categorical

- Nominal (named categories): profession, sex, ethnicity.
- Ordinal (named and ordered categories): attitudes to suicide prevention scale (ASP), scored 1–5.

Quantitative

- Interval/ratio (measurement with equal units/intervals between data points): age (years), number of years in profession, confidence in assessment and management of clients (100 mm VAS, scored 0 for 'no confidence' to 100 for 'very confident').

Figure 22.1   An example of study variables and their levels of measurement

level may be assumed (McDowell and Newell, 1996). The Barthel Index is a rating scale comprising 15 items (revised version) that was developed to monitor performance of people with chronic conditions and to estimate how much nursing care was required (McDowell and Newell, 1996). Scores on individual items are summed to produce a total score. Many researchers treat the resultant data as being measured at an interval level.

Careful consideration should be given to the meaning of results from analyses on data collected using these types of tool since, for some, the overall score might not satisfy all the common rules of arithmetic that are used in many statistical analyses. In all instances, however, results are meaningless when data lack validity (that is, when the data do not measure what they purport to measure) and reliability (that is, when the data are not reproducible or consistent) and, therefore, judicious choice of measurement tools is essential.

It is evident that the type of data is an important consideration in the choice of descriptive and inferential statistics used for the analysis of quantitative data. Figure 22.1 lists the variables collected in a study by Gask et al. (2006), and considers their type and level of measurement.

Descriptive statistics: techniques for describing quantitative data

The aim of the first part of the results section in any study is to give the reader a 'picture' of the data collected. The numerical data are organised and summarised to portray or describe important features. This description usually involves numbers and percentages that are presented in words (for example, the percentage of bedridden patients who have bed sores), tables and/or **charts**. A few meaningful numbers (called 'summary statistics') are presented to summarise the overall data set. Summary statistics include: sample size; counts or frequencies (often expressed as percentages for comparison purposes); maximum and minimum values, and values such as percentiles and quartiles; **measures of central tendency** (**averages**); and **measures of dispersion** or spread of data (variability). A measure of central tendency provides a value around which data cluster, and a measure of variability provides a value indicating how closely the data cluster around this central value.

Summary statistics would enable the reader to gain a rough idea of the comparability of participants in different groups. This would be of particular interest when two different groups of people are involved, for example when comparing the characteristics of the intervention group with the control group at the beginning of a randomised control trial (RCT) (as, for example, Table 2 in Chan and Lam, 2006). The statistics should be seen to be similar, so that any conclusions reached after intervention are not due to a difference in values at the start. If there are some differences, these should be noted by the author and allowed for in the analysis and discussed in the discussion section.

Choice of summary statistics depends on the level of measurement of the data, as outlined above. Table 22.1 summarises some appropriate summary statistics dependent on the level of measurement of the data, and definitions of some summary statistics are given in Figure 22.2.

Table 22.1   Summary statistics associated with different levels of measurement

	Nominal (named categories)	Ordinal (named and ordered categories)	Interval/ratio (measurement with equal units/intervals between data points)
Averages (measure of central tendency of data)	Mode	Median* Mode	Mean* Median Mode (not so useful)
Variability (measure of dispersion or spread of data)		Range* Interquartile range (IQR)*	Standard deviation (SD)* Range IQR

Note: * most useful measure for a given level of data.

Correlation

A **correlation coefficient** is a measure of the strength of association between two variables and can take values between 0 (no correlation) and ±1 (perfect correlation).

Averages:

- Mode = most frequently occurring value
- Median = middle value, when all data are placed in order
- Mean = sum of all values divided by the number of values

Other location measures:

- Lower quartile = middle value of the ordered data from minimum to median value
- Upper quartile = middle value of the ordered data from median to maximum value

Measures of variability (dispersion) of data:

- Range = maximum value – minimum value
- Interquartile range (IQR) = upper quartile – lower quartile
- Standard deviation = an 'average' distance of all values away from the mean
- Variance = (standard deviation)^2

Figure 22.2   Definitions of some summary statistics

(Further properties of these measures can be explored in the resources listed at the end of the chapter.)

Correlations can be positive (that is, both variables increase or decrease together, for example blood pressure increasing with older age) or negative (that is, as one variable increases, the other decreases; for example physical agility decreasing with longer duration of rheumatoid arthritis).

A Pearson's coefficient of linear correlation (usually denoted by r) is often used when the data are measured at an interval/ratio level. This correlation assumes that proportionate changes occur in the two variables being considered. The researcher can check whether this assumption is reasonable by plotting one variable against the other on a graph called a 'scatter diagram'.

When the data have been collected at an ordinal level of measurement, strength of association can be measured using Spearman's coefficient of rank correlation (usually denoted by r_s). This variation of Pearson's coefficient does not assume that a linear association exists between the two variables and, therefore, can also be used to measure association between two variables when the data have been collected at interval/ratio level and a scatter diagram indicates non-proportionate changes on the two variables.

Tables and charts

Tables can be used when it is important that the reader has the exact figures for reference purposes, say. They often contain basic demographic information about the sample, and/or summary statistics for the variables under study; for example, Maag (2006) reports geographical location against age, gender and academic level of nursing students taking part in a study about their attitudes to using technology. Percentages can be useful for comparison purposes, but it is important to give the actual numbers too. After all, 70 per cent conveys a sizeable quantity, but when it refers to a sample of size 10, this is only 7 people.

Charts give an instant visual representation of the relative size of figures – it is said that 'a picture tells a thousand words'. Suitable charts for summarising data include: pie and bar charts for categorical data (for example, a bar chart for the number of nurses who work in different specialist areas); histograms, box and whisker plots (for example, a box plot of pain scores for people with different types of arthritis); and line graphs for quantitative data (especially when the data are collected over time). Pollard et al. (2004) use box and whisker plots to compare attitudes of students from ten different disciplines to interprofessional learning at the start of their undergraduate course. A scatter diagram allows the relationship between two variables to be explored; for example, a scatter diagram of cholesterol level and age.

All charts should have certain elements to aid interpretation of information presented in them. Figure 22.3 lists some of these features:

All charts should:

- Have a relevant and succinct title.
- Have clearly labelled axes, showing any measurements used.
- Use a careful choice of scale – often multiples of 2 or 5 are used, rather than multiples of, say, 3 or 7.
- Use scale breaks for 'false origins' – particularly when the vertical axis does not start at zero.
- Use carefully chosen plot symbols and connecting lines – more importance appears to be given to a solid line than to a dashed line, for example. See Takase et al. (2006: 755) for a clustered bar chart using different line styles.
- Show all relevant study information, e.g. sample size.

(Chatfield, 1995)

In addition, they should:

- 'Stand on their own' without the need for reference back to the text – there is the possibility of figures being taken out of context and misinterpreted, for example.
- Use of 3-D charts on paper should be avoided, as they are mathematically incorrect, although many modern computer packages allow the use of interactive charting to 'move around' a 3-D plot, thus permitting exploration of 3 variables.
- 2 or 3 charts are preferable to 1 'busy' one.

Note: See Watson et al. (2006: Ch. 4) for a good discussion about data presentation and an exploration of potentially misleading charts.

Figure 22.3   Chart checklist

Inferential statistics

Researchers who collect quantitative data through an experimental design or a survey usually do so with the intention of making inferences about a wider population of people (or institutions, objects or events) on the basis of data collected from a sample of people. For example, Chan and Lam (2006) randomly assigned 1,483 mothers of young, sick children who were at risk of passive smoking to an intervention group (receiving a simple nursing education intervention) or a control group (receiving no intervention). The aim was to evaluate the effectiveness of the intervention to decrease passive smoking exposure for sick children (that is, to generalise findings from this sample of mothers to all mothers with sick children at risk of passive smoking).

In practice, generalisation is influenced by several aspects within a study protocol, including: research design, sampling method, inclusion and exclusion criteria, recruitment strategy, willingness of participants to volunteer, conditions pertaining to any intervention under study, sample size, data collection tools and their administration, completeness of the collected data, and data analysis. Inferential statistics use sample data to make generalisations about a population of which the sample is representative, through testing statistical hypotheses.

Statistical hypotheses

In the study by Chan and Lam (2006), the researchers conducted the research because they believed that the nursing education intervention would decrease passive smoking exposure for sick children at risk. This prior belief (or assumption) is called a 'research hypothesis' and is stated at the design stage in a study (see Chapter 6).

At the data analysis stage, the research hypothesis is translated into two statistical hypotheses, called the 'null' and 'alternative' hypotheses:

- *Null hypothesis*: The nursing education intervention has no effect on passive smoking exposure for sick children at risk.
- *Alternative hypothesis*: The nursing education intervention has an effect on passive smoking exposure for sick children at risk.

The statistical hypotheses are part of the analysis method. They describe the two possible and complementary situations in the population from which the sample was drawn and of which it is representative. The alternative hypothesis states that the intervention has an effect in the population – implying that differences between groups in the data are due to a real effect in the population. Although unlikely, the intervention might have increased passive smoking exposure and not decreased it, hence the non-directional wording (named 2-tailed or 2-sided) of the alternative hypothesis. If, however, some theory or substantial prior evidence existed that precluded a situation in which the intervention might increase passive smoking exposure, then a directional alternative hypothesis would be stated (1-tailed or 1-sided):

- *Directional alternative hypothesis*: The nursing education intervention decreases passive smoking exposure for sick children at risk.

The null hypothesis represents the prior assumption in **statistical hypothesis testing**. This is usually the situation that the researchers believe to be false. It is an assumption of no effect or no change – implying that differences between groups in the data are due to chance or random error and are not due to a real effect in the population.

Sampling variation

By definition, a sample is a subset of the population from which it was selected (Chapter 19). Hence, differences between groups in the data collected from a sample are unlikely to be identical to the effect in the population. Differences between the sample statistic and the population effect are called 'sampling error'. Further, the observed difference between groups is likely to be different when calculated from a second sample randomly selected from the same population. This difference across samples is called 'sampling variation'. The theory of sampling variation is the basis on which statistical hypothesis tests are developed.

Statistical hypothesis testing

Conventional statistical hypothesis tests are based on the prior assumption that the null hypothesis is true. This statement can be verified or refuted using data from a random sample drawn from the population of interest. Large differences between groups in the data provide evidence that the null hypothesis is false, whilst small differences cast no doubt on its truth. The dilemma lies in determining what magnitude could be considered to be sufficiently 'large' to support a decision to reject the null hypothesis in favour of the alternative hypothesis, in the existence of sampling error.

Statistical hypothesis tests (such as those in Figure 22.6) enable the researcher to make a decision about the null hypothesis and to state a probability that the decision is wrong. These wrong decisions are the Type I and Type II errors that are reported in the literature. There are two possible statistical decisions:

- Reject the null hypothesis in favour of the alternative hypothesis.
- Do not reject the null hypothesis in favour of the alternative hypothesis.

	Situation in the population	
	No effect (null hypothesis is true)	**An effect exists** (null hypothesis is false)
Reject null hypothesis	Incorrect decision Type I error (significance level)	Correct decision (✓) (Called the 'power')
Do not reject null hypothesis	Correct decision (✓)	Incorrect decision Type II error

Decision on the basis of data from a random sample

Figure 22.4   Statistical decision against 'true' situation

These decisions are illustrated in Figure 22.4, against the 'true' situation in the population.

The null hypothesis is rejected when the chance (or probability) of obtaining at least as extreme an outcome as the observed data is smaller than some selected value. Otherwise, the null hypothesis is not rejected (Figure 22.5). The computed value of chance is the p-value reported in research studies and the selected cut-off value for decision making is the significance level. The choice of significance level is based on tradition or importance of a Type I error and should not be influenced by the data in a study. Hence the significance level is specified at the design stage. Conventionally, it is set at 5 per cent, and is associated with a p-value of 0.05 for making a decision.

Types of statistical hypothesis tests

In general, statistical hypothesis tests may be termed **parametric** or non–parametric methods. Their use requires certain assumptions to be satisfied, as summarised below for frequently used hypothesis tests:

- *Parametric methods*
  For example: t-test of difference between mean values of two populations, one-way ANOVA (analysis of variance) test of differences between mean values of two or more populations:

  - data measured on at least an interval level
  - data (in each group) constitute a random sample from a normally distributed population, i.e. data is distributed mostly around a central value with a few lower and higher values, forming a bell-shaped pattern
  - equality of group variances (called homogeneity).

- *Non-parametric methods*
  For example: chi-squared test of independence between two attributes used to classify the data, Mann-Whitney U test of difference between median values in two populations:

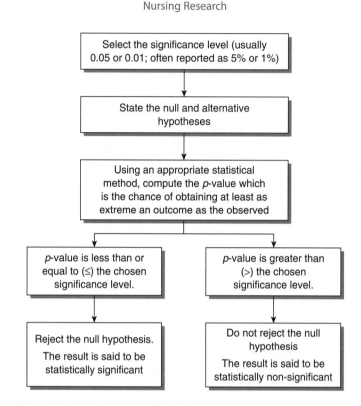

Figure 22.5   Steps in making a statistical decision

– data measured on at least a nominal level
– does not require assumptions of normality and homogeneity
– requires independence between cases.

Interpretation of results from statistical hypothesis tests

When the null hypothesis is rejected, the data provide evidence of an effect that is larger than expected by chance. However, the magnitude of the observed effect might or might not be of importance in clinical practice. There is a difference, then, between a result that is *statistically significant* and one that is *clinically important*. The practitioner needs to decide the order of magnitude of an effect that is clinically important. Statistical methods cannot do this.

The size of a minimal clinically important effect must be decided at the design stage. From this, a sample size can be determined (using statistical techniques) that enables an effect of clinical importance to be detected as statistically significant. An effect that is not statistically significant might have occurred by chance and, therefore, provides no evidence to inform practice.

An alternative approach to statistical hypothesis testing is to estimate the magnitude of effect in the population through a 'confidence interval' that is computed from the data in the sample. A confidence interval is stated as a lower value and an upper value that bound the magnitude of effect in the population with a stated confidence. In this way, it indicates how small or how large the effect might be in the population.

Choosing a statistical method for data analysis

Choice of an appropriate test is dependent upon:

- Research question:
  - association (for example, relationship between variables)
  - difference (for example, between groups in an experimental design)

- Type of data collected:
  - level of measurement

- How many factors (one or more):
  - variables or attributes that are deliberately controlled in an experimental design, for example, amount of analgesic (1 'factor'); type and amount of analgesic (2 factors); frequency, intensity and duration of exercise within a particular programme (3 factors)
  - attributes or characteristics across which certain outcome variables are to be compared – usually within a survey, for example, gender (1 characteristic or factor); type of health professional and management approach for a specific condition (2 attributes or factors)

- How many groups (two or more):
  - levels of a factor, for example, 250 mg, 500 mg of analgesic (2 groups within a factor 'amount of analgesic'); low, medium, high doses of an analgesic (3 groups within a factor 'amount of analgesic')
  - sub-classification within an attribute or characteristic, for example, male, female (2 groups within a factor 'gender'); rheumatoid arthritis, osteoarthritis, ankylosing spondylitis (3 groups within a factor 'type of arthritis')

- Same or different participants in each group.

Figure 22.6 shows a decision chart from which to choose an appropriate hypothesis test linking the above elements. The tests are not exhaustive of all statistical techniques or research questions, but represent some of the more frequently used tests of association and differences.

Instruction for use: Start from the top, answer the questions and follow the appropriate lines until you reach one of the test boxes.

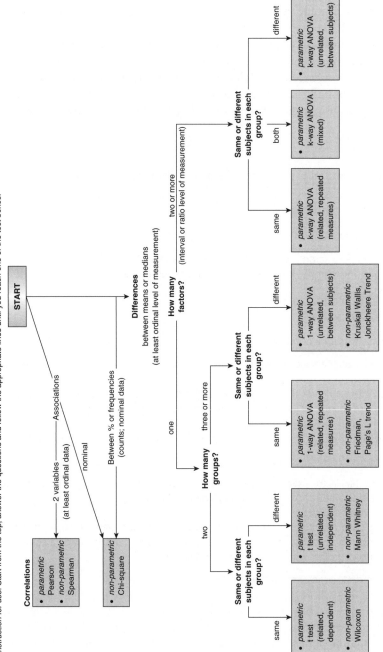

Figure 22.6   Hypothesis testing decision chart

Source: Adapted from Greene and D'Oliveira 1999

Using computer software for analysis

Most researchers use computer software to conduct analyses of quantitative data. This is due to the advent of menu-driven packages and the increased availability of data-handling software, such as SPSS. The use of computer software enables the emphasis of statistical analysis to be placed on appropriate techniques and interpretation of results. Accuracy of calculations is assured, provided that the data have been entered correctly. However, a computer will conduct any techniques requested of it, regardless of their lack of suitability, as, currently, computers are not programmed to ask a series of questions to ensure that the analysis that has been requested is appropriate. Hence the researcher needs to think carefully about what statistical analyses are requested and how the data need to be input.

MS Excel (or other 'spreadsheet' package) is another program that may be used to produce basic charts and simple statistical analyses; for example, calculation of means and standard deviations. Excel is more versatile than SPSS for creating some charts, such as clustered bar charts. Some researchers prefer to enter data into Excel, from where it is possible to transfer the data into SPSS. It is important to appreciate that charts drawn using software packages can be edited, so that the default output from the computer does not have to be accepted. Most aspects of a chart can be altered to be consistent with points raised earlier in the chapter.

Data preparation, input, verification and cleaning

Data need to be transferred from the data collection tool (for example, form, questionnaire or equipment output) into a format that is suitable for analysis. This often takes the form of a grid, with participants or cases in rows and responses to variables in columns. Before any analysis takes place, it is important to check the accuracy of the data and to deal constructively with any missing values.

Data preparation

Prior to transfer, the data may need to be coded. Answers to closed questions in a questionnaire, for example, provide single or multiple responses, the latter arising from 'tick as many as apply'. These can be coded with numbers for ease of data handling. A single response creates one variable. For example, a question requiring a 'no' or 'yes' response could simply be coded as 0 or 1 respectively, and the appropriate code recorded. For questions with more than two alternatives, more codes would be allocated. For example, marital status according to single, married, living with partner, separated, divorced and widowed could be coded with numbers 1 to 6 for each category respectively. Often this coding can be seen on a questionnaire in small print next to questions. Otherwise, it can be added manually down the right-hand margins on receipt of the questionnaire.

If more than one response may be ticked, each of the multiple responses will need to be regarded as 'not ticked'/'ticked' and hence become 'no'/'yes' variables. Therefore, if a question has ten responses, any number of which may be ticked, this translates into ten variables, each with an answer 'yes' if ticked but 'no' if not, and coded 1 or 0, as above.

A further consideration occurs if the respondent is asked to indicate, in order, the three most important concerns in relation to an issue. This translates into three variables, indicating first, second and third choices. Responses to quantitative variables, for example, height or a mark on a VAS, are recorded with none or some decimal places, as required.

Data input

Data can be written on squared paper and totals counted by hand, but, ideally, a data set can be entered directly into a data analysis package (e.g. SPSS, SAS, Minitab), or at least a spreadsheet (e.g. MS Excel), to allow speedy formulation of frequency tables and some summary statistics and charts. Data are input carefully, according to an agreed coding, into an already structured database (see software instructions to achieve this). Online questionnaires and some equipment provide an option to import data directly into a computer package, thus saving data input time.

Data verification

Once the data have been entered into the computer package, they need to be checked carefully for accuracy. Verification is an attempt to ensure that errors do not occur when transferring data from one source to another; for example, from questionnaire to database, or from one computer package to another. Strategies to achieve this include proof-reading, checking 10 per cent of data entry and 'double entry', when data are entered twice, and compared for agreement.

Data cleaning

Inputting errors need to be corrected. For example, if scoring on a Likert scale can range 1 to 5, a value recorded as 6 will need investigating. A negatively worded statement on a Likert scale scoring from 1 to 5 will need its responses to be reverse-scored; that is, 1 will become 5, 2 will become 4 and so on. In addition, decisions need to be made as to how to code missing data, and data need to be checked that they are within sensible limits. Once this data set is prepared, it should be carefully stored or saved to disk as a raw data file, and another copy becomes the 'working file' that is used for subsequent analysis.

Decisions need to be made on how to deal with missing data. The most direct approach is to eliminate any missing observations, known as 'listwise deletion'. However, although simple, this does reduce the effective sample size. 'Pairwise deletion' only excludes missing values for particular calculations. Another approach is to make some sort of estimate of the missing value(s).

For example, if you are asking participants to respond to several statements with a range of options, say from '1 = low' to '7 = high', it is acceptable practice to 'impute' the mean of the reported responses to obtain an overall scale score provided that at least 50 per cent of scores have been completed. An alternative approach is to substitute the group mean of available responses to a particular variable, although this is no longer considered to be good practice. Newer, less biased methods for estimating missing values, for example, 'multiple imputation', are being developed all the time. It may be possible to deduce responses to one missing question by a response to another. For example, it might be known that all the patients in one ward, where data have been collected, are female, so that a missing gender response may be completed. However, absolute honesty and openness must be adhered to at all times. It is recommended that advice about estimating missing numbers be sought from experienced researchers. The best solution is to maximise response rates, thus avoiding missing values altogether!

Ethical considerations

Ethical issues that might arise with regard to the analysis of quantitative data include anonymity, confidentiality, deception, exploitation and risk of harm (see Chapter 5).

Data from individual participants are combined during statistical analyses and results are reported as numerical values, so anonymity and confidentiality are unlikely to be infringed. However, it is good practice to use a unique number to identify data from each participant rather than their name (especially in a computer database) and to store a list of identifiers and participants' names in a different location from the data.

Deception and exploitation might arise in several ways. In theory, deception and exploitation of participants occur when data are used for a purpose other than that stated or inferred on the participant information sheet or consent form. Whilst this would not cause harm to the participants, if the data were manipulated to fit requirements for a different purpose (or the design or data collection methods were inappropriate for the other purpose), the resultant findings might be erroneous with potential to mis-inform decisions based on them. The consequence could be risk of harm (physical, psychological, social or economical) to future patients, health professionals or other groups of people. A similar situation might arise when:

- results are obtained through inappropriate statistical methods (for example, incorrect level of measurement, assumptions not satisfied)
- data cases are omitted from analyses without sound justification and the researchers do not report this in a clear and honest manner
- outcome measures are not valid for the population of interest in the study
- the primary outcome is chosen after the data have been analysed to ensure that a statistically significant result can be reported
- the sample size is too small to enable differences (or changes) of clinical importance to be detected as statistically significant
- the statistical findings are incorrectly interpreted, with too much or incorrect emphasis on statistical significance and little discussion on clinical relevance.

Chapter summary

- Statistical methods are used to organise and summarise large quantities of numerical data.
- Statistics are used to portray or describe important features in the data, either graphically or by calculation of a few meaningful numbers called 'summary statistics' (often presented in tabular form).
- Statistical methods use data collected from a (random) sample of a population of interest to draw inferences about that population.
- Statistical methods aim to generalise findings to a population of which the sample is representative.
- Statistical methods are applicable for all experimental studies (for example, RCTs) and for many surveys and comparative studies.
- Statistical methods use probability theory.
- Statistical methods are 'deductive' in that they test a prior assumption (or hypothesis) about the population, are based on specific assumptions (a method is valid only when its assumptions are met) and used ethically and honestly.

References

Chan, S. and Lam, T.H. (2006) 'Protecting sick children from exposure to passive smoking through mothers' actions', *Issues and Innovation in Nursing Practice*, 54 (4): 440–9.

Chatfield, C. (1995) *Problem Solving: Statistician's Guide*, 2nd edition. London: Chapman & Hall.

Gask, L., Dixon, C., Morriss, R., Appleby, L. and Green, G. (2006) 'Evaluating STORM skills training for managing people at risk of suicide', *Nursing and Healthcare Management and Policy*, 54: 739–50.

Greene, J. and D'Oliveira, M. (1999) *Learning to Use Statistical Tests in Psychology*, 2nd edition. Buckingham: Open University Press.

Maag, M. (2006) 'Nursing students' attitudes towards technology', *Nurse Educator*, 31 (3): 112–18.

McDowell, I. and Newell, C. (1996) *Measuring Health: A Guide to Rating Scales and Questionnaires*, 2nd edition. New York: Oxford University Press.

Pollard, K.C., Miers, M.E. and Gilchrist, M. (2004) 'Collaborative learning for collaborative working? Initial findings from a longitudinal study of health and social care students', *Health and Social Care in the Community*, 12 (4): 346–58.

Takase, M., Maude, P. and Manias, E. (2006) 'Role discrepancy: is it a common problem among nurses?', *Journal of Advanced Nursing*, 54 (6): 751–9.

Watson, R., Atkinson, I. and Egerton, P. (2006) *Successful Statistics for Nursing and Healthcare*. Basingstoke: Palgrave Macmillan.

Wright, C.C. (2002) 'The role of statistics in research in healthcare', *British Journal of Therapy and Rehabilitation*, 9 (4): 146–50.

Suggested further reading

Altman, D.G. (1991) *Practical Statistics for Medical Research*. London: Chapman & Hall/CRC.

Campbell, M.J. and Machin, D. (2004) *Medical Statistics: A Textbook for the Health Sciences*, 4th edition. Chichester: Wiley.

Fowler, J., Jarvis, P. and Chevannes, M. (2002) *Practical Statistics for Nursing and Health Care*. Chichester: Wiley.

Harris, M. and Taylor, G. (2005) *Medical Statistics Made Easy*. London: Taylor & Francis.

McKillup, S. (2006) *Statistics Explained: An Introductory Guide for Life Scientists*. Cambridge: Cambridge University Press.

Munro, B.H. (2005) *Statistical Methods for Healthcare Research*, 5th edition. Philadelphia, PA: Lippincott Williams & Wilkins.

Pallant, J. (2007) *SPSS Survival Manual: A Step-by-step Guide to Data Analysis Using SPSS v15*, 3rd edition. Buckingham: Open University Press.

Pett, M.A. (1997) *Nonparametric Statistics for Health Care Research: Statistics for Small Samples and Unusual Distributions*. Thousand Oaks, CA: Sage.

Salkind, N.J. (2004) *Statistics for People Who (Think They) Hate Statistics*, 2nd edition. London: Sage.

Schmuller, J. (2005) *Statistical Analysis with Excel for Dummies*, Hoboken, NJ: Wiley.

Scott, I. and Mazhindu, D. (2005) *Statistics for Health Care Professionals: An Introduction*. London: Sage.

Swinscow, T.D.V. and Campbell, M.J. (2002) *Statistics at Square One*, 9th edition. London: BMJ Books.

Watson, R., Atkinson, I. and Egerton, P. (2006) *Successful Statistics for Nursing and Healthcare*. Basingstoke: Palgrave Macmillan.

Wood, M. (2003) *Making Sense of Statistics: A Non-mathematical Approach*. Basingstoke: Palgrave Study Guides.

Websites

Exploring data website from Central Queensland University: http://exploring data.cqu.edu.au/

SurfStat Australia from the Australian National University: www.anu.edu.au/nceph/surfstat/surfstat-home/surfstat.html

23

QUALITATIVE DATA ANALYSIS TECHNIQUES

Qualitative data analysis can often commence at the start of the project and the researcher will continue analysis throughout the period of data collection and beyond. In a grounded theory approach, for example, the qualitative researcher in nursing will engage in data analysis as soon as the first data are collected. Analysing data throughout the data collection period supports a constant comparative method used in grounded theory research (see Chapter 14). In this research approach the researcher will be looking for evidence of themes and revising research questions to support theory development as the project progresses (Corbin and Holt, 2005). Engaging in data analysis throughout the data collection process contrasts with the approach to quantitative data analysis we described in Chapter 22. When working with quantitative data, the researchers tend to collect all of the data before starting data analysis.

Those new to analysing qualitative data often find the process complex. Qualitative data analysis processes can raise far more issues than seen in the analysis of quantitative data. This arises as the process of preparing and analysing qualitative data relies on the individual judgements and interpretations of the researcher. Mechanisms can be built into the process that can aid the 'objectivity' seen in qualitative analysis. These can include 'member checking', where the research participants are involved in verifying the interpretations of the researcher, corroborating the analysis. Other validation strategies can be employed, such as the provision of an 'audit trail'. This presents the research journey and approaches taken to the analysis of the data (Lincoln and Guba, 1985). Such strategies aim to support the trustworthiness of data analysis and should be an integral part of any data analysis process.

Polit and Beck (2006) suggest further challenges to the nurse researcher, including the volume of effort required in the analysis of lengthy narrative materials and the presentation of the data in a concise form that maintains meaning and value. Quantitative data is often presented in tabular or graphical form. This affords the presentation of copious amounts of numerical data in a concise space. In contrast, the presentation of narrative, often as verbatim quotes of the spoken word extracted from interview transcripts, can be challenging. The researcher must select specific data for presentation that will support the key issues arising from the interpretation of the vast quantities of textual data.

In this chapter we discuss the methods employed in the analysis of qualitative data. Chapter 14 presented some of the approaches used in qualitative research and identified that qualitative data was often derived from field notes generated as part of participant observation, personal diaries and the verbatim transcriptions from interviews. The discussion below reviews how researchers manage qualitative information, drawing interpretations from text-based and visually presented data.

Learning outcomes

This chapter is designed to enable the reader to:

- **Appreciate the processes involved in preparing qualitative data for analysis**
- **Understand how qualitative data is interpreted**
- **Understand how computer packages can assist the process of data preparation and analysis**
- **Appreciate the need to establish rigour in the process of analysis**

KEY TERMS

Computer-assisted data analysis, Content analysis, Data coding, Discourse and conversation analysis, Interpretation of qualitative data, Narrative analysis, Preparation of data, Qualitative data analysis, Rigour, Trustworthiness

---

Analysis of qualitative data

There is no one approach that should be used when analysing qualitative data, but an array of methods is available. Back in 1990, Tesch reported 26 possible strategies for analysing textual data. These might be employed in the analysis of transcripts from interview or focus-group data, field notes or documents (see Chapter 21). Qualitative data can also include digitally recorded visual images, such as photographs, video and pictures. The analysis of images would draw on further analytic frameworks. In selecting the method of analysis, Coffey and Atkinson (1996) advise the researcher to explore the variety of methods available, selecting an approach that would enable the interpretation of data through a rigorous approach.

The analysis of qualitative data should be embedded in the research process, often integral to the period of data collection. This allows the process of analysis to be reflexive and iterative. The analysis of data collected initially can then inform further data collection. Within action research and participatory enquiry (see Chapter 17), data analysis is seen as an ongoing process occurring as part of reflective processes within data collection. In action research approaches, the development of practice and implementation of change are based on the initial research findings and followed by further data collection and analysis as the outcomes of new actions are evaluated (Noffke and Somekh, 2005).

Reflexivity is part of nursing practice and needs to be a consideration within nursing research, particularly where the researcher may have the dual role of practitioner. Researching as an 'insider' being part of the culture of nursing should be acknowledged by the researcher, who will have predetermined experiences and thoughts about practice. These can have an impact on the approach taken to the analysis of findings and requires the validation of interpretations. Researchers can attempt to 'bracket' themselves (see Chapter 14 for explanations on the use of 'bracketing' in phenomenology), trying to ensure their personal experiences are acknowledged, limiting any researcher bias in the **interpretation of qualitative data**. Researchers can also validate their interpretations externally by returning original data to participants for clarification of meaning or through the involvement of independent researchers in the process of analysis.

It is also worth noting that the analysis of qualitative data can be viewed as a series of tasks, whereas for others it is an act of interpretation, where meaning is drawn from the data. Hollway and Jefferson (2000) suggest that researchers with large amounts of unstructured data often resort to imposing structure upon it, by breaking it into manageable segments through **data coding** and retrieval methods. They criticise **computer-assisted date analysis** packages for fragmenting data in this way. However, Miles and Huberman (1994) offer one approach to **qualitative data analysis** that encompasses data reduction, display and conclusion drawing and verification.

Qualitative data analysis is viewed as continuous. Data is selected, simplified from the initial field notes or transcriptions. Codes, themes or clusters are identified, transforming the data. This process involves analysis, and data is displayed or organised to allow conclusion drawing. The explanations or propositions are tentative, developing as data collection continues. When more develop, these conclusions are tested through verification processes, such as returning to the 'raw data' or gaining outside opinion. The following sections examine more closely the **preparation** of qualitative data for content and **narrative analysis**.

It should also be remembered that qualitative data, though generally in text format, could be pictorial and visual. The analysis of photographic images can be based on key observational questions such as the weather, the scenery, the interactions taking place, or can include measurements of the number of trees or number of people. Video can be used to record skill acquisition, allowing more detailed analysis of learning by more than one researcher. For example, Whitfield et al. (2003) videoed the public using automated external defibrillators when attending a collapsed casualty who had had a suspected heart attack. The actions recorded on the video were analysed against a pre-determined schedule that included the steps in the skill of basic life support with automated external defibrillator use. The team was able to judge the learning that had taken place by identifying accurate demonstration of the steps in the skill and areas where the skill was less well accomplished.

Preparing the data

The nurse researcher will collect raw data, which could encompass text, tape/digital recordings or visual data such as photographs and video. The types of textual data available will reflect the data collection processes involved. They could include notes taken in the field (field notes), participant diaries or documents. The researcher may have collected verbal data through tape-recording individual interviews or focus-group discussions. This data is initially prepared through verbatim transcription, providing a written record of the conversation to include all verbal interactions noted between the participants and interviewer. Visual data can be in the form of still photographs, pictures or moving images. Initially, whatever the form of data, it will exist in copious amounts and require preparation prior to analysis.

The researcher will need to have a system of storing data that enables easy retrieval. This may be a computer-based system, depending on the type of data being held. For example, digital photographs can be held in online files, whereas printed photographs, accessed from historical records, will need indexing into a document-based filing system, perhaps by month and year the image was recorded, or by location. If using a computer program for analysis, the data may need specific preparation to enable its use.

Field notes and transcripts of interviews or focus-group discussions are more likely to be available electronically as word-processed documents. Field notes may need reading through before organising into more coherent notes. Detailed notes can be stored in electronic files for easy access. Following data collection at interview or focus group, the researcher will have taped or digitally recorded conversations that require transcription. Transcription can be a lengthy process, taking a number of hours to transcribe one hour of recorded interaction. There are different schools of thought regarding the approach that should be taken. One view suggests transcription can be undertaken by support staff and need not occupy the researcher's time. Another view would suggest that there are enormous benefits gained through the researcher taking time to transcribe the recordings. These relate to the opportunity afforded for immersion in the data, from listening to the recording and word processing its content. However the process is facilitated, the researcher must ensure that the data is prepared to allow analysis. Once the data is stored in easily accessible and identifiable files, be they electronically or physically based, the researcher can retrieve it for further analysis.

One approach used by Ward and Moule (2007) aided analysis by a team of researchers. The transcription was presented using the layout in Figure 23.1. This presentation of the data enabled the research team members to identify key information about the focus-group conversations. It provides space for the researcher to record interpretations alongside the text. In numbering the lines of data transcript, the researcher was able to identify specific quotes for use in later stages of analysis and presentation of data. These electronic documents were then shared with other team members and the participants to support verification.

Using computer software for analysis

Given the vast amounts of data generated in qualitative research, computer-assisted qualitative data analysis software (CAQDAS) can support the nurse researcher in analysis. A number of packages are available for use, offering differing levels of support. Some packages merely code and retrieve, others are able to start to make connections between categories, and finally there are packages that have theory-building capacity. This said, none completely analyses the data without researcher input. The researcher needs to identify the codes required and suggest the links that should be identified across the data.

The most commonly used packages include ETHNOGRAPH, ATLAS Ti, Nvivo, HyperRESEARCH and NUD*IST. ATLAS Ti, NUD*IST and HyperRESEARCH are examples of packages that are described as having theory-building capability. All these packages have 'coding' ability, retrieving data that relates to specific codes, which can then be arranged to show relationships as determined by the researcher.

The benefits of using computer-assisted data analysis aren't necessarily linked to time-saving, but there are advantages to the researcher in the way packages organise and store information. The electronic storage and retrieval of information within the programmes is superior to that offered through paper-based working or basic word-processing packages. They facilitate access by members of the research team working in different locations, supporting ongoing interpretation across national and international boundaries if required. There is scope to copy material and store a number of versions as analysis develops.

Project title: How do student nurses use computers in clinical practice?

Date of focus group: 21.02.2006

Focus group transcript number: Focus group 3

Site: A

Facilitator(s): Pam Moule

Number of participants: 8

Pseudonyms used: Diane, Warwick, etc.

Line no.	Speaker	Comment	Analysis
1 2	Interviewer	Can you tell me about your experience of using computers in clinical practice?	
3 4 5	Diane	I don't really use computers in the workplace, well only for finding out patient information, records and stuff like that.	Uses computers to access patient information.

Figure 23.1   Example of a transcription template (adapted from Ward and Moule, 2007)

There are, however, some concerns that the use of packages may reduce researcher immersion with the data as the process becomes more mechanical, less cognitive and more detached (Polit and Beck, 2006). These concerns arise because the researcher is one step away from handling the data, as the processes of analysis are managed within the programme. This said, the use of computer-based packages to support qualitative data analysis within nursing research is increasing. Changing practices may reflect the development of packages, with new versions offering greater scope and enhanced usability. It should be remembered that new versions are regularly produced and each one is more sophisticated in its functions than its predecessor. ATLAS Ti version 5, for example, supports the analysis of video and textual data, whereas version 4 analysed still images and text. Additionally, nurse researchers are developing their computer-based skills. This reflects an increased use of computer packages in other aspects of research, including computer employment in data collection and dissemination. Nurse researchers also have access to a range of training materials and courses to enable their use of computer-based packages. For example, there is supportive information on the use of CAQDAS provided by the Economic and Social Research Council through their Networking Project, www.caqdas.soc.surrey.ac.uk.

Content analysis

As part of analysis data is organised and managed, the researcher is able to retrieve key areas of information. The process of analysis is therefore one of making sense of the data. **Content analysis** is the simplest form of data processing. It is a process that involves labelling the data for retrieval.

The nurse researcher starts with the textual or visual data. Taking interview transcripts as one example of textual data, the researcher will have a number of pages of data to analyse. The content of the data is explored, reducing the data by the process of 'coding'. This can be approached using one of a range of computer packages, or through manual processes. The process of coding is one where the researcher is retrieving the data, which can then be organised into categories and themes or constructs. Thus the process relates to Miles and Huberman's (1994) interpreting and conclusion-drawing. Different researchers may approach the process of coding in different ways.

Moule et al. (2008) analysed interview data by initially reading through the transcripts and identifying key words to reflect their individual interpretations of the data. These initial thoughts were then shared with other members of the researcher team. This was achieved by each member noting key issues onto Post-it® notes. These were then arranged on a wall and reviewed by the team. The researchers then attempted to develop the codes into categories and themes, linking codes in ways that were meaningful. This research explored mental health nurses' experiences of using computer-based learning in the clinical setting. A team of three researchers analysed two focus-group transcripts. Initially the researchers were provided with electronic copies of the transcripts for coding. Each researcher read through the transcripts, identifying key words to describe the content, producing a list of about 30 codes. The team then met to share their initial coding, which was presented on flip-chart sheets. It was clear from this stage of analysis that there was some consistency across the team, with a number of the key areas being identified across, though often different terminology was used to present the same issues. The team then agreed a common terminology and reviewed areas where there were differences in the interpretations. Links across the data were then explored, building the coded data into categories and then these into themes. Box 23.1 an example of the coded data from this research that relates to one theme, 'Meeting individual learning needs', with examples of data relating to two categories shown, flexibility of use (B1) and revision aid (B2).

Box 23.1 Example of transcript data (Moule et al., 2008)

Interviewer: Okay then? So really what we wanted you to talk about was em, because you've already used the learning approach in relation to the basic life support with automated external defibrillators, we wanted to get a feel of your experience of using that, so …

Laura: I suppose from my point of view I'm quite experienced in using computers and IT so I found that using the actual e-learning fairly simple. I don't know if everybody would though, and that's one thing I noted. I found it quite easy to use, it ran quite freely to some extent. There was some difficulty. In some of the e-learning when I was doing it, some of the video work was sticking, or not coming through quite properly and I suppose it's not downloading properly and it made it quite difficult to follow. **B2** But luckily I knew what I was doing anyway so I wasn't a new learner, I'm quite experienced in basic life support and AED's so, I knew what I should be seeing so I can kind of guess what should be happening, so that was a bit awkward …

Sophie: **B1** I went and did it at home because I felt that it would just be easier for me and quieter ……

[Additional text removed]

Sophie: **B1** I actually took a whole afternoon off to do mine and very much the same I felt that when my … because when you are staring at that computer screen it can be a bit tedious, so I felt I could go off and have a cup of tea or walk around the garden whenever I felt like it, or re-go over bits I don't quite understand. So I think that was quite good, and you know you can read it at your own pace, I found it quite good for that reason.

[Additional text removed]

Liz: **B1** I did it all in one hit so I was a bit sick really. [*laugh*] With the … on the background the fact that I had my diary off to do it in one hit and I found that the easiest way to do it. I'm a bit more different, a) I know the subject, but b) once I start something I kind of like to complete it really. I found it quite easy.

At the initial stage of analysis the researchers had coded the sentences in Box 23.1 as data that showed the computer-based learning was flexible to use (B1) and that the package had been used as a revision tool (B2). Looking across the transcript there were several examples of data that could be coded in this way, as shown in the three areas of text highlighted as (B1) above. Further analysis enabled the researchers to look at the coded areas for links. In the example above, the coded areas of 'revision of learning' and 'flexible way of learning' were seen to link, as supporting the way the individual staff were learning. Thus they were presented as categories of a theme, 'Meeting individual learning needs'. The research included two focus groups as part of its design and therefore with the team choose to use manual analysis rather than a computer-assisted data analysis package. Had a computerised package been used, the researchers would have specified the links that should be made between the categories and themes, getting the programme to retrieve the data within this hierarchical structure rather than approaching this manually.

Narrative analysis

Narratives and stories are collected through open interviews as part of research approaches that seek to understand the lived experience of participants. Narrative may also be generated in the field naturally as part of participant observation (see Chapter 21).

Those undertaking narrative analysis are concerned with the structure of the story, rather than focusing on the content. They will review how the story was organised. They will be interested in how the story was started and progressed, reviewing why it was told in a particular way, how the story was developed and brought to a conclusion. Transcriptions of the story will be read several times to identify the structure and facilitate analysis. Narrative analysis can form part of the analysis of textual data within research.

Box 23.2   Example of the use of narrative analysis

Carter et al. (2004) explored what people living with terminal illness felt were priorities in their lives. Ten participants were interviewed, with analysis including principles of grounded theory and narrative analysis. Initially the interview transcripts were thematically analysed, identifying more than 30 categories that were then collated into five themes. These included personal/intrinsic factors, external/extrinsic factors, future issues, perceptions of normality and taking charge. The findings concentrated on presenting the themes, though alluded to the individual stories within demonstrating how the patients were feeling.

In the example in Box 23.2 the researchers employed grounded theory (see Chapter 14), which seeks to develop theory from the data obtained. Analysis within grounded theory approaches often involves coding as seen above, followed by theoretical saturation and constant comparison (Strauss and Corbin, 1998). In the process of analysis the researchers will reach a point when the categories that have emerged have sufficient data to support them. No further data collection is required. The data is examined as part of constant comparative method, ensuring the data supports the themes and theory development.

Discourse and conversation analysis aim to make sense of conversations. Conversation analysis can be employed to interpret audio or video recordings. Tapes are transcribed and analysed in detail to show overlaps in conversation, pauses and intonation. Conversation analysis describes and analyses the language of social interaction that takes place in conversation between people. Discourse analysis also seeks to make sense of conversation, but is interested in broader issues of the rules of conversations, mechanisms guiding discussion, power issues and gender positions. This form of analysis might be used to explore discourse between nurses and patients or members of the interprofessional healthcare team within the workplace. There is a range of approaches that researchers can use to analyse discourse which may involve some coding to facilitate management of the data, though the emphasis is on using evidence from the discourse to support interpretations rather than basing them on prior assumptions (Potter, 2004). Conversation and discourse analysis are often used by ethnomethodologists such as Heritage (2004) who are concerned with questions about how people function in their everyday lives. Communication is viewed as the basis of maintaining social order and is therefore analysed in order that roles, relationships and social norms might be understood.

Interpreting the findings

This chapter has given some examples of how qualitative data can be stored and retrieved to enable its interpretation. As mentioned, there are a number of frameworks available to support the nurse researcher in the interpretation of qualitative data. Colaizzi (1978) provided such a framework, now frequently used, that provides a set of steps that can be applied in the analysis of phenomenological data that recounts the lived experience of the participant (see Box 23.3 and Chapter 14). Colaizzi (1978) advises a process of analysis that involves six main steps:

1   Reading the transcripts to identify the content and 'get a feeling for them'.
2   Extracting initial key data as statements.
3   Formulating meaning from the statements.
4   Looking for links in the data that are clustered into themes.
5   Ensuring that the themes represent the entire data set.
6   Validating the themes by returning the interpretations to the participants.

Further analytical frameworks used within phenomenology include those of van Kaam (1966) and Giorgi (1985).

Strauss and Corbin (1998) offer a comprehensive analytical framework to support the interpretation of data within a grounded theory approach (see Chapter 14). The method includes three types of coding:

- Open coding: data are broken into parts and compared for similarities. This generates the categories that are similar actions, events and objects that are grouped together.
- Axial coding: Categories and sub-categories are linked around the axis of a category.
- Selective coding: The integration and refining of the theory.

Box 23.3   Example of the use of Colaizzi and constant comparison

Scannell-Desch (2005) researched pre-bereavement and post-bereavement struggles and triumphs of midlife widows aged between 35 and 60 years. Interview tape recordings were listened to several times. Significant statements that related to the investigated topic were extracted from the interview transcript. Each new unit of information was compared to previous units of information. Continuous comparison of the data allowed the organisation of data into emergent themes that related to struggling and triumphing. Data were compared across and within potential themes. The transcripts, significant statements and themes were examined by two experienced researchers to validate the appropriateness of the themes, credibility of the data within the themes, and interpretations.

These frameworks are amongst many including that previously mentioned, developed by Miles and Huberman (1994). This framework includes three interrelated activities that can occur concurrently (see Table 23.1).

Operationalising this process involves the researcher coding the data to identify data that enters the display. Further data reduction may be required as more categories emerge and the initial conclusions are drawn. This may lead to further data collection to verify the conclusions.

Lockyer et al. (2008), when analysing focus-group data, employed this approach to data analysis. Nursing staff in surgical settings completed online-based learning in cancer care and were then asked to discuss their experiences. The excerpt in Box 23.4 shows how the data was displayed as a verbatim transcription. The complete transcript was read and re-read to gain initial understanding of the data. The data was then coded, reducing the data to support initial conclusion-drawing. A further focus group was conducted and the data displayed and coded in the same way. Once both were coded, links were established across the data from both transcripts. This process again involved reducing the data and

Table 23.1 Framework for qualitative data analysis (Miles and Huberman, 1994)

Activity	Description
Data reduction	Working with field notes or transcriptions, the data is subjected to selection and simplification. There is focus, as part of analysis, with transformation of the data. This process is continuous, occurring throughout the project.
Data display	The organisation of the data, displayed to allow conclusion-drawing. This can be as text, verbatim quotes, graphs, charts or diagrams that show links and interrelationships.
Conclusion-drawing/verification	Starting at the data collection stage, the researcher begins to draw meaning from the data. Initial patterns in the data are noted, regularities and irregularities, possible explanations are outlined, causation patterns outlined. Final conclusions are made when data collection is complete and the research verifies these through confirming the conclusions.

producing new displays to support ongoing conclusion-drawing. Further data reduction took place with three key themes emerging, with sub-themes.

Box 23.4 Example of a focus group transcript

Interviewer:	Tell me about the experience you have had of the online cancer nursing course. If you could just … just tell me, maybe, what the experience has been – whenever you want to start.	
Jane:	I was just going to say, I think it was quite daunting at first because I looked at it and thought,	Daunting
	Oh my God but when I actually worked through it and kind of studied the questions, I thought Oh, well I do know some of the things, and then kind of – you know – go through all the the internet questions and – you know – reinforcement –	Reinforced learning
	also learned new as well, but just sort of – pre-empted what I did know, and I didn't really realise I did this.	New learning
Sue:	I was just going to say exactly the same thing. The thought of it was actually … the thought of it was actually more work than it actually was …	
Interviewer:	Thank you very much. [*nervous laughter*]	
Sue:	I kept thinking I would have to put hours to one side to do it, so I put it off and put it off, thinking this is going to take ages, but then actually you could just dip in and dip out, you didn't have to spend hours and	Daunting Flexible learning

	hours doing it each time. So then, kind of ... it was just the thought ... the thought of ...	
Jane:	When you first put the first bit through, it was about five pages wasn't it? – of the questions,	Daunting
	and you think – crikey! And I don't know this many ... vignettes and bits you'd be able to do and then bits you wouldn't. It's going to take ages. Probably be able to do another lot – you know – do a second lot, but actually, it was quite ... the actual site itself was quite user friendly and it didn't take as long as I thought. You know when you went to it and it said 'username' and 'password' and I thought my God, I can't do any of this, and then I realised it was just the number, and again it wasn't as daunting as I thought it was going to be – I thought it would be a lot more complicated.	User friendly
Interviewer:	Right. And that is ... sort of ... the beginning part. Were you talking about the programme ...	

Theme/sub-theme structure:

Learning experience	– student centred (flexibility, new learning, reinforced learning)
	– need for preparation (daunting)

Chapter summary

- Qualitative data analysis often occurs throughout the project.
- Researchers are often working with vast amounts of data.
- A number of methods/frameworks exist that can support the researcher in data analysis.
- Audio data is prepared for analysis through transcription.
- A number of computer packages exist that can code and retrieve data and facilitate theory-building following researcher instruction.
- Textual data can be subjected to 'coding' or narrative analysis.
- The interpretation of findings can be verified through expert review or member checking.
- Verification processes support the maintenance of **rigour** and **trustworthiness**.

References

Carter, H., MacLeod, R., Brander, P. and McPherson, K. (2004) 'Living with terminal illness: patients' priorities', *Journal of Advanced Nursing*, 45 (6): 611–20.

Coffey, A. and Atkinson, P. (1996) *Making Sense of Qualitative Data*. Thousand Oaks, CA: Sage.

Colaizzi, P. (1978) 'Psychological research as a phenomenologist views it', in R. Valle and M. Kings (eds), *Existential Phenomenological Alternative for Psychology*. New York: Oxford University Press. pp. 48–71.

Corbin, J. and Holt, N. (2005) 'Grounded theory', in B. Somekh and C. Lewin (eds), *Research Methods in the Social Sciences*. London: Sage. Chapter 5, pp. 49–55.

Giorgi, A. (1985) *Phenomenology and Psychology Research*. Pittsburgh, PA: Duquesne University Press.

Heritage, J. (2004) 'Conversation analysis and institutional talk: analysing data', in D. Silverman (ed.), *Qualitative Research: Theory, Method and Practice*. London: Sage. pp. 161–82.

Hollway, J. and Jefferson, T. (2000) *Doing Qualitative Research Differently: Free Association Narrative and the Interview Method*. London: Sage.

Lincoln, Y. and Guba, Y. (1985) *Naturalistic Enquiry*. Newbury Park, CA: Sage.

Lockyer, L., McGuigan, D. and Moule, P. (2008) 'Web-based learning in practice settings: Nurses' experiences and perceptions of impact on patient care', *Electronic Journal of E-learning*, Special Issue: e-Learning in Health Care, 5 (4): 279–86.

Miles, M. and Huberman, A. (1994) *Qualitative Data Analysis*, 2nd edition. Thousand Oaks, CA: Sage.

Moule, P., Albarran, J., Bessant, E., Pollock, J. and Brownfield, C. (2008) 'A comparison of e-learning and classroom delivery of basic life support with automated external defibrillator use: a pilot study', *International Journal of Nursing Practice*, 14: 427–34.

Noffke, S. and Somekh, B. (2005) 'Action research', in B. Somekh and C. Lewin (eds), *Research Methods in the Social Sciences*. London: Sage. Chapter 10, pp. 89–96.

Polit, D. and Beck, C. (2006) *Essentials of Nursing Research: Methods, Appraisal and Utilization*, 6th edition. Philadelphia, PA: Lippincott Williams & Wilkins.

Potter, J. (2004) 'Discourse analysis as a way of analysing naturally occurring talk', in D. Silverman (ed.), *Qualitative Research: Theory, Method and Practice*. London: Sage. pp. 144–60.

Scannell-Desch, E. (2005) 'Prebereavement and postbereavement struggles and triumphs of midlife widows', *Journal of Hospice and Palliative Nursing*, 7 (1): 15–22.

Strauss, A. and Corbin, J. (1998) *Basics of Qualitative Research: Techniques and Procedures for Developing Grounded Theory*, 2nd edition. Thousand Oaks, CA: Sage.

Tesch, R. (1990) *Qualitative Research: Analysis Types and Software Tools*. London: Falmer.

van Kaam, A. (1966) *Existential Foundations of Psychology*. Pittsburgh, PA: Duquesne University Press.

Ward, R. and Moule, P. (2007) 'Supporting pre-registration students in practice: current ICT use', *Nurse Education Today*, 27: 60–7.

Whitfield, R., Newcombe, R. and Woollard, M. (2003) 'Reliability of the Cardiff test of basic life support and automated external defibrillation version 3.1', *Resuscitation*, 59 (3): 291–314.

Suggested further reading

Coffey, A. and Atkinson, P. (1996) *Making Sense of Qualitative Data*. Thousand Oaks, CA: Sage.

Li, S. and Seale, C. (2007) 'Learning to do qualitative data analysis: an observational study of doctoral work', *Qualitative Health Research*, 17 (10): 1442–52.

Miles, M. and Huberman, A. (1994) *Qualitative Data Analysis*, 2nd edition. Thousand Oaks, CA: Sage.

Rogers, B. (1998) 'Teaching computer-assisted qualitative data analysis to new users: NUD.IST demonstrations and workshops', *Health Informatics Journal*, 4 (2): 63–71.

Website

Information on the use of CAQDAS provided by the Economic and Social Research Council through their Networking Project: www.caqdas.soc.surrey.ac.uk

24

PRESENTING AND DISSEMINATING RESEARCH

The dissemination of research findings to the nursing and healthcare professions is a key component of the research process and one that unfortunately cannot be neglected. Those nurses completing research need to plan their dissemination strategy as part of the research process, considering how to present the research to a range of interested audiences. This may include a final written report, often required by those funding the research. Researchers often produce papers written for academic and professional audiences and can undertake international, national and local dissemination through presentation at conferences and research meetings. A range of options is therefore available to the researcher and different approaches may be taken to dissemination that reflect the scope of the research. Employing a dissemination strategy will ensure that the research findings are presented in the public domain and are accessible to practitioners.

In this chapter we discuss the most common methods of dissemination. The main approaches to communicating research results through the written word include the final research report, academic and professional journal papers and short research reports. Research findings are also presented verbally through conference papers, spanning international to local arenas and through virtual hosting online.

Learning outcomes

This chapter is designed to enable the reader to:

- **Identify the key components of a research report**
- **Appreciate how to develop a paper for publication**

- **Understand the publication process**
- **Discuss how to develop and deliver a conference presentation and poster**
- **Understand the range of methods available to use in disseminating research**

KEY TERMS

Conference presentation, Publication, Research papers, Research reports

---

Dissemination of research

The research report

The **research report** is the presentation of the research journey. A report is usually required by the research funding body and may need to be written to a specified brief. It would usually include detail of the research process, outcomes and recommendations for future practice. A report may be required for local, unfunded or small-scale research, though the scope of this may vary and alternative forms of output may be acceptable, such as a published paper in a peer-reviewed journal.

If a report is required, the research team should understand what is expected, when it should be produced and to whom it should be sent. Though report structures may vary, commonly the headings suggested in Table 24.1 are used. When completed, an International Standard Book Number (ISBN) can be obtained through the library or administration staff, which gives a unique identifying number to the report. These are usually 13 digit numbers presented as a barcode that enables ease of identification and tracking.

Alternative modes of presentation

As mentioned above, the final research report remains a requirement for many funded research projects. It provides key information about the research journey for the funder and other audiences. There are, however, some areas of research where different modes of presentation are becoming more acceptable or being offered as alternatives to the final report. It may well be the case that small-scale projects are looking for other outputs as part of the dissemination process.

Alternative outputs might include the **publication** of a **research paper** in a peer-reviewed journal, electronic publication of web pages or CD-ROM, a podcast (verbal

Table 24.1   Suggested research report structure

Heading	Content
Executive summary	Provides an overview of the report content, including main findings and recommendations for practice. This could be developed at the start to aid thinking about the report content and then revised once the report is completed.
Introduction	Should include the rationale for the study, research aims questions/hypotheses should be stated here (see Chapter 6).
Literature review or background	The key literature including background policy should be included here. This may encompass current and previous knowledge. The depth of presentation will depend on the audience, with some funders requiring minimal information (see Chapter 18).
Research design	The overall research design is presented (see Chapters 11–17).
Ethical approval	Any ethical approval processes involved should be presented, including reference to ethics committee approval, information provision, informed consent (see Chapters 4 and 5).
Sampling	The sampling approach used, sample size and any power calculations guiding this should be included. Any sampling issues should be discussed here and raised as part of the study limitations. The composition of the final study sample should be presented (see Chapter 19).
Data collection	The approach to data collection is presented, including presentation of data collection tools used, location and processes.
Data analysis	The handling of data is discussed, how it was stored and processed, including the use of any statistical tests, processes of qualitative analysis and rationale for these (see Chapters 22 and 23).
Results	The presentation of quantitative results in the form of charts, tables and graphs is included in the report, either in total or as a selection. Qualitative findings are presented within the discussion.
Findings/discussion	In reports presenting qualitative data, this section will present the findings as part of a discussion. In reports presenting quantitative research, this section will discuss an interpretation of the results, providing evidence for support where available in the current literature.
Limitations	Here the authors should refer to any limitations of the research design and process, identifying how these might affect the interpretation of the results.
Conclusions	The author discusses what the findings mean for further research and practice.
References	All literature referred to in the report is included here.
Appendices	These are included as appropriate, such as sample raw data, data collection tools.

presentation that can be downloaded onto mobile devices such as a mobile phone) or the dissemination of any products of the research such as teaching materials or guidelines. Such outputs are being requested by some funders of educational research where the dissemination and sharing of newly produced teaching materials or other research outputs are prioritised above a traditional report. Nurse researchers must be clear at the outset of the research what the desired outputs are, and plan to deliver these on completion of the project. Calls for project proposals will often outline specific deliverables that may encompass more than a final report (see Chapter 10).

Dissertations and theses

Nurses studying at undergraduate (BSc), Masters (MSc) and Doctoral level will often be required to present their research as a dissertation or thesis. The dissertation can be the final written assessment of a BSc and MSc programme, written to meet specific learning outcomes and to certain criteria. For example, a dissertation can address research questions through a literature review or primary research, presented with an abstract and chapters that include the background, methodology, discussion of findings to answer the research question and a concluding chapter that presents implications for nursing practice and further research.

The thesis is a more in-depth piece of written work presented as part of the written examination of a professional Doctoral programme, such as an EdD (Doctorate in Education) or Doctoral studies (PhD, Doctor of Philosophy). A number of texts are written specifically to guide those producing a thesis (see Murray, 2002; Walliman, 2004; Oliver, 2008). The length of a doctoral thesis varies between 40,000 and 100,000 words and can be written over a period of two to five years. The structure of the thesis will be determined by the research approach taken, but is likely to include chapters on the background literature, research design, data collection, data analysis, discussion of results, theoretical development, conclusions and recommendations for practice and research.

Writing up research papers

Dissemination strategy

The dissemination strategy should be conceived by the authors of research reports and papers at an early stage and this should include publications, conference and other presentations. Erlen (2002) and Graf et al. (2007) highlight a number of potential key issues that need addressing at an early stage of the research process to avoid potential conflicts and issues. It is suggested that issues such as the authorship should be considered. In writing the paper the authors must be confident of the integrity of the publication content, avoid plagiarism and present the results in such a way as to protect anonymity and confidentiality. Any possible conflicts of interest that exist for the author must also be considered. The authors must also avoid simultaneous submission of a paper to a number of journals for publication.

A dissemination plan can be conceived prior to commencing the research, as part of an application for funding or support. If this is not the case, then the team should discuss and develop a dissemination strategy early in the research process and identify the authorship of papers. This should include mapping the potential publications and authors' contributions, which may allow for more novice writers to work alongside more experienced writers and will enable time for negotiations and agreement of authorship that reflect the contributions made, avoiding later conflict. Albarran and Scholes (2005) remind us that journals often require disclosure of each author's contribution to a paper prior to acceptance. This enables publishers to determine whether those credited with authorship have made a significant contribution to the paper and the development and implementation of the research. Authors are also asked to return a completed copyright assignment form, often at the stage of submission. This ensures the reviewing journal has the right to publish the paper should it be accepted, and prevents simultaneous submission to a number of journals. The submission process can involve authors making statements regarding the research ethics of a project. These can be additional to those placed in the paper itself and can involve confirming whether the study was presented to an ethics committee, the outcomes of this and any processes involved such as provision of written information and securing of informed consent (see Chapters 4 and 5).

Editors are also expecting to receive a paper that assigns credit to other authors and funders where needed and presents accurate findings, to include any data presented (Erlen, 2002). Authors should ensure that any presentation conforms to acceptable ethical practices, being honest in its content and presentation. This will require careful construction and proofreading, involving the statistician if required and team members. Team members should also declare any conflict of interest (Oermann, 2002) and identify any funding received on the paper, and may need to include this in the submission information provided for the editor. This again links to the need for integrity in the presentation that avoids any bias that may favour the research funder.

What, who for, where?

One of the main ways of disseminating research findings is through publication. Research papers may also present other aspects of the research such as the literature review, methodology and ethical discussions. The process of publishing multiple journal papers from one piece of research is known as 'salami slicing'. The decision as to what should be written may come early in the research process, or develop as the research continues and is completed.

Table 24.2 Possible journals to consider

Focus	Journals
Cancer care practitioner	*Journal of Cancer Care*
	European Journal of Cancer Care
	(www.blackwellpublishing.com/journal)
Education	*Nurse Education Today*
	(www.elsevier-international.com/journals/nedt)
	Nurse Education in Practice
	(http://intl.elsevierhealth.com/journals/nepr/)
Research	*Journal of Advanced Nursing*
	(www.journalofadvancednursing.com)
	Nurse Researcher
	(www.nursingstandard.co.uk/nurseresearcher/)

The nurse researcher will need to consider the target audience for the research, as this will help determine suitable journals for publication. A number of audiences may be interested in various elements of the research. For example, research in the field of cancer care education could have three potential key audiences: practitioners in cancer care, educationalists in universities and healthcare settings, and researchers. Each paper should be presented differently, with the emphasis tailored to the target audience, and can be submitted to journals that reflect this (see Table 24.2). There may also be a requirement among some professionals to write for those journals that have high academic ranking. This is particularly the case for nurses attached to academic institutions who are active researchers likely to be submitted by the institution as part of an exercise that measures research quality. Formerly this has been the Research Assessment Exercise (RAE) and from 2009 is likely to be as part of the Research Excellence Framework (REF). In the RAE the quality of published research was graded by national and international experts and further research funding was awarded according to the institutional grading achieved. In the future a system that includes metrics of recorded citations and peer review is likely, though currently under development. More experienced nurse researchers in universities will be able to give advice on this when the time comes.

The range of publications available is vast, and unless the researcher is familiar with the journals in the field an initial search is required to include a review of the aims, objectives, philosophy and journal contents.

Following contributors' guidelines

Having identified the target journal for a particular paper, the researcher needs to obtain a copy of the guidelines for authors and use these to inform the writing.

Guidelines can be available in published journals and are usually held online. In relation to the above journals (see Table 24.2), key information is available on the websites identified. Prior to writing, all authors should have access to these guidelines, have agreed different writing responsibilities and timeframe for the work and have dealt with any ethical issues of writing as discussed below. There are a number of publications available to support authors in writing (see www.man.ac.uk/publish/index.htm; Albarran and Scholes, 2005). Novice writers will benefit from the support of more experienced authors drawn from within the team or from supervisors and research advisers. It is vital to check through the paper for errors prior to submission, and all referencing should be checked for accuracy.

Paper submission

Contributors' guidelines should also state how to submit a paper. Papers are usually submitted electronically via the journal website. As part of the submission process authors may need to provide information such as authorship details and evidence of ethical approval. A statement is often needed to authenticate author contributions; this may need to be faxed or sent by post separately if it requires signatures from all those involved. Receipt of the submission will be confirmed by the journal and then the process of review is commenced. This may start with initial consideration by the editor and can lead to an immediate rejection decision. If acceptable at this stage, the paper will be forwarded for two independent reviews. This process can take a number of weeks and is usually anonymised. Reviewers are often academics or practitioners, who are provided with a set of key questions to guide the review process. The types of questions reviewers are asked to address include:

- Does the paper meet the aims and scope of the journal?
- Are the presentation criteria met?
- Is the content accurate and up to date?
- Is there scientific rigour in the research?
- What contribution does the paper make to the field?
- Should the paper be published in the journal?

Revise or rethink

There are generally four possible outcomes from the review of an academic paper:

- Acceptance without change (this is rare).
- Acceptance with minor revisions (requires changes and resubmission to the editor).

- Acceptance with major revisions (requires changes and possibly resubmission to reviewers as well as to the editor).
- Rejection (the reviewers feel the paper is not appropriate for publication in the journal).

Depending on the outcome, there will be various actions required. Acceptance without change will result in you receiving 'galley proofs' of the paper at some stage to check and return. This is important, should be done carefully and is often to a tight publication deadline. These proofs are a copy of those that will appear in print, so they need to be accurate. It may be several weeks before the paper appears in the journal, though in the interim electronic versions may be made available online. Acceptance with minor or major revisions requires some thought. Feedback from the reviewers will be helpful in identifying what amendments are needed, and the authors need to agree who will make these changes prior to resubmission. These should be done as quickly as possible and checked carefully before resubmission.

Rejections are common and the feedback should help the researcher make decisions about how to develop the paper and take dissemination forward. Difficulties with presentation and content will need addressing prior to forwarding to other journals. The research team may also need to review the emphasis of a paper or reconsider the target audience.

Preparing conference presentations

Conference abstracts

Conference calls appear throughout the year, often advertised online and through mailings. Conferences are held internationally, nationally and locally. They vary in audience and style. A novice researcher may want to select a conference where new presenters are supported and perhaps deliver their presentation to a small audience. Some conferences offer a themed approach and place common papers together in small groups. The presenters are able to get to know each other throughout the conference as they deliver their papers within their small group settings. Often this kind of environment is supportive and less threatening than conferences where larger audiences are expected. It is important when selecting a conference to ensure synergy between the intended presentation and conference themes outlined in the call. Many conferences are focused on particular specialisms, such as critical care, cancer care, nursing education or nursing research and will invite abstract submissions related to specified themes. For example, the British Association of Critical Care Nurses hosts an annual conference and invites calls for specific themes such as evidence-based practice, clinical practice and education.

When submitting an abstract, thought needs to be given to the probable content of the presentation. If presenting at a research-focused conference the methodology or ethical issues are likely to be emphasised, whereas practitioners attending a clinical conference may prefer to hear about the research results. The abstract needs to be presented as specified in the conference call. As an example, the abstract shown in Figure 24.1 was submitted and accepted at the Royal College of Nursing of the United Kingdom Annual International Nursing Research Conference. It includes a title, presents research under key headings that reflect the research process and includes two references.

The conference call information should include the following to help presenters:

- Key practical information:
  - the conference dates
  - location of the conference
  - accommodation
  - travel
  - payment.
- Specific information:
  - aims of the conference
  - themes for presentation
  - abstract content and presentation, suggested headings, reference use, word limit
  - instructions for submission
  - review process
  - dates of notification of reviewer's decision will be given
  - criteria for selection that should adhered to closely.

Any submission not addressing specified criteria is unlikely to be successful. There will also be information on how to submit the abstract; often electronic online submission is required. A presenter profile may be requested as well as information on employing organisations, funding and evidence of ethical approval for any study presented.

Oral presentations

If the abstract is selected for an oral presentation the conference organisers will contact the presenter, providing details of the date, time and location of the presentation. There should also be details of the facilities available. Commonly, presenters use PowerPoint presentations to provide key information, though overhead projection can still be used, and a verbal presentation of a paper or other text, such as poems, may be presented. If Internet access is needed, this should be requested. Flipchart and whiteboard access should also be requested if required.

The content of the presentation needs to be developed to reflect the detail of the accepted abstract, and consideration should be given to the amount of time available for the presentation and questions. A 20-minute time slot will allow for the presentation of

---

A COMPARISON STUDY OF E-LEARNING AND CLASSROOM DELIVERY OF RESUSCITATION SKILLS

Purpose of the study

Investment to provide mandatory resuscitation skill updating for healthcare providers is problematic, being resource intensive and requiring absence of staff for training (Moule and Albarran, 2002). Alternatives to classroom delivery are increasingly being explored, including the use of electronic packages. The purpose of this study was to compare resuscitation knowledge and skill development after either e-based or classroom delivery, measuring the effect size between the two groups according to specified outcome criteria.

Materials and methods

Eighty-four healthcare providers from one mental health institution were randomised to one of two training groups. Classroom delivery of six 1-hour sessions was completed by 53 staff, the remainder completed an online programme with practice support. Content reflected current guidelines. Knowledge was assessed through pre- and post-tests. Using VAM software and the validated Cardiff Test (Whitfield et al., 2003), we measured skill performance on a calibrated Laerdal© skill meter manikin. Pre- and post-test scores and data from the manikin software were compared for effect size, to determine any differences in knowledge and skill attainment across the two groups.

Results

Preliminary data suggests that knowledge is improved in both groups regardless of training method. Initial analysis suggests there are no statistically significant differences in overall skill performance between the groups, including the use of the automated external defibrillator.

Conclusions

There appear to be no differences in the knowledge and skill acquisition between e-learning and classroom delivery. As a consequence, e-learning may offer a viable mode of developing these essential skills. For many institutions this mode of provision has the potential to provide resource savings in training costs and manpower hours. Using e-technology can ensure standardised delivery of evidence-based and regulated content, optimising accessibility to a wider community.

References

Moule, P. and Albarran, J.W. (2002) 'Automated external defibrillation as part of BLS: implications for education and practice', *Resuscitation*, 54: 223–30.
Whitfield, R., Newcombe, R. and Woollard, M. (2003) 'Reliability of the Cardiff Test of basic life support and automated external defibrillation version 3.1', *Resuscitation*, 59 (3): 291–314.

Authors: Pam Moule, John W. Albarran, Elizabeth Bessant

Figure 24.1   Example of a conference abstract

approximately ten PowerPoint slides, provided they present only key headings and words. A PowerPoint presentation would include an opening slide, with the logos of any funding bodies and the presenter's employer, and should follow a corporate design if one exists. PowerPoint presentations allow for the use of images, video and, if Internet connection is available, the ability to demonstrate and link to the Web. Given the limited scope of the presentation, it is unlikely that the entire research project will be presented, but emphasis will be placed on certain aspects of the research dependent on the audience. The content may emphasise the research methodology, ethical issues or findings.

Some conference organisers request access to the PowerPoint slides ahead of the conference. In these cases the slides will be loaded and available in the appropriate conference room for presenter access. Alternatively, the conference organisers may request the presentation on arrival or expect the presenters to load the PowerPoint onto the conference room computer, downloading from a CD or flash pen. Whatever the process, it is recommended that presenters visit the conference room to be used ahead of the presentation to familiarise themselves with the surroundings, ensure access and functioning of the PowerPoint presentation and availability of other equipment needed.

More novice presenters may wish to enrol colleagues to listen to the presentation prior to the conference. Alternatively, there may be an opportunity to present the work informally to a local audience ahead of the conference. This will give an opportunity to check the timing, slide content, and refine the presentation if needed. It can be useful to have feedback on your style of presentation and mannerisms. Presenters can also take printed versions of the PowerPoint presentation, gauging the number of copies needed on the expected audience size. Presenters should have the presentation on at least one flash pen or CD-ROM, even if it has been emailed ahead.

Poster presentations

Posters form a significant part of nursing and healthcare conferences, with a number awarded prizes for innovative presentations. Many organisers allocate specific time slots in a conference programme for viewing posters, as well as setting coffee and lunch breaks around the displays. Presenters should be available to discuss the poster content at these times. Some conferences provide opportunities for presenters to deliver a verbal presentation of the poster content.

Presenters often leave contact information with posters for delegates to take, such as business cards, pdf versions of the poster, and/or an abstract with contact details. Taking such steps ensures contact information is available for the delegates when the posters are left unattended.

Applications to present a conference poster follow the same process as that outlined above, with an abstract being submitted in a particular format. Successful presenters will receive specific information from the conference organisers. This will include: the required poster size; whether the design should be presented as landscape or portrait; when the poster is expected to be displayed; where it will be displayed; and if a verbal presentation is required, this will be indicated. The times of scheduled poster viewings should also be identified.

Poster presentations have been a popular method of displaying research findings at conferences for some time (see example in Figure 24.2). Given the longevity of their use, there has been a development of the style and quality of presentation, aided by the advent of computerised desktop publishing software. Many nurse researchers will have access to design and production services within their organisations, or can access these services from high street printers. There is often a charge for these services that can be considerable. This may be justifiable if the poster is likely to be used more than once, and can be displayed in workplace or education settings following use at conference. The poster may need to present a corporate image if one exists for the presenting university, hospital or employing organisation. Usually a poster will include the logo of any funding body and employing organisation(s), as well as having details about the content authors and place of work.

The design of the poster needs consideration. Often, less is more. Presenting key images and text can be the most effective. Designers should remember that the content of the poster needs to be digested in five minutes (Ryan, 1989), and consideration should be given to the colours used, eye-catching use of pictures or design, the use of headings and essential text (Moule et al., 1998).

In designing the poster, transportability also needs thought. The most popular presentation is a poster of A3 size and above, laminated for protection, and rolling to enable transport in a lightweight and waterproof carrying tube. Preferably the tube should travel as hand luggage if flying, though it may have to be placed in the aircraft hold.

Conference organisers may provide materials to enable display of the poster; however, it is recommended that presenters take a supply of adhesive velcro, drawing pins or other adhesive materials and a mechanism for displaying pdfs, abstracts and business cards, such as an A4 plastic wallet.

Chapter summary

- A dissemination strategy should be decided as early as possible in the research process and agreed by members of the research team.
- A research report is often required by funders and would usually include details of the research process, outcomes and recommendations for future practice.
- There are a number of alternative methods of dissemination that include presentations, research papers, provision of online materials, podcasts and making available the products of research.
- Research students are usually required to present their research as a dissertation or thesis.
- Researchers need to follow contributors' guidance when producing papers and abstracts for conference presentation.
- Novice researchers may benefit from gaining feedback on submissions and presentations and can benefit by working with more experienced writers and presenters initially.

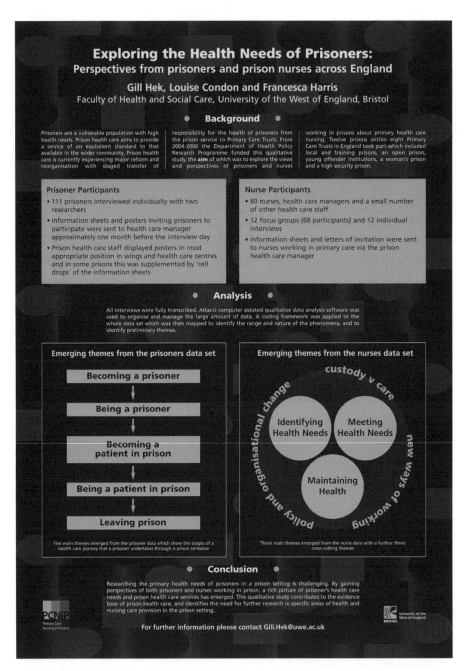

Figure 24.2 *Example of a conference poster* (Reproduced with kind permission of Louise Condon and Francesca Harris)

References

Albarran, J. and Scholes, S. (2005) 'How to get published: seven easy steps', *Nursing in Critical Care*, 10 (2): 72–7.

Erlen, J. (2002) 'Writing for publication: ethical considerations', *Orthopaedic Nursing*, 21 (6): 68–71.

Graf, C., Wager, E., Bowman, A., Fiack, S., Scott-Lichter, D. and Robinson, A. (2007) 'Best practice guidelines on publication ethics: a publisher's perspective', *International Journal of Clinical Practice*, 61 (1152): 1–26. Available at www.blackwell-synergy.com/doi/pdf/10.111/j.1742-1241.2006.01230, accessed 5 May 2008.

Moule, P., Judd, M. and Girot, E. (1998) 'The poster presentation: what value to the teaching and assessment of research in pre- and post-registration nursing courses?', *Nurse Education Today*, 18: 237–42.

Murray, R. (2002) *How to Write a Thesis*. Buckingham: Open University Press.

Oermann, M. (2002) *Writing for Publication in Nursing*. Philadelphia, PA: Lippincott.

Oliver, P. (2008) *Writing Your Thesis*. London: Sage.

Ryan, N. (1989) 'Developing and presenting a research poster', *Applied Nursing Research*, 2 (1): 52–5.

Walliman, N. (2004) *Your Undergraduate Dissertation: The Essential Guide for Success*. London: Sage.

Suggested further reading

Canter, D. and Fairbairn, G. (2006) *Becoming an Author: Advice for Academics and Other Professionals*. Maidenhead: McGraw-Hill.

Cormack, D. (1994) *Writing for Healthcare Professions*. Oxford: Blackwell.

Hadfield-Law, L. (1999) *Effective Presentations for Healthcare Professionals*. Oxford: Butterworth-Heinemann.

Jones, A. (2000) 'Changing traditions of authorship', in A. Jones and F. McLellan (eds), *Ethical Issues in Biomedical Publication*, Baltimore: Johns Hopkins University Press. pp. 1–19.

Lynn, M. (1989) 'Poster sessions – a good way to communicate research', *Western Journal of Nursing Research*, 11 (4): 477–85.

McCarthy, P. and Hatcher, C. (2002) *Presentation Skills: The Essential Guide for Students*. London: Sage.

McVeigh, C., Moyle, K., Forrester, K., Choboyer, W., Patterson, E. and St John, W. (2002) 'Publication syndicates: in support of nursing scholarship', *Journal of Continuing Education in Nursing*, 33: 63–6.

Oermann, M. (2002) *Writing for Publication in Nursing*. Philadelphia, PA: Lippincott.

Oliver, P. (2008) *Writing Your Thesis*. London: Sage.

Palmer, R. (2002) *Write in Style: A Guide to Good English*, 2nd edition. London: Routledge.

Smith, R. (1997) 'Authorship is dying: long live contributorship', *British Medical Journal*, 315: 696.

Van Emden, J. and Becker, L. (2004) *Presentation Skills for Students*, Basingstoke: Palgrave.

Walliman, N. (2004) *Your Undergraduate Dissertation: The Essential Guide for Success*. London: Sage.

Website

Guidance on getting published in nursing and healthcare journals: www.man.ac.uk/ publish/index.htm

25

USING RESEARCH IN PRACTICE

Research is important for every nurse, and nursing research is needed to inform nursing practice. The evidence provided by research helps to ensure that care is safe and effective and, to some extent, enables nurses to describe and explain nursing practice.

The emphasis on practice being evidence-based has altered the way nursing research is regarded and it has become every nurse's responsibility to engage in research in some way. The expectation is that, at the very minimum, nurses will have an awareness of research. Awareness in this context requires nurses to access, read, appraise and apply research that is relevant to their practice. In other words, it is expected that nurses utilise research as part of their professional practice.

There is, however, also a need to recognise that it is not always easy to implement research findings and that the existence of a gap between research and practice in healthcare has long been recognised. Back in 1601 the benefits of limes and sauerkraut to prevent scurvy were discovered, but the British Navy did not introduce rations containing vitamin C until 1795. It then took a further 70 years for the British Board of Trade to order citrus fruits to be provided on merchant ships; a total of 264 years between evidence and practice (Berwick 2003). Then in the 20th century, in a speech to the World Health Organisation in 1968, Lord Rothschild stated:

'If for the next 20 years, no further research were to be carried out, if there were a moratorium on research, the application of what is already known, of what has already been discovered, would result in widespread improvements in world health.' (in Peters, 1992: 68)

Since then the volume of research has increased and there is even more of a drive to implement research findings into practice with the advent of National Service Frameworks, the Commission for Health Improvement (CHI) and the National

Institute for Clinical Excellence (NICE), which have sought to promote the notion of evidence-based practice amongst healthcare practitioners as well as the recipients of healthcare. Associated with this has been an increasing public awareness of healthcare research in terms of the way it can lead to increased health benefits and the areas where there is still a need for more research. However, actually implementing change, getting research into practice or improving the quality of patient care is complex and can be very demanding (Rycroft-Malone et al., 2002). This chapter discusses issues concerned with getting research into practice, how nurses and healthcare consumers influence the research agenda and research roles for nurses.

Learning outcomes

This chapter is designed to enable the reader to:

- Appreciate the need for research to be implemented into practice
- Have an understanding of some of the barriers for getting research into practice
- Understand the difference between evidence-based practice and research utilisation
- Have an appreciation of the different roles for nurse researchers
- Have an appreciation of the role of healthcare consumers in research

---

KEY TERMS

Evidence-based practice, Healthcare consumer, Nursing research, Research utilisation

---

Why should we use research in practice?

The impetus to use research in practice can be arrived at from a number of sources but essentially it is driven by the need to deliver care that is efficacious, patient orientated and cost effective. Some of this is because healthcare resources are limited, both in terms of financial and staff resources but also in respect of the level of knowledge of how to restore or maintain health. The imperative is for healthcare professionals to meet the challenges of delivering healthcare in the best way possible and to ensure that we actually think about the care that we provide and appreciate the expectations of our patients. Furthermore, it is illogical to spend time, effort and resources on research only to have the findings ignored and continue to practise on the basis of experience rather than rely on information that should improve the outcome and quality of care. As Clifford (2004) remarked, using research is not an optional extra, but rather it is an integral part of professional practice.

Getting research into practice, or **research utilisation**, is about applying research findings from one or more studies into practice and is unrelated to the original research (Polit and Beck, 2006). This recognises that completing a research study is not sufficient; that both nurse researchers and practitioners have responsibilities. For nurse researchers these responsibilities focus on ensuring that their research has relevance for practice. This is not saying that nursing research has to have a clinical orientation, but simply that the focus is on problems that practitioners identify as being relevant to them professionally and to the practice of nursing. Researchers also need to ensure that their research is based on rigorous methods and, where appropriate, is multi-centred. Associated with this is the need to consider whether studies need to be repeated to confirm findings, either with different patient groups or within different settings, to ensure that findings are robust. The role of the nurse researcher is not, however, simply about doing research. Nurse researchers also have a responsibility to ensure that their findings are published and taken to a wider audience so that they can be implemented in practice once a study has been completed.

The responsibilities of nurses in practice in relation to research focus on the utilisation of findings into their own practice and the practice of others, including healthcare assistants, learners and other healthcare professionals. This requires nurses to keep themselves up to date by reading research reports and attending conferences where research findings are reported. In addition, they then need to apply, appropriately, their research-based knowledge in practice. These responsibilities are related, primarily, to the development of an evidence-based practice culture in healthcare, as well as being connected with the need for nurses to accept a personal responsibility for professional development and a sharing of knowledge with other healthcare practitioners.

This need for research utilisation is not specific to nursing or healthcare and, as has already been indicated, is not even a contemporary issue. However, the need to put research findings into practice has taken on more significance because of the pressures on healthcare resources alongside societal demands for 'best practice' in terms of healthcare delivery. It is, however, important to recognise that research utilisation is not synonymous with evidence-based practice (see Chapter 1).

Evidence-based practice has been described as the integration of best research evidence with clinical expertise and patient values (Sackett et al., 2000). Evidence-based practice involves making clinical decisions on the best evidence available. The best evidence is primarily gleaned from rigorous research, but also uses other sources of credible information such as clinical expertise, patient input and resources available for practice.

Barriers to research utilisation and getting research into practice

Not all practice can be research based

The difference between research utilisation and evidence-based practice highlights that fact that not all practice can be research based and that nursing expertise and experience also have a role to play in the delivery of good-quality care. However, as Closs and Cheater suggest, 'the nature of many research projects is such that direct changes to practice are inappropriate – rather they may extend the way that nurses think about what they do, how they relate to the people they care for, and generally stimulate more reflecting and questioning attitudes' (1994: 512). In other words, research may act as the prompt that stimulates a review of practice where direct implementation of findings may be inappropriate or difficult to achieve in a given situation. It also relates to the expectation that all nurses have a role in research. This role can be that of the active researcher, but for many it will simply be making the best use of research findings in their own practice by applying these appropriately.

The scope and lack of nursing research

Another criticism of nursing research has been that it tends to be wide ranging and thus gives rise to the potential of a plethora of individual studies that reduces development of depth in knowledge about practice (Closs and Cheater, 1994). Some of this may be due to the fact that much nursing research has been, and still is, undertaken in order to fulfil the requirements of a degree programme rather than in the context of funded research. This may lead to there being only a limited amount of research available on a topic. Furthermore, it should be noted that until relatively recently much of the nursing research has not been practice orientated but focused on managerial, educational issues and descriptive rather than evaluative (Wilson-Barnett et al., 1990).

In the UK, until relatively recently there has been no strategy to influence the research and development agenda for nursing. This should now be changing with the *Making a Difference* (DoH, 1999) document and an action plan to ensure that the nursing contributions to key health priorities is properly researched, evaluated and supported by robust evidence and that the research and development agenda is properly informed by nursing expertise (DoH, 2000). Whilst the HEFCE (2001) report suggests that the lack of a scientific base for nursing is a consequence of the relative youth of nursing as a profession, together with inadequate funding and career structures. Part of this strategy also gives more of a focus, and a commitment to funding, for nurse researchers and to improving the research links between academic nurses and practice.

This may take the form of facilitation by which experienced nurse researchers can help novice and less experienced researchers to become active researchers (Rycroft-Malone et al., 2002). However, it has to be noted that this is not an exclusively British problem. A 2005 Sigma Theta Tau International position paper looking at nursing research priorities from an international perspective highlighted gaps between research and practice and a need to develop transnational nursing research and the evidence-practice base alongside the capacity of nursing research.

There is also the difficulty of actually being able to research complex issues of nursing and healthcare practice. This may be because of ethical issues and perceptions held by many nurses that gaining ethical approval for research is very difficult. But also, in nursing research the outcome criteria can be hard to define, for example how to measure quality of nursing care of patients where communication is difficult, as would be the case with some chronically mentally ill patients or terminally ill patients. Similarly, in some practice areas some interventions need to be so person-specific that they can never be entirely research based. For example, giving details of a need for palliative care to patients with cancer has a sound research base, but the needs of an individual patient for pain reduction and other symptom relief can only be met by a nurse who delivers care based on an amalgam of knowledge.

Inappropriate research utilisation

Linked with the lack of an extensive body of nursing research is the problem of inappropriate use of research. As has already been stated, not all research is appropriate for utilisation in practice. There is, however, also a risk that with the increasing emphasis on evidence-based practice there will be a tendency to implement research without due consideration of the quality, generalisability and applicability to a given practice setting (McDonnell, 1998). For example, in most situations it would be inappropriate to implement a change in practice on the basis of a single study unless it was of a high quality and involved large numbers. Rather, recommendations for practice from a single study that appear to be applicable to your own practice should encourage a critical appraisal of the study to ascertain its quality and validity. Then there should be a consideration of the need for replication of the study to confirm the outcomes. Again, this highlights the need for all nurses to have some understanding of research and an ability, and willingness, to critically appraise research.

Accessibility of research findings

In a study, *Nurses' Use of Research Information in Clinical Decision Making* (Cullum, 2002), one of the barriers identified was lack of accessibility to research findings.

Some of this was associated with a perception that interpreting and working with research outcomes was 'too complex', 'academic' and overly statistical. Some of this may simply be a perception that the 'language' of research is not 'nurse friendly', but is also linked with negative attitudes that see research as not really related to practice (Polit and Beck, 2006). This places a responsibility on nurse researchers to ensure that their results are presented in a way that practitioners can readily understand them. It may lead to nurse researchers publishing or presenting findings in a range of settings and publications that they would not ordinarily consider appropriate, for example presenting results of a study on the uptake of breast or cervical screening at Women's Institute meetings.

Accessibility also refers to the fact that not all research is published and, therefore, not readily available to the nursing population as a whole. It is not uncommon for research findings to be reported at a conference rather than being published in a journal, and so will only reach a limited audience. For some nurses, access to research findings may be associated with difficulties with actually getting the opportunity to read reports. This could be for variety of reasons, including lack of, or limited, library/IT facilities; location of library or inconvenient opening hours, and being unable to gain access in the clinical setting. Simple strategies like establishing a journal club or lunchtime discussion groups where the content of a recently published research report can be discussed may go some way to addressing these issues. In some NHS healthcare institutions the implementation of evidence-based practice has resulted in the establishment of working groups where specific areas of nursing care, such as patient privacy, have facilitated nurses being given the time and opportunity to consider the research evidence available and thence initiate research-based changes for practice. Other strategies could include having local nursing conferences where nurses can present their own innovations in practice to other nurses working in their locality. Such conferences could include presentations from nurse researchers and provide opportunities for networking and interaction between practice and research. This can be very useful in enabling practitioners to get advice and support from experienced nurse researchers about how to evaluate the effectiveness of a practice innovation. An increasing trend is also for academic nurses/researchers to have formal links or joint appointments with healthcare institutions. In this way practitioners can have direct contact with researchers who can provide support, advice or guidance at the level needed by practice.

Professional barriers

There has been until relatively recently, and persists in some areas, a perception that nurse researchers are academic and not practically orientated. This perception arose because much of the early nursing research was not clinically focused (Wilson-Barnett et al., 1990). In addition, there was only limited interaction between clinical nurses and researchers, and what contact there was tended to be transient (Polit and Beck, 2006). The increasing reliance on evidence-based practice has helped to highlight the need for research and the role of nurse researchers but, unfortunately, many practitioners still identify research as something others do. A recent personal experience of working as a research facilitator in practice illustrates an advantage of being able to change these perceptions. A Diabetes Clinical Nurse Specialist (DCNS) had developed an online referral system and was eager to publish her innovation in a specialist journal. Assistance was sought on the writing-up of the project, and in the ensuing discussions a need for formal evaluation of the project was identified. The DCNS had stated at the first meeting that, although she had an interest in research, she did not feel that she had the capabilities or time, as a lone worker, to get involved in research herself. By the time the article was submitted for publication the DCNS was eager to start an evaluation research project and had even more ideas for further research around her role. From being a relatively research-naïve practitioner, this nurse specialist has started on the process of becoming research active and, even more encouragingly, is also talking with other nurses and encouraging them to seek assistance from the Research in Practice Facilitator.

Professional barriers also include individual perceptions about abilities to understand and critically appraise the research literature. In theory at least, these barriers should be lessening. But a UK study looking at the utilisation of research findings by graduate nurses and midwives (Veeramah, 2004) reported that nurses wanted more help with searching the literature, developing critical appraisal skills and implementing research findings into practice. The inference from this is that even graduate nurses still lack confidence in connection with research. However, it is important that any nurse lacking the confidence to get involved with research should recognise his or her own limitations and seek assistance (Clifford, 2004). Just as important is for nurse researchers to be available and willing to offer advice and assistance.

Organisational barriers

Very closely associated with professional barriers to research are organisational barriers. Every organisation has its own culture, but there will inevitably be different perspectives that influence attitudes towards the implementation of research into the clinical setting. There may be resistance to change or a perception that research utilisation will disrupt the status quo. There may be a reluctance to expend resources on a research utilisation project, for example the time required to train staff in a new way of working, despite the fact that in the longer term it will result in more cost-effective care delivery. However, unexpected prompts may act as facilitators of research into practice, such as a directive from organisations like the National Patient Safety Agency that can provide impetus for the implementation of research-based innovations which would not necessarily have been given the required organisational support. Unfortunately some staff may associate research and research utilisation with time away from patient care and therefore inappropriate when there are many pressures on healthcare. This may be a fault on the part of nurse researchers and wariness about interacting with the clinical setting, but it does highlight the need to investigate how best research can be translated into practice.

Research utilisation needs the support and commitment of management and recognition that it takes time to implement changes to practice. Overcoming organisational barriers is not just about getting a commitment to support and fund research initiatives at a senior management level. It means getting a commitment at practice level so that any nurse who has a research idea gets the necessary support to take it forward. The support needed may be something as simple as facilitating time in the library or IT access in order to search the literature and identify whether there has been any other research undertaken on the topic. More tangible support may be necessary for some nurses in the form of experienced nurse researchers readily available to guide and encourage. Or the option of being able to get small grants locally that could, for example, 'buy out' practitioner time to facilitate data collection/analysis or purchase time from statistician.

Consumer involvement in research

The developing role of consumers in health research represents a change and alters the relationship between researchers, participants and potential users of research findings. There is now an expectation, and in some respects a requirement, that researchers involve consumers in a research process that sees them as 'partners' at all stages of the research process (CNHSRSU, 2000).

The need to involve consumers in research has been associated with the changing expectations of patients, linked to increasing understanding of what healthcare can actually provide, and consequently more awareness of problems of healthcare outcomes and healthcare delivery (Goodman, 1996). In many areas this has also been accompanied by a rise in the number of patients' groups and developments in the role of these groups to one where they are consulted and involved in service delivery and policymaking. Almost inevitably attention has also focused on research and a desire to influence not only healthcare, but also research and the research agenda.

The term 'consumer' is controversial but has come to be accepted in the way that patients are now often referred to as 'service users' (Hill, 2007). This change of terminology is also linked with the broadening of the remit for healthcare to have more of a focus on prevention and health promotion, and when referring to individuals, how

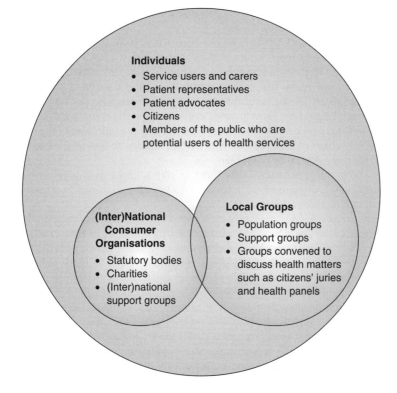

Figure 25.1   Classification of consumers in health research (adapted from Boote et al., 2002: 217)

they can access or be targeted as patients or clients. This does, however, mean that there is a need to define consumers, and for research involvement, in particular, to explain the differing ways that consumers can expect to be involved. Boote et al. (2002) suggest a classification for consumers in health research (see Figure 25.1). This gives an indication of the different perspectives that consumers can provide for healthcare research, but does not explain the level of involvement and where in the research process consumers could expect to be involved.

In the UK, the Consumers in NHS Research and Support Unit (CNHSRSU, 2004) suggests that consumers can be involved at all stages of the research process, although there will be a range of ways for consumers to be included. Essentially, involvement can be categorised as being involved in basic research, clinical research, public health research and health services and health systems research (Hill, 2007):

- *Basic research* is research that happens in the laboratory and does not directly involve individuals, except that they can donate items such as cells, ova, sperm or organs (removed during surgery). It is expected that consumer involvement at this level is primarily concerned with research policy and ethical issues.

- *Clinical research* is probably that main area that consumers would associate with healthcare research and also where there is most likely to be the greatest amount of consumer involvement. This type of research can be either laboratory based or in healthcare institutions, and is usually linked with research into the causes of disease and ill health.

  Again consumers can be involved with policy and research prioritisation. This could include them helping to identify what outcomes are the most appropriate, or how research findings may best be disseminated to potential beneficiaries of the research. For example, consumers may suggest ways of getting findings to potential beneficiaries that had not been considered by the researchers.

  More commonly, consumer involvement in clinical research is where they become active participants or 'guinea pigs' in research studies; for example, in drug trials or in evaluation of care research projects.

- *Public health research* is concerned with research into communities and populations that aims to reduce levels of ill health and risks. Again, the expectation is for consumers to be involved, offering advice at policy level or raising issues of concern, particularly in the development of programmes to help change practice, such as participating in action research projects; for example, helping to develop different ways for risk populations to access community-based hypertension clinics and advice centres.

- *Health services and health systems research* aims to improve the delivery of healthcare and may focus on issues such as access, equity, healthcare cost effectiveness and efficiency. The expectation is that consumers involved with this level of research will be able to offer a different perspective from that of healthcare professionals, for example suggesting variations for accessing healthcare services and adding a consumer voice when developing training programmes.

Obviously, it is expected that benefits will accrue from the involvement of consumers in healthcare research. From the researcher perspective, these are essentially associated with being able to get a different perspective on research. From my own experience, having consumers involved at the research proposal stage of a study investigating the management of constipation in palliative care (Goodman et al., 2003) helped to identify what would be an acceptable way of assessing levels of constipation. Consumer involvement can also assist the research community in setting priorities, which can be very beneficial when there are competing claims for the resources available, though it must be recognised that consumer priorities can be very different from those of healthcare practitioners and will not always make the decision-making process of exactly what research to prioritise easy.

From a consumer perspective it has to be acknowledged that benefits will not necessarily be as direct as those gained by the research community. However, benefits have been associated with improving the level of patient-centred care (Brown and Zavestock, 2004) and raising the the profile of the need for research in certain spheres, for example research involving women and HIV/AIDS. It can also be argued that increasing consumer involvement in turn increases awareness and the willingness of individuals to become involved in research projects themselves, and the possibility of obtaining properly informed consent (Moynihan, 2005). Other benefits include a change of research priorities for studies that focus on patient-centred outcomes, such as quality-of-life and treatment outcomes, that reflect patient preferences rather than disease-oriented outcomes (Hill, 2007). It has also been suggested (Tallon et al., 2000) that giving consumers a voice in research has led to more attention being paid to their rights and to research ethics alongside influencing the research agenda so that it is more likely to reflect current and potential patient needs.

It does, however, need to be acknowledged that involving consumers in research may slow down the research process, but that the benefits that can be achieved by their involvement will usually mitigate any delays.

Nurse research roles

According to the Department of Health's (2000) strategy for nursing research and development, there is no clear picture of the numbers of nurses with research skills and qualifications; about the number of nurses who research training or career patterns, aspirations and destinations. There is also confusion amongst the nursing research community about differing roles for nurses in research. The DoH strategy sets out aims that should help to increase the contribution of nurses to healthcare research and to help expand the nursing research-active community.

Anecdotally, it seems that there are a many nurses working in clinical trials units who are primarily research co-ordinators with differing levels of expertise in the conduct of research and who do not actively undertake their own research, though some nurses working in these roles will be actively involved in conducting their own research alongside the clinical trial with which they are involved.

Some nurse researchers have a role that is primarily to facilitate other nurses to undertake research and provide them with advice and support. As a consequence, their active involvement in research may be limited, although getting many other nurses to become active researchers probably outweighs any disadvantages associated with being less research active themselves. Other nurse researchers work in departments or organisations that enable them to focus almost entirely on research which may or may not be practice orientated. More importantly, it should be recognised that there is a variety of opportunities, current and proposed, that make it possible for more nurses to become research active. There may not, as yet, be a recognised career structure available for nurses wanting to pursue a career in research, although in the UK there are now more opportunities, such as with Research Networks. It is, however, also incumbent on all nurses to remember that practice cannot be divorced from research and that research can extend the way they think about their practice and stimulate more reflective and questioning attitudes that will enhance their contribution to patient care.

Chapter summary

- Getting research into practice is about applying research findings from one or more studies into practice and is unrelated to the original research, that is, closing the gap between the knowledge generated by research and using it in clinical practice to improve patient care.
- Evidence-based practice involves making clinical decisions on the best evidence available; it is not the same as research.
- Not all practice can be research based; where there is research evidence it should be incorporated into practice.
- The current base of clinical nursing research is relatively limited, but a strategy has been proposed (DoH, 2000) that should help to improve the contribution nurses can make and increase the numbers of research-active nurses.
- Care needs to be taken to ensure that research utilisation is appropriate.
- Nurses need to recognise that research has an important role in improving patient care and be aware of when they need to seek assistance.
- Experienced nurse researchers should expect, and endeavour, to encourage and facilitate colleagues to become research active.
- Healthcare organisations should promote a research culture that is inclusive for nurses.
- Involving consumers in research can be time-consuming, but should improve the applicability of research and make it more patient-centred.
- There is a variety of roles for nurses in research, but all nurses should endeavour to utilise available research in their practice.

References

Berwick, D. (2003) 'Disseminating innovations in health care', *Journal of the American Medical Association*, 289: 1969–75.

Boote, J., Telford, R. and Cooper, C. (2002) 'Consumer involvement in health research: a review and research agenda', *Health Policy*, 61: 213–36.

Brown, P. and Zavestock, S. (2004) 'Social movement in health: an introduction', *Sociology of Health and Illness*, 26 (6): 279–94.

Clifford, C. (2004) 'Research and development in practice', in C. Clifford and J. Clark (eds), *Getting Research into Practice* Edinburgh: Churchill Livingstone. Chapter 12.

Closs, S. and Cheater, F. (1994) 'Utilization of nursing research: culture, interest and support', *Journal of Advanced Nursing*, 19 (3): 151–5.

CNHSRSU (2000) *Involving Consumers in Research and Development in the NHS: Briefing Notes for Researchers*. Eastleigh: Consumers in NHS Research Support Unit.

CNHSRSU (2004) *Getting Involved in Research: A Guide for Consumers*. Eastleigh: Consumers in NHS Research Support Unit. Available at www.invo.org.uk.

Cullum, N. (2002) *Nurses' Use of Research Information in Clinical Decision Making: A Descriptive Analytical Study*, Vol. 2008. York: University of York.

Department of Health (1999) *Making a Difference: Strengthening the Nursing, Midwifery and Health Visiting Contribution to Health and Healthcare.* London: DoH.

Department of Health (2000) *Towards a Strategy for Nursing Research and Development: Proposals for Action.* London: DoH.

Goodman, M.L. (1996) 'Can we afford palliative care?', in MA thesis, 'Philosophy', Keele: University of Keele. p. 116.

Goodman, M.L., Wilkinson, S. and Lowe, J. (2003) *A Study of the Management of Constipation in Palliative Care across the Marie Curie Centres.* London: Marie Curie Palliative Care Research and Development Unit.

HEFCE (2001) *Research in Nursing and Allied Health Professions, Report of the Task Group 3.* Bristol: HEFCE.

Hill, S. (2007) 'Involving the consumer in health research', in M. Saks and J. Allsop (eds), *Researching Health: Qualitative, Quantitative and Mixed Methods.* London: Sage. Chapter 19.

McDonnell, A. (1998) 'Factors which may inhibit the application of research findings in practice and some solutions', in P. Crookes and S. Davies (eds), *Research into Practice.* Edinburgh: Baillière Tindall.

Moynihan, R. (2005) 'The marketing of a disease: female sexual dysfunction', *British Medical Journal*, 330: 192–4.

Parahoo, K. (2006) *Nursing Research: Principles, Process and Issues.* Basingstoke: Palgrave Macmillan.

Peters, D. (1992) 'Implementation of research findings', *Health Bulletin,* 50 (1): 68–77.

Polit, D. and Beck, C. (2006) *Essentials of Nursing Research: Methods, Appraisal and Utilization.* Philadelphia, PA: Lippincott Williams & Wilkins.

Rycroft-Malone, J., Harvey, G., Kitson, A., McCormack, B., Seers, K. and Titchen, A. (2002) 'Getting evidence into practice: ingredients for change', *Nursing Standard*, 16 (37): 38–42.

Sackett, D.L., Straus, S.E., Richardson, W.S., Rosenberg, W. and Haynes, R.B. (2000) *Evidence-based Medicine: How to Practice and Teach EBM*, 2nd edition. Edinburgh: Churchill Livingstone.

Sigma Theta Tau International (2005) Resource paper on global health and nursing research priorities. Available at www.nursingsociety.org/about/position, accessed February 2008.

Tallon, D., Chard, J. and Dieppe, P. (2000) 'Relation between agendas of the research community and the research consumer', *Lancet*, 355: 2037–40.

Veeramah, V. (2004) 'Utilization of research findings by graduate nurses and midwives', *Journal of Advanced Nursing*, 47 (2): 307–13.

Wilson-Barnett, J., Corner, J. and De-Carle, B. (1990) 'Integrating nursing research and practice – the role of the researcher as teacher', *Journal of Advanced Nursing*, 15 (5): 621–5.

GLOSSARY

Accidental sampling: see Convenience sampling.

Action research: a research approach that involves planning, implementing and evaluating change in practice.

Anonymity: refers to the way we attribute information from a specific person. Participants are likely to give researchers large amounts of very personal information if they are assured that they cannot be identified if it is quoted.

Audit: a methodological review.

Average: a numerical value around which collected data values cluster; a measure of central tendency, for example, mean, median, mode.

Beneficence: literally means 'doing good'. The moral principle is the moral obligation to do good, to remove and prevent harms and weigh possible goods against the costs and possible harms of an action.

Capability building: developing the ability to undertake research.

Capacity building: developing an ability to appreciate and use research for practice.

Case study: a research design that focuses on specific groups or populations, often one, and collects data using a number of methods. The case is defined and limited.

Chart: pictorial summary of numerical data that displays patterns in collected data; a graph of data values, for example bar chart, box-and-whisker plot, histogram.

Cluster/multi-stage random sampling: a cluster or multi-stage random sample includes the sampling of clusters that are used to draw further samples.

Computer-assisted data analysis: analysis of research data using computer packages.

Conference presentation: presentation of a poster or academic paper at a conference gathering.

Confidentiality: relates to the way information gained from participants is treated and the assurances given that it will not be revealed to anyone outside the research team.

Confirmability: a measure of the objectivity of the data, the extent to which data and interpretations reflect the phenomena of study.

Consensus technique: the consensus method involves a panel of multi-disciplinary experts who meet face to face to discuss and develop practice. Gaps in knowledge and resultant research priorities can also be identified as part of consensus knowledge-building.

Construct validity: the degree to which a questionnaire or scale reflects the construct that is being measured.

Content analysis: analysis of textual data content, often produced as part of qualitative research, to identify key themes.

Content validity: the degree to which a measure, such as a question in a questionnaire, can collect data about the phenomena under study.

Convenience/accidental sampling: a convenience or accidental sample is usually taken from the local population convenient to the researcher and team.

Correlation coefficient: is a measure of the strength of a relationship (association) between two variables, and lies between 0 and 1 for positive correlation or between 0 and -1 for negative correlation. Positive correlation implies that values of both variables increase (or decrease) together, whereas negative correlation implies that as values of one variable increase, the other decreases (or vice versa).

Credibility: a study has credible findings if they reflect the experience and perceptions of the participants. Those who read the report and any published journal articles must also view the findings as credible.

Criterion-related validity: the results obtained by a measure can be validated by comparing them with those results obtained through another validated questionnaire.

Critical analysis: is a structured process of identifying and evaluating the merits and/or value of research.

Critical appraisal: is a structured process of identifying and evaluating the merits and/or value of research.

Critical incident technique: the technique involves asking participants about key events they have experienced, and collects observations of human behaviour in defined situations.

Critique: exercising careful judgement or evaluation.

Data coding: the researcher applies codes to the data as part of the process of interpretation and conclusion drawing.

Data Protection Act 1998: sets out how to handle and process personal information and data collected through research.

Data security and storage: data must be stored safely and with due regard to issues of confidentiality and anonymity.

Deductive reasoning: principles or theories are applied to a particular situation.

Delphi technique: a form of survey that collects the views of experts on a particular issue. The experts are invited to respond individually to issues and rank statements or concepts according to priority. A series of rounds of review and revision continue until a consensus is achieved.

Dependability: establishing dependability can be seen as a parallel process to that of confirming reliability in quantitative data. An audit trail of the research may assist in establishing the dependability.

Diaries: researchers can use diaries as part of qualitative research designs to ask participants to record current events, keeping a record over time of feelings, experiences, events, actions and reflections.

Discourse/conversation analysis: the analysis of discourse, which includes verbal, non-verbal and written communication. This approach attempts to understand interactions between people.

Dual role of researcher and nurse: there are potential conflicts of interests associated with the dual role of practitioner and researcher. Nurses must ensure that participants understand the role of the nurse in a research study.

Emic perspective: gaining the insider view.

Epidemiological research: research that measures the prevalence and incidence of disease in populations.

Ethical principles: refer to moral norms that are basic for biomedical ethics. Ethics is a generic term for various ways of understanding and examining the moral life.

Ethnography: a qualitative research approach developed by anthropologists to guide the study of culture and cultural groups. Ethnographers observe behaviour, customs, rituals, interaction and practices.

Etic perspective: entering the culture from the outside.

Evaluation outcomes: have to be appropriate to the question being asked and can be qualitative or quantitative or a mixture of both. Outcome indicators can be classified as patient-, carer-, staff- and service-based.

Evaluation research: is a form of applied research that is designed to address current issues or questions about the way a service functions or the impact of services, care programmes or policies.

Evidence-based practice: use of current best evidence in making decisions about nursing care delivery and practice.

Experimental design: a quantitative research design that tests a hypothesis through applying a treatment or condition to an experimental group. The outcomes are usually compared with a control group.

Feminist research: research conducted for the benefit of women.

Focus group: discussions with one or more researchers and between two and nine participants.

Follow-up studies: involve seeing patients following a particular intervention or treatment to monitor progress.

Full economic costing: the costing and charging of research undertaken by universities.

Good Clinical Practice: in research is an international ethical and scientific quality standard, and compliance with the standard should provide public assurance that the rights, safety and well-being of research participants are protected and that the clinical research data are credible.

Grounded theory: a qualitative research methodology that aims to support the generation of theory through a process of simultaneous data collection and analysis.

Hawthorne effect: occurs as a result of research participants knowing they are involved in a study.

Healthcare consumer: a controversial but now accepted term for 'patient'.

Hermeneutics: understanding the human experience.

Heterogeneity: variability in the characteristics of the sample of individual studies.

Hierarchy of evidence: placing evidence in a hierarchy based on the rigours of the approach taken to collect the information, with evidence from a systematic review of multiple well-designed randomised controlled trials being at the top and personal, professional and peer expertise and experience at the bottom.

Historical data: research data used by historical researchers that can be text-based, visual or numerical.

Historical research: a research approach that examines past events to increase understanding and gain new knowledge to inform current and future practice.

Human Tissue Act 2004: for anyone involved in research with organs or tissue, the full legislation of the Human Tissue Act must be consulted and particular reference made to the consenting process.

Hypothesis: attempts to answer a question which has emerged from a research problem, usually in the form of a statement of the relationship between variables.

Inductive reasoning: principles or theories are developed from a situation or observation.

Informed consent: refers to the process of gaining agreement from an individual to participate in a research study, based on having been given all relevant information, in a manner that is appropriate for that individual, about what participation means, with particular reference to possible harms and benefits.

Interpretation of qualitative data: processes undertaken by the researcher to draw meaning and interpretation from qualitative data such as text.

Interval level: data is named, ordered and measured on a scale marked in equal intervals, for example body temperature in °C.

Interviews: a data collection technique that includes gathering information through verbal communication. Interviews can be managed in one-to-one situations, groups, over the telephone and face to face.

Intuition: developed insight gained through experience.

In vitro: physiological measures conducted without the presence of the participant, for example, in a laboratory.

In vivo: physiological measures made in the presence of the participant, for example, recording a pulse.

Justice: refers to the moral obligation to be 'fair' and requires that preference is not given to some participants over others in respect of morally relevant equalities and inequalities.

Life history: life histories and biographical material report individual life experiences, often accessed through in-depth interviewing.

Likert scale: a measurement scale that requires the participant to give an opinion on a series of statements.

Literature review: is the selection of available documents (both published and unpublished) on a topic and the effective evaluation of these documents in relation to the research being proposed.

Literature search: aims to identify the most appropriate sources to answer a question within a field of study.

Longitudinal designs: these designs are used to measure the effect of changes over time. They involve the collection of data at various points, sometimes from the same participants.

Measure of central tendency: see Average.

Measure of dispersion: numerical value that indicates how closely collected data values cluster around the average; a measure of scatter or dispersion around the average, with smaller values indicating data values clustered closer to the average, for example, standard deviation, range.

Mental Capacity Act 2005: researchers can undertake research with vulnerable participants or those who lack capacity to give consent provided that the requirements of the Act are fulfilled. The act sets out duties to ensure that individuals who lack capacity are treated with due respect and their rights protected.

Meta-analysis: is a statistical amalgam of the findings of a number of research studies that have been carried out on a specific topic and is usually regarded as secondary analysis of original data.

Mixed methods: using different data collection methods within one study. Usually qualitative and quantitative methods are combined.

Multi-stage random sampling: see Cluster sampling.

Narrative analysis: can form part of the analysis of textual data within research. Those undertaking narrative analysis are concerned with the structure of the story rather than focusing on the content.

Narrative review: selection of literature about a topic, often addressing a broad range of issues, to give a descriptive overview.

Naturalistic observation: observation of phenomena in naturally occurring contexts.

Network/snowball sampling: network or snowball sampling is the approach used when nurse researchers are aiming to select hidden samples. The researcher will need to draw on networks to identify the sample, often involving a third party.

Nominal data: can be classified into named categories, which have no inherent order attached, for example, male or female.

Nominal group technique: a technique of data collection where the participants meet face to face to try to achieve a consensus through a process of ranking and refining responses to key issues.

Non-maleficence: is the principle of 'doing no harm'. For research participants there is a duty to prevent harm (physical, psychological, emotional, social and economic) and do good; to protect the weak and vulnerable; and the weak, vulnerable or incompetent should be defended.

Non-probability sampling: non-random methods are used to select elements for inclusion in non-probability sampling. This means the researcher is unable to state the chances of elements of the population appearing in the final sample.

Nursing research: systematic gathering of information to answer questions and solve problems in the pursuit of creating new knowledge about nursing.

Observational methods: can be used to examine phenomena such as communication, non-verbal interactions and activity in practice settings. Researchers observe practice and may record this activity in a structured or unstructured way.

Ordinal data: can be classified into named categories, which do have an inherent order attached, for example, strongly agree down to strongly disagree.

Outcome: refers to the effectiveness or impact of any intervention in relation to individuals and communities.

Panel studies: use the same participants over a given time.

Parametric methods: make certain assumptions about the distribution of data (for example, data measured on at least an interval level and follows a normal distribution), whereas non-parametric (distribution-free) methods do not.

Participant information: should be presented in manner that is comprehensible to potential participants, and should explain what question the research is trying to answer and what a participant will have to do.

Personal knowledge: individual knowledge shaped through being personally involved in situations and events in practice.

Phenomenology: a qualitative research approach that aims to understand human experience. Researchers focus on individuals' interpretations of their lived experiences.

Population: a group of people, documents, events or specimens the researcher is interested in collecting information or data from.

Preparation of data: preparing the 'raw data' which could encompass text, tape/digital recordings, numerical data or visual data such as photographs and video for analysis.

Probability sampling: all units in the sampling frame have more than a zero chance of being included in the final sample.

Process: refers to the activities themselves and how services are organised and delivered.

Publication: a process of preparing research papers for publication in academic journals.

Purposive/purposeful sampling: the researchers use their own judgement and knowledge of the potential participants to support recruitment.

Qualitative approaches/research: a term for research designs and methods that collect non-numerical data that is often textual.

Qualitative data analysis: the analysis and interpretation of data obtained through qualitative research approaches, which might include textual data from interviews.

Quantitative approaches/research: a term for research designs and methods collecting numerical data that is analysed using statistical methods.

Quasi-experiment: an experimental design where the research does not meet all three criteria of a true experiment. An intervention is always present, but randomisation and/or a control group may not be used.

Questionnaires: a data collection instrument that includes questions requiring written responses. These can be administered via the post, Internet, in person or left for respondent collection.

Quota sampling: an approach to sampling where the researcher pre-determines the numbers required in each group and selects according to these specified characteristics. For example, the researcher can select the sample to meet gender and age requirements.

Randomised controlled trial (RCT): this design is the true experiment, with a control group, randomisation and an intervention. RCTs are usually conducted in clinical practice settings.

Ratio level: data is named, ordered, measured on a scale marked in equal intervals and has an absolute zero, for example, weight of adults in kg.

Reading analytically: is an active process concerned with learning to think.

Reliability: is the consistency with which a tool measures what it is intended to. The nurse researcher is interested in three measures of reliability that include the stability of a measure, its internal consistency and equivalence.

Replication studies: focus on the group used to test the tool/questionnaire.

Research aims: describe the overall purpose of a project.

Research design: a map of the way in which the researcher will engage with the research subject(s) in order to achieve the outcomes needed to address the research aims and objectives.

Research ethics: refer to the principles that underpin ethical research. Nurses in research are expected to be guided by the principles of veracity, justice, non-maleficence, beneficence, fidelity and confidentiality.

Research Ethics Committees: consider applications from researchers wishing to undertake healthcare research; scrutinise research protocols; and determine whether the study is ethical. Research studies in healthcare cannot be started until ethical approval has been given.

Research Governance Framework: sets standards; defines mechanisms to deliver standards; describes the monitoring and assessment arrangements; and aims to improve research quality and safeguard the public.

Research hierarchies: a kind of league table where some types of research are classed as being of better quality than others.

Research literate: having the ability to interpret research findings, an essential skill for knowledge-led nursing practice.

Research objectives: describe the individual tasks that need to be carried out in order to meet the research aims.

Research papers: published papers written to disseminate the research findings.

Research problem: a broad topic area of interest that has perplexing or troubling aspects which can be 'solved' by the accumulation of relevant information or evidence.

Research process: a series of steps or stages undertaken by researchers in order to address research questions.

Research proposal: outline of the research to be undertaken, detailing research aims, methods, costing and ethical issues.

Research question: is a concise description of exactly what issues the research intends to acquire information about.

Research reports: a research report is often required by funders at the end of a project and would usually include details of the research process and outcomes and recommendations for future practice.

Research utilisation: is about applying research findings from one or more studies into practice.

Respect for autonomy: autonomy is the capacity to make deliberate or reasoned decisions for oneself and to act on the basis of such decisions. Respect for autonomy is the norm of respecting the decision-making capacities of autonomous persons.

Rigour: the accuracy and consistency of a research design that gives a measure of its quality.

Safety of researchers: may include providing taxis, special training, counselling, mobile phones, working in pairs, overnight accommodation.

Sample: is a subset of the population, selected through sampling techniques.

Sample size calculation: a mathematical calculation used to determine the size of the sample required in quantitative research, in order that the study can be powered to enable a clinically important difference to be detected as statistically significant.

Sampling frames: developed to include all of the possible members of the population who might be eligible for inclusion in the final sample.

Scientific knowledge: knowledge developed and verified through systematic and rigorous enquiry.

Secondary research/analysis: includes systematic reviews because new data is not collected and makes use of previous findings.

Simple random sampling: a simple approach to sampling that draws on the sampling frame to select a random sample as a subset of the population.

Snowball sampling: see Network sampling.

Statistical hypothesis testing: methodical process that uses the laws of chance to test an explicit assumption about characteristics in a population (or of differences in values across more than one population) on the basis of data collected from a sample of people drawn from that population (or populations), for example, when researching the effectiveness of different approaches to managing pain.

Statistics: formally collected numerical data, for example number of patients on a waiting list; numbers that summarise specific features in a sample of collected data, for example mean; methods used to collect, analyse and interpret numerical data, in particular to inform decision making, for example when researching the effectiveness of different approaches to managing pain.

Storage: see Data security and storage.

Stratified random sampling: the researcher separates the sampling frame into sub-sections, such as gender groups, age groups, professional disciplines, before randomly selecting an agreed number from each group for inclusion in the study.

Structure: the organisational framework for an activity or care-giving environment.

Structured observations: a data collection method used where actions or events are observed and recorded in predetermined categories or checklists.

Survey/survey design: a design that collects descriptive or correlation data from a sample of population (such as the census that includes the entire population).

Synthesis: is the rearranging of elements derived from analysis of the literature to idenfiy relationships not previously noted.

Systematic random sampling: this approach sees the researcher drawing a random sample by selecting units from a list at predetermined set intervals. Every unit has an equal chance of inclusion in the sample.

Systematic review: is a review of a clearly formulated question that uses systematic and explicit methods to identify, select and critically appraise relevant research, and to collect and analyse data from studies that are included in the review.

Tacit knowledge: developed through practice and experience over time.

Theoretical sampling: involves the determination of the sample on the basis of the themes that emerge from the data analysis and the researcher then explores these themes in more depth and/or develops a theory from these data. It is frequently used in grounded theory.

Thick description: an analysis of the group culture, a view of its patterns of working, member relationships, meanings and functions.

Tradition: ongoing use of past actions or customs which may or may not continue to have relevance and currency.

Transferability: the extent to which the research findings can be transferred from one context to another by providing a 'thick description' of the data, as well as identifying sampling and design details.

Trend studies: explore how patterns change over time.

Triangulation: the use of two or more research approaches, data collection methods or analysis techniques in one study.

Trustworthiness: a term used in the appraisal of qualitative research when describing credibility, dependability and transferability.

Unstructured observations: a data collection method used where actions or events are observed and recorded without predetermined categories or checklists.

Validity: a measure of whether a data collection tool accurately measures what it is supposed to. A measure is unlikely to be valid unless it is also reliable.

Vulnerable participants: individuals who may have compromised capacity to give informed consent due to physical, mental or psychological debility.

INDEX

Entries in **bold** represent glossary definitions